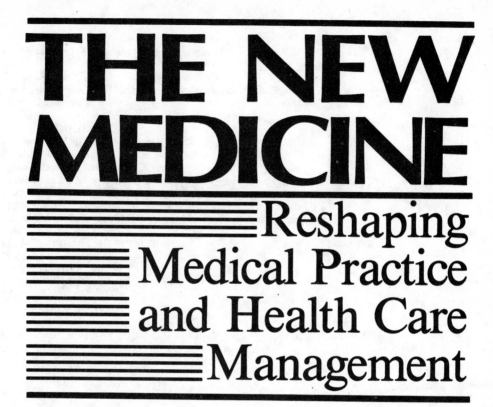

THE NEW MEDICINE

Reshaping Medical Practice and Health Care Management

Russell C. Coile, Jr.

President
Health Forecasting Group
Alameda, California

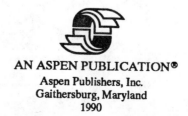

AN ASPEN PUBLICATION®
Aspen Publishers, Inc.
Gaithersburg, Maryland
1990

Library of Congress Cataloging-in-Publication Data

Coile, Russell C.
The new medicine: reshaping medical practice and health care management /
Russell C. Coile, Jr.
p. cm.
"An Aspen Publication."
Includes bibliographical references.
ISBN: 0-8342-0103-8
1. Medicine—Practice—United States. 2. Health services
administration—United States. 3. Medical policy—United States.
4. Medical care, Cost of—United States. I. Title.
[DNLM: 1. Delivery of Health Care-trends-United States. 2. Medicine-
trends-United States. 3. Practice Management, Medical-trends-United States.
W 84 AA1 C58n]
R728.C57 1989 362.1'0973-dc20
DNLM/DLC
for Library of Congress
89-17636
CIP

Aspen Publishers, Inc., grants permission for photocopying for limited
personal or internal use. This consent does not extend to other kinds of
copying, such as copying for general distribution, for advertising or
promotional purposes, for creating new collective works, or for resale. For
information, address Aspen Publishers, Inc., Permissions Department,
200 Orchard Ridge Drive, Gaithersburg, Maryland 20878.

Editorial Services: Marsha Davies

Library of Congress Catalog Card Number: 89-17636
ISBN: 0-8342-0103-8

Printed in the United States of America

3 4 5

*Dedicated to the memory of
Hank Koehn, futurist,*

*with thanks for the inspiration of my parents,
Russell C. Coile
and
Margaret L. (Peg) Wallace,*

*and the resident family intellectual,
Bess L. Zeigler.*

Table of Contents

Preface

We won't have to wait long for the future of medicine.

Change is coming and the future is here. Not since the debates over Medicare 25 years ago has medicine been in such ferment. Just look at the signals of change:

- The Harvard Relative Value Scale (RVS) study may establish national physician prices.
- National health insurance is back on the policy agenda.
- Rationing of medical care is state law in Oregon.
- National expenditures for physician services are rising at a 10 percent rate.
- Medicare spending on physician services is rising at an 18 percent rate.
- A federal "cap" on physician payments is likely.
- Outcomes of medical care are published in newspapers.

Medicine is in flux today, and tomorrow is uncertain. The purpose of *The New Medicine: Reshaping Medical Practice and Health Care Management* is to (1) highlight the trend lines and future directions of the changing health care environment and (2) suggest strategic implications for physicians and their hospitals.

The future of medicine will be the central story of the U.S. Health industry in the 1990s. Physicians still control an estimated 80 percent of hospital utilization and direct the majority of health care expenditures. Doctors are at the pivot point when it comes to changing tomorrow's health system. Hospitals are retreating from marketing health services on the retail model. They made an important discovery about health care marketing in the 1980s: Physicians still control patients and drive the health system. That fundamental truth is becoming widely recognized by hospitals, insurance companies, managed care plans, and government officials. All reforms to be made in tomorrow's health industry will involve changing physician behavior. Physicians occupy the high ground at the mouth of the channel, and any alterations of the U.S. health system must take this into account. That is why the future of medicine is so important.

ECONOMICS + TECHNOLOGY = FUTURE

Medicine's future will be driven by economics as well as technology. The assumption here is that each physician's practice is an enterprise in a world the economists call a market. Shifting market trends require a strategic response. Of course there are options. That is the underlying reason why this book was written. All physicians must be their own strategists, charting their preferred future in this sea of sometimes unfathomable change.

Another key assumption is that the future is neither remote nor mysterious. Major trends that will affect doctors and their hospitals are widely evident. Every physician and health care organization is making assumptions about the future. Think of this book as a "second opinion" about those assumptions.

THE ORGANIZATION

The structure of *The New Medicine* is simple. Part I is an overview of the near and midrange future. It presents the key market trends that will drive medicine and health care in the decade of the 1990s, including

- medicine's new economics
- the new consumer
- age wage
- continuum of care
- new technology
- managed care
- behavioral medicine
- AIDS, ethics, and economics

Health care's response to these trends is forecasted in Part II, including

- physician bonding
- medical enterprise
- physician channeling
- restructuring hospital–physician relations
- service line strategy
- contract management
- innovation and enterprise
- marketing innovations

- outcomes management
- health care as a designed experience

The epilogue presents four alternative scenarios for the future of medicine in the year 2000.

A suggestion to readers: This book is designed to be "grazed," like the appetizers in today's ultramodern restaurants. Read any chapter in any order. The book does not have to be read from front to back or cover to cover. Each chapter stands alone. The reader's interest should determine the order in which the chapters are explored. The reader may come back to particular chapters as the information and insights are needed—whether next month or next year.

THE AUDIENCE

This book is for and about doctors. The physician practice is the basic strategic unit in planning for the future of medicine. Doctors are encouraged to consider this book a resource in planning for their future. The assumption is that a strategically managed practice will outcompete all those that simply drift with the trends. There are too many rocks in the whitewaters of change ahead for physicians to simply float with the current.

This book is also for hospitals. Physicians are the single most important strategic resource of any hospital for its future. Health care executives are vitally concerned with the future of medicine and will play an active role in shaping it. That explains why the title refers to "reshaping medical practice and health care management." An understanding of the changes medicine is undergoing is fundamental for the development of a new and symbiotic relationship between hospitals and physicians. That relationship will be the linchpin of all important strategic moves that U.S. hospitals plan for the decade ahead.

For both physicians and hospitals, remember the underlying philosophy of this book: *Futures management*. Reduced to the essence this means "You manage the future or the future will manage you."

Acknowledgments

A number of physicians were inspirational in the development of this book. Dr. Daniel Lang is developing physician leadership programs to bridge the chasm between medicine and hospitals under the auspices of the National Health Foundation of the Hospital Council of Southern California in Los Angeles. Dr. Paul Torrens of the UCLA School of Public Health is both historian and futurist in laying out the lines of change for U.S. medical care. Dr. Arnold Relmen of the *New England Journal of Medicine* is an articulate voice for progressive ideals in medical practice. Dr. Everett Koop, the most widely recognized surgeon general of modern times, is an energetic advocate for the public's health without prejudice or regard to status. Dr. Dennis O'Leary is transforming the once staid Joint Commission on Accreditation of Healthcare Organizations (Joint Commission) into one of the most influential institutions in shaping the U.S. health care system. Dr. Paul Ellwood, having established the HMO industry, is now transforming quality assurance from a paper exercise into "outcomes management" on the model of American industry. Dr. Roger Shenke is building the Association of Medical Executives into one of the fastest-growing professional organizations in U.S. health today. Dr. Bruce Spivey, who concurrently directs San Francisco's Pacific Presbyterian Medical Center and the American Academy of Ophthalmology, is an example of the medical executive of tomorrow. Dr. James Sammons is emblematic of the many physicians who ably represent organized medicine to policy makers and payers at the national, state, and local levels.

This list could obviously be extended. So many physicians are making contributions to the future of medicine today—in medical research, medical practice, medical policy making, and medical economics. An enormous number of young physicians are entering the profession today, by joining groups or HMOs, taking hospital positions, engaging in scientific research or biomedical engineering, and establishing independent practices. Clinician, scientist, entrepreneur: Today's doctors are all three, and more. They must be strategists who can see the future and plan so as to achieve it.

The New Medicine: Reshaping Medical Practice and Health Care Management is also dedicated to America's hospitals, which provide workshops and laboratories for medicine. The future of U.S. hospitals is fundamentally linked to the future of medicine. Physicians and hospitals will share that future. Their relationship is still experimental and evolving. Its degree of success will determine how well the transition of American health care will go in the 1990s.

In the preparation of this book, many people provided advice and encouragement. Aspen Publishers deserves much credit for the publication of the book, and it has my appreciation for its permission to use information from my Aspen-based newsletter, the *Hospital Strategy Report* (formerly the *Hospital Entrepreneurs' Newsletter*). Many thanks to Russ Pottle, Steve Mautner, Mary Taylor, Marsha Davies, and Martha Carnahan at Aspen for their patience and support. Michael Doody, Dru Konen, Al Woods, Kate Grant, and Dave O'Malley of Consolidated Catholic Health Care (CCHC), Westchester, Illinois, deserve grateful mention for their contributions to some of the seminal themes of this book, which were developed in special reports for the CCHC Futures Program.

My friends and colleagues Dennis Strum, Lois Green, and Kimi Mann of UniHealth America (formerly Lutheran Hospital Society of Southern Society) have encouraged my development as an independent futurist specializing in the health field.

A major contributor to my growth as a health care forecaster has been Katherine E. Johnson of the Healthcare Forum. As sponsor of my columns "FutureTrack" and "The Leading Edge," *Healthcare Forum* is frequently cited in this book as a source of ideas and information on future trends.

My deep appreciation also goes to my friend Chuck Lauer, publisher of *Modern Healthcare*, and to Clark Bell, editor, and Karen Petite, managing editor, and to their excellent journalists. As the business magazine of the health industry, *Modern Healthcare* is the source of many case studies of medicine and health care in change. Similar thanks are due to Russ Jackson, editor of *Managed Care Outlook*, and to Pamela Taulbee and Marie Robertson of *Health Care Competition Week*, who have kept me current with news from the "front lines" of health care.

For the help and inspiration of all those cited above, I am much appreciative. For any biases regarding these often controversial topics, as well as for errors of omission or commission, I take personal responsibility. This book contains opinionated research that is presented for comparison with your own assumptions of what may lie ahead for America's physicians and their hospitals. There is nothing inevitable about the trends discussed below. May we all face the 1990s with a belief that individuals and organizations can change the future.

Part I

Time of Transition

Chapter 1

Health Care 1990: Outlook for the Decade Ahead

The ten-year transition of medicine and health care is almost over. Call the past before 1983 *cost reimbursement*. Only a handful of services such as acute psychiatric care are still paid on this basis. Think of the recent past (1983–1989) as the era of *competition*. Health care has learned to compete on price, give discounts to major buyers, diversify the product portfolio, and master the art of marketing. Next comes the future—the era of *managed care* (see Figure 1-1). When more than 50 percent of the population is enrolled in a managed care plan, a level of market penetration that should be reached in the early 1990s, then the transition will be complete.

TEN LEADING HEALTH CARE TRENDS FOR THE 1990s

What's next for physicians, hospitals, and the health industry? While the old assumptions fade into history, new patterns are taking shape that will drive health care into the 1990s. The future is starting now. Transition into the 1990s will be accompanied by volatility and uncertainty. On the following page are the

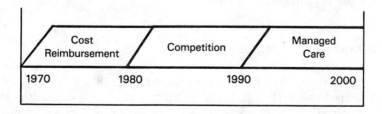

Figure 1-1 Transition of the Health Care Economy 1970–2000

top ten trends that will shape the future of hospitals and the health industry in the next decade.

Trend 1: Declining Reimbursement and Expanding Revenues

The year 1989 was a very difficult one for America's physicians and hospitals. Is the worst over? Or will 1990 be worse? And 1991? The short answer is that health care payment rates will go down but revenues will go up. Reimbursement (per visit, per procedure, per diem, and per case) will continue to shrink another 1–2 percent, but inpatient revenues will increase 3–5 percent and ambulatory revenues will rise 5–8 percent or more. For physicians with declining practice incomes and for financially pressed hospitals, the early 1990s will be the "best of times, and the worst of times." As for Medicare payments for the same period, few forecasters believe that Health Care Finance Administration (HCFA) reimbursement rates will increase more than a token 1–2 percent per year. Medicare funding will certainly not keep pace with soaring MD practice expenses or hospital wage costs. Double-digit hospital cost increases, which started in 1988, will continue into the 1990s, driven by a continuing upward spiral of wage raises. Cost increases should begin to slow by 1990, as nursing "wage wars" play out. By the early 1990s, the 1989–1991 "spike" of high inflation should end, and inflation will probably hold at 7–9 percent through the mid-1990s as managed care becomes a national phenomenon.

Inflation in the medical care component of the consumer price index (CPI) should continue to rise towards double-digit levels in 1989–1991 (see Table 1-1). Hospital charges will be the number one cause of health care inflation in this three-year period, but physician fees will move upwards at double-digit rates as well. Physician service costs will increase 10–12 percent from 1990 to 1993, even as hospital inflation begins to ease below 10 percent by 1990. Physician fees will fall below 10 percent by the mid 1990s as "national physician fee schedules" are adopted by HCFA and other third-party payers based on the Harvard RVS study completed in 1988. Other health care cost components, including pharmaceutics, supplies, long-term care, and home care, will experience 7–9 percent inflation in the 1990s.

Trend 2: Inpatient Renaissance

The five-year slump in acute inpatient care ended in 1988. Nationally, length of stay bottomed out in 1988 and may increase as much as a half day in 1989 before leveling off. This estimate is supported in a new forecast of market conditions by *Healthcare Forum Journal's* national panel of 500 health care experts (Table 1-2).

Table 1-1 Inflation Forecast for 1989–1991: Medical Care Component of Consumer Price Index (CPI)

Medical Care Index	Compound Annual Rate for One Year Ending September 1988	1990 (Estimate)
Professional	6.9	7.0–8.5
Physician	7.8	8.0–10.0
Hospital & Related Services	11.3	11.5–13.0
Hospital Room	11.8	12.0–13.5
Other Inpatient Services	11.9	12.0–13.5
Outpatient Services	8.8	8.5–10.0
Total Medical Care	7.2	8.5–10.0

Source: Consumer Price Index, Bureau of Labor Statistics, September 1988; estimates provided by Health Forecasting Group, Alameda, California.

The renaissance of acute inpatient care which began in 1989 will be driven by *longer lengths of stay* and *rising hospital admission rates*. After five years of decline, inpatient admissions began to rebound 0.5–1.0 percent in 1988, and the trend will continue in 1989 and on into the early 1990s, with 1–2 percent annual increases. 1988 was the turning point. Finally, all those who could be treated as outpatients have been screened out of inpatient care by their payers, resetting the balance between supply and demand for hospital beds. The aging of the population is the "rising tide that will lift all boats," as the growing number of U.S. seniors translates into higher numbers of inpatient admits. Although the admission rate for those under 65 continues to decline by 0.5–1.0 percent, the rate for adults 65 and above is on the rise.

As inpatient care recovers, better hospitals and public hospitals will experience *bed shortages* in the 1990s. To date, bed crunches have been spotty, but the trend is accelerating. Critical care units in many hospitals will run at consistently high occupancy rates in the future (80–95 percent). This will result in a growing number of temporary emergency room closures due to lack of beds in critical care for acutely ill patients. Emergency room nurses reported in 1988 that as many as 13 percent of U.S. hospitals closed their emergency rooms at least briefly in the month surveyed.

Trend 3: Ambulatory Hospitals

Ambulatory care is still a high-growth market and will grow at rates of 7–15 percent in the 1990s, depending on the service. Expect double-digit growth for

Table 1-2 Forecast 1989: Delphi Survey of Healthcare Forum Panel of 500 Experts

	AGREE[a]	DISAGREE
1. More than 20% of U.S. hospital executives will turn over in 1989.	59.5%	27.4%
2. Managed care plans (HMO/PPO) will enroll 50% of U.S. population by 1991.	46.2	42.5
3. Hospitals will cut 25% of top and middle managers by 1991.	74.5	13.2
4. Wage costs for all hospital personnel—not just nursing—will rise at twice the rate of consumer price index.	59.5	38.6
5. Despite higher wages, labor shortages in health care will get worse.	85.9	7.5
6. Hospitals will double spending for new information systems and high-tech substitutes for labor costs.	85.7	8.5
7. Hospitals will cut operating budgets by 3–5% in 1989.	77.3	15.1
8. Inpatient stay rises by ½ day due to higher case severity.	80.1	16.0
9. Hospital occupancy rises 1–2% on a national basis.	74.5	17.9
10. Health care inflation continues at double-digit levels in 1989, despite efforts of payers and government.	82.1	11.3

Source: "Forecast 1989," Delphi survey by Health Forecasting Group, *Healthcare Forum*, Association of Western Hospitals, © November/December 1988.
[a]Percentages do not include "no opinion" responses.

laser surgery, ophthalmology procedures, urology procedures, plastic surgery, and MRI scanning in the short run (1989–1991). Many hospitals will have a ratio of 50:50 inpatient to outpatient surgery by 1990. In that year, another milestone is likely to be reached. There will be as many ambulatory surgery centers as hospitals.

This does not mean that all physicians will see more patients, but the downward trend in office visits should bottom out, and there will probably be a rise in the 1990s for the many clinical specialities that treat older adults. As the number of elderly approach 15 percent of the population by the year 2000, physician visit rates will be pushed upwards. Doctors whose patients are children or women of childbearing age can expect gradually declining numbers in the 1990s, as the Baby Boom generation ages and the "Echo Boom" consisting of their children comes to an end.

A few small and well-diversified hospitals are beginning to experience 50:50 inpatient revenue to ambulatory revenue. The five-year period 1990–1995 will be a watershed time for ambulatory care. Ambulatory care has cut the umbilical cord that tied it to inpatient care. The growth of ambulatory care is no longer dependent upon shifting inpatient procedures to an ambulatory basis. Most inpatient procedures have already been shifted by changing medical practice and payer policies.

Beginning in 1989, the first generation of "ambulatory hospitals" is testing the concept of clustering ambulatory care services off hospital campuses. Health care guru Jeff Goldsmith is developing, in conjunction with the Sutter Health System of Sacramento, California, and other sponsors, "integrated medical campuses" that embody the ambulatory hospital concept. Some of these ambulatory hospital projects will be designed as "medical malls" but without a hospital as the anchor tenant.

A variation on the concept of the ambulatory hospital has potential for rural hospitals. The Montana legislature enacted in 1988 a new level of hospital licensure, the *medical assistance facility*. More than 30 of Montana's small and rural hospitals serving low-density populations will qualify for hospital payment but under scaled-down regulations for facilities and staffing. The key to this experiment will be HCFA approval of Montana's request for a waiver to pay medical assistance facilities for Medicare services. A number of other state legislatures have contacted Montana for information on this innovative idea.

Trend 4: Speciality Niches

The war of competition among hospitals and among physicians will be fought in the "techno-niches" of clinical specialties. Hospitals and MDs will increasingly use technology for market advantage. The market focus will be on specialized high-tech facilities ("centers of excellence") that the average community hospital will use to compete in a crowded marketplace. Every hospital over 200 beds will have at least one specialty (see Table 1-3 for a list of the top clinical niches for the 1990s).

Recruiting *medical superstars* is, for specialty niches, a shortcut to market dominance. The stakes are high. When Good Samaritan Medical Center of Los Angeles in 1987 recruited Southern California's top cardiac surgeon from St. Vincent's, it swung 400 open-heart surgical procedures to Good Samaritan in the first year. St. Vincent's, which had been California's busiest cardiac program, lost 33 percent of its revenues in one year. Good Samaritan's revenues soared 15 percent in 1988.

Techno-niche programs that feature high-tech procedures have today's highest profit potential, programs such as laser surgery. Demographics are driving the growth—or decline—of niche markets. As the Baby Boom generation moves into its postreproductive years, obstetrics and children's services will

Table 1-3 Clinical Niches: Rating the Specialties for the 1990s

Clinical Niche	Profit Potential	Time Frame
AIDS	Low/losses	2–10 years
Alzheimer's	Low	1–10 years
Cancer	Growing	3–10 years
Cardiac care	High	1–5 years
Diagnostic imaging	Medium	1–10 years
Eye surgery	Declining	Last 5 years
Infectious diseases	Low	1–10 years
Laser surgery	High	Immediate
Lithotripsy	Growing	1–7 years
Lung & respiratory diseases	Medium/low	2–10 years
Neonatal intensive care	Low/losses	1–5 years
Neurosurgery	High	1–10 years
Obstetrics	Medium/low	1–5 years
Occupational medicine	High	Immediate
Otology & cochlear implants	High	2–10 years
Orthopedics & joint replacements	High	1–10 years
Pediatrics	Low	1–5 years
Pediatric cardiology	Medium	1–10 years
Rehabilitation	High	Immediate
Urology	High	1–10 years

decline. The growing number of elderly will create an increasing demand for specialty services such as rehabilitation, lithotripsy, oncology, and urology.

Trend 5: Managed Care

By the beginning of the 1990s, it should be clear that managed care is not a West Coast phenomenon but the shape of things to come. The insurance concept is dead. Indemnity health plans will be virtually unavailable by 1995. Health insurers are reconceptualizing and restructuring their health care book of business on the PPO model. Smaller insurers will use third party administrators to develop private PPO networks in local markets. Managed care will dominate medicine and health care in the 1990s.

Managed care enrollment—in HMOs, PPOs, and EPAs (exclusive provider arrangements)—should be equal to at least 50 percent of the non-Medicare population by 1995. The trend is beginning to impact America's hospitals. Expect that managed care will contribute 5–15 percent of the admissions to hospitals and patients to physicians located in metropolitan areas in 1990, increasing to

20–35 percent by 1995. On the West Coast, the rise will be to 35–45 percent. Rural areas, with smaller employers and low-density populations, will be the last to feel the impact of managed care.

And this is not including Medicare! The managed care percentage will rise still higher as Medicare HMOs and Medicare PPOs begin to enroll significant numbers of the elderly in the 1990s. Seniors are more likely to prefer the PPO option because of its flexible physician choice. Managed care plans could enroll 50 percent of Medicare beneficiaries by 1995. That means discounted Medicare fees for physician services from the Medicare HMO and PPOs, a problem that could be compounded if Congress enacts "mandatory assignment" and acceptance of Medicare fees as payment in full.

The growth of managed care means U.S. physicians and hospitals will be put on a diet of *fixed-price revenues*. When managed care is added to Medicare, many MDs and hospitals will find that 60–75 percent of inpatient revenues are prospectively set. The trend toward physician "fee bundling" with hospital reimbursement probably means less revenue for both MDs and hospitals on inpatient care. Worse yet, a high percentage of physician services and inpatient admissions will be priced at or below cost, depending on how large a discount was negotiated by managed care buyers, how well the hospital is coping under DRGs, and how well the MD's specialty was treated by the new Harvard RVS.

How far away is the managed care era? Not far. California, the bellwether state, had 69.7 percent of its non-Medicare population enrolled in managed care plans at the beginning of 1988, with 7 million HMO members and 11 million PPO enrollees. The Twin Cities of Minnesota are not far behind.

Watch for *blurring boundaries* between HMOs and PPOs in the 1990s. The fastest-growing kind of HMO today is the "open-ended HMO," which works something like a PPO. Enrollees decide whether to use the HMO or PPO option every time they get sick and pay a high deductible for selecting the PPO option to use their personal physicians or non-HMO hospitals. Open-ended HMOs enrolled 350,000 new members in the first quarter of 1988, according to InterStudy in Excelsior, Minnesota. Half of those signed up for Prudential's open-ended option.

EPAs are redefining the concept of preferred provider. Major insurance companies and employers will begin to channel patients into hospitals that have an exclusive contract to provide specialized services such as open-heart surgery and transplants. Prudential Insurance and Honeywell have recently selected a short list of hospitals that will be the exclusive providers of high-tech specialized services. The competition for such arrangements will be won on quality, not price. Hospitals must put into place systems like MediQual to demonstrate their quality and effectiveness to buyers. In the 1990s, watch HMOs, PPOs, and insurance companies follow a similiar pattern of contracting only with selected medical groups and preferred MD specialists.

Trend 6: Age Wave

Older Americans will become the main customers of U.S. hospitals and physicians. Hospitals will see an increasing number of older patients in 1989 and the decade ahead. The "age wave" that gerontologists Ken Dychtwald and Mark Zitter forecast is arriving. Their company, Age Wave (of Emeryville, California), is well-named. The average community hospital will experience a 35–45 percent Medicare caseload in 1989, and a growing number of hospitals will break through the 50 percent Medicare level by 1991. A sign of the times occurred in 1988: A new association was formed that consists of hospitals with over 75 percent of their patients on Medicare. The association was created by Saddleback Community Hospital (in Laguna Hills, California) and more than 15 other hospitals for the purpose of articulating their special problems to Congress and to HCFA. Saddleback is adjacent to Leisure World and draws heavily from its older residents. Most other members of the 75-percent club are either small and rural or located within inner cities.

Hospitals will intensify development of the *continuum of care* of elderly services. The Medicare length of stay may rise by 0.5 days in 1989, after a 5-year decline. Hospitals will need long-term care alternatives to minimize costly extra "administrative days" needed by Medicare patients. Expect a growing number of hospitals (1) to convert underused beds to subacute and extended care and (2) to buy nursing homes in the 1990s. Demand for continuing care retirement centers (CCRCs) is slowing; the market is glutted now, but the demand will return by the early 1990s.

Laventhol & Horwath predicts the next trend will be *assisted living facilities* (ALFs). These facilities provide assistance with activities of daily living but no "health" services, and they are licensed by welfare, not health, departments. Most ALFs are small, family-owned operations. The new generation of ALFs will be co-located with nursing homes, providing another level of care.

Senior membership plans (SMPs) will be sponsored by more than 50 percent of U.S. hospitals by 1990. Peter Yedidia, of San Francisco-based Geriatric Health Systems, and Edita Kaye, of Kaye Associates in New York, believe senior membership plans may be the single most important marketing initiative for hospitals to use in tapping the senior market. As competition rises among SMPs, each hospital must differentiate its plan from those offered by rival hospitals. Senior discounts, free health screenings, Medicare copay write-offs, newsletters, and incentives will be offered, and more. A good strategy neglected by most hospitals is to have a senior activity center. More than 50 percent of all seniors use activity centers at least monthly.

New *federal funding for long-term care* will be enacted by the next Congress. President Bush took a stand supporting expanded federal support of health services for older Americans. He was responding to the "senior lobby," today's most potent political voter bloc. Representative Claude Pepper's $40 billion proposal to expand home care and long-term care did not pass, but Senator Ted Kennedy and Representative Henry Waxman have legislative proposals with price tags of $20 billion to $25 billion that have a better chance of providing long-term care services to the elderly. Long-term care will be a major legislative battle zone in the 1990s.

Trend 7: Hub-and-Spoke Networks

Like the airlines, America's hospitals and physicians are restructuring to form hub-and-spoke networks. Such networks are being constructed on a national, regional, and local basis. Many hospitals will belong to networks at all three levels.

National networks (i.e., service alliances and purchasing organizations) are enrolling hospitals rapidly. Niche-oriented national alliances, such as Consolidated Catholic Health Care and Premier Alliance, both located in Westchester, Illinois, are developing a national membership base. Established national alliances, such as VHA and American Healthcare Systems (AHS), will sharpen their focus on their base businesses (group purchasing and member services) and scale back diversification efforts. VHA may sell its share of the Partners health plan. By 1995, more than 90 percent of U.S. hospitals will be affiliated with a national alliance or purchasing group.

Regional networks are gaining market clout. At the regional level, alliances such as SunHealth and purchasing organizations such as AmeriNet are member-driven and expanding rapidly. They will make some inroads among clients of VHA and AHS, and AmeriNet of St. Louis is expanding into the national market. Regional alliances such as Virginia Mason's multistate network in the Northwest and VHA's regional "clusters" are being established around VHA shareholder hospitals. The VHA regional hub-and-spoke networks are formalizing clinical relationships to channel tertiary care patients and are marketing regionally distributed managed care plans. SunHealth is organizing similiar networks at the state level. Cooperating multihospital systems are beginning to establish managed care networks on a regional basis, such as the PPO Alliance sponsored by UniHealth America and the Adventist West systems in southern California.

Local networks will be the next trend. Hospitals will develop local networks to manage local markets by establishing a dominant market presence. Major medical centers will take the initiative to organize their own local hub-and-spoke networks. Local networks will include hospitals, medical groups, and preferred medical specialists. Most are now organized for managed care contracting (HMOs and PPOs) and to control flows of patients for specialized services. Many small and rural hospitals are joining networks to gain access to group purchasing, financial services, sophisticated information systems, marketing, and clinical support. Management agreements tighten the bonds between the small hospital and the network's core hospital. Physicians will be brought into the loop using systems like Magliaro and McHaney's remote practice network or Baxter Health-care's physician computer networking system. Computerized physician referral services like the "Ask-A-Nurse" system developed by the Referral Systems Group of Roseville, California, provide an overlay that reinforces the bond between physicians and hospitals.

Among physicians, a similiar trend is developing. Large group practices of 25–100 doctors will become commonplace in major metropolitan areas. These "supergroups" will be multisite, be electronically networked, and have large managed care contracts and caseloads for which the doctors are "gatekeepers." Although some groups are expanding by direct acquisition of smaller practices, most groups are scaling up through voluntary affiliation (merger) or by increasing the number of salaried physicians (internal growth).

Trend 8: Service Line Management

Product line management has not caught on with hospitals, but this will change in the 1990s. The reason is simple. In 1988–89, hospital inpatient volume rose while profits fell. There is no longer any necessary relationship between activity and profitability in U.S. hospitals. If occupancy rises again, so may losses. That means that every service, unit, and program is a minibusiness, with its own customers, market, demand, ability to pay, medical staff, cost structure, staffing, and competitors. Each service and department is a strategic business unit largely independent of other units.

Reconceptualize the hospital as *health care mall* with a series of medical boutiques. Service line management is the way hospitals will respond, by clustering related services under a single manager for clinical and market management. This puts enormous pressure on department heads and program directors to become small business owners and entrepreneurs. Most are untrained for service line management and lack many important business and marketing skills. Nothing in preparing the annual budget based on "plus or minus 5 percent" has given department heads the skills they will need. And top management will put enormous pressure on every service unit to be profitable in tomorrow's climate of shrinking payments for inpatient services.

The result will be high levels of *middle management turnover*—in the range of 15–30 percent in the early 1990s. Managerial stress will be high and morale low in middle management ranks unless hospitals move to strengthen skills and give service line managers the backup they will need in finance, business planning and marketing.

Trend 9: Service Excellence

The shortest route to high performance and profitability is quality *service*. Gaining a service advantage over competitors is much cheaper than buying high-cost technology, and it is also a strong factor in repeat business. Customer service guru Ron Zemke, of Minneapolis-based Performance Management Associates, has a new book, *The Service Edge: 101 Companies that Profit from Consumer Care* (1989), which includes three hospitals among these exemplary service companies.

These three are among the top hospitals in America, all of which are beginning to experience the wave of *bed shortages* that will crest in the 1990s. What makes these hospitals magnets for patients and physicians is the quality of their care and their caring. What makes these hospitals tops in service? Customer-driven CEOs like Duffy Watson, who heads the 125-bed Henry Mayo Newhall Hospital in Valencia, California. Watson walks his hospital's corridors on weekends, pocket dictating machine in hand, and notes any deviations from perfection in the hospital's environment or service. Monday morning memos to Henry Mayo's management team are called "Shazzams!" after the lightning bolts in comic strips. After ten years of his high-visibility concern for service, Duffy Watson needs to send fewer Shazzams each year. The entire hospital knows his concern, and superior customer ratings demonstrate the impact.

Large physician groups are discovering "guest relations" as they expand the scope of practice marketing. A rolodex may be a doctor's most valuable marketing tool. No doctor can take patients' loyalty for granted today. To maintain high rates of return business, physicians are turning to customer relations programs that go well beyond "charm school" for physician office staff. Managing the service dimension of medical practice begins with an understanding of customers. Physician marketing consultant Randall Elliott, of Dynamic Solutions (based in Littleton, Colorado), underscores the need for MDs to practice "relationships management" with their patients. Today's health care consumers want choices, information, and doctor and office staff responsiveness.

Trend 10: Outcomes Management

In a managed care, market-driven world, physicians and hospitals with the best-managed quality outcomes will be the *preferred providers*—preferred by managed care plans, insurance companies, employers, physicians, and consumers. Five major forces are converging to propel quality to the fore:

1. *Managed care buyers* (employers, HMOs, PPOs, and insurance plans) will select hospitals and physicians based on their quality and effectiveness.

2. *Federal and state governments* are increasing public disclosure of morbidity and mortality rates.
3. *Major employers* and employer health care coalitions are developing regional data bases, implementing comparative quality assessment systems like MediQual, hiring quality consultants to pick superior providers, and entering into exclusive provider arrangements with select hospitals and MDs for specialized services.
4. *Consumers* are asking for second opinions, reading books like *The Best Hospitals in America* and *The Best of Medicine*, and shopping for quality and value.
5. *Voluntary certifying bodies* such as the Joint Commission are widening the range of facilities they review for quality, extending certification to HMOs, and pilot-testing the first sets of outcome criteria that will be added to the hospital certification process in 1991–1993.

In response, the health industry may create a new profession, *outcomes manager*, according to health care guru Paul Elwood, M.D., of InterStudy in Excelsior, Minnesota. Outcomes management is more than a mindset, it may be a new profession, believe health care recruiters, Miller and Moore, an executive search firm in San Diego, California. Inspired by an article by Ellwood in a recent issue of the *New England Journal of Medicine*, Miller and Moore is developing job descriptions and a profile of the knowledge, skills, and experience needed by outcomes managers, whose positions may range from program director in a community hospital to vice-president in a major medical center or multihospital.

The concept of outcomes management has potential. Multihospital systems can scrutinize outcomes in their units from their corporate perspective. HMOs and PPOs will use outcomes to identify preferred providers and create screens to routinely monitor and manage quality across their provider network. Major employers can use outcomes managers to oversee employee health, focusing on high-cost procedures given to employees, dependents, and retirees.

The result will be an increased focus on *quality* in the 1990s, with stepped-up programs for risk management and quality assurance and closer attention paid to customer ratings. Hospital-based risk management programs will be extended to physician offices. Expect hospitals to experiment with the position of outcomes manager, coordinating the activities of risk management, quality assurance, environmental monitoring, regulatory and certification compliance and reporting, occupational health and safety, and customer ratings.

STRATEGIC IMPLICATIONS FOR PHYSICIANS

1. *Every physician must be a forecaster*. The future is too important to leave to chance. Physicians must be continuously concerned about the future,

tracking the trends impacting their patients, practice, medical specialty, hospitals, and the professions.

2. *Organized medicine needs an organized environmental assessment program.* Every medical specialty society, in cooperation with the American Medical Association, should prepare an annual forecast of key trends in the specialty for its practitioners and disseminate the report widely. The process can be repeated every three years, with a less sweeping review of past trends and predicted changes conducted annually.

3. *Physicians must take the leadership in hospital-planning processes.* Ideally, physicians would co-chair every hospital planning committee in America. Their high-level participation is essential, both to advance the interests of medicine and to add the clinical viewpoint to the decision-making process with regard to strategic issues of importance to hospitals.

4. *Physicians must learn the skills of medical futuring.* Trained in the reductionist methods of science, clinicians are only half-trained when it comes to strategic thinking and managing their future. Physicians must expand their awareness and set of skills to include the methods of forecasting and futuring.

5. *Medical visionaries should be encouraged.* Medicine needs to reaffirm the importance of the role of medical visionary. To advance clinically and economically, medicine must develop its own vision. Medical visionaries can communicate new images of what the future may bring medicine and thus advance the debate and improve medicine's readiness to manage its future.

STRATEGIC IMPLICATIONS FOR HOSPITALS

1. *Every health care executive must be a forecaster.* The job descriptions of America's health executives should contain a new role: forecaster. No one knows better what the future will bring to a hospital than its senior executives. They know local market conditions best and can "read the tea leaves" of industry change from the perspective of local experience.

2. *"Industry trends" need to be placed in a broader socioeconomic context.* Health industry trends must be interpreted in light of broader socioeconomic patterns affecting regional and local markets. Every market is unique. Think of forecasts by industry experts as second opinions on the judgments of local executives, which are hopefully buttressed by the opinions of local medical staff, trustees, and managers. Ideally, all will share a sense of what lies ahead for the hospital and the community health care marketplace.

3. *Assumptions about the future should be explicit and tested often.* These future assumptions need to be spelled out clearly. They will guide all major

strategy, market, capital investment, budget, and operations decisions for the coming years. In a period of rapid change, it will be important to continuously recheck the key assumptions used by the hospital in planning its strategic future.

4. *Annual "State of the Union" forecasts should be developed.* Here is a suggestion to hospital executives and senior strategists for a New Year's resolution: Publicize your views on the market outlook for the year ahead on January 1. Hospital execs should prepare a State of the Union white paper on the outlook for health care and the institution in the year ahead. The forecast should be widely shared and presented to trustees, medical staff, management, and employees in January and February. This will set the stage for the annual budgeting cycle in the spring.

5. *Forecasting is a symbolic leadership act.* Preparation of an annual market forecast could be one of the most important symbolic management acts the hospital executive will perform all year. It confirms the role of the executive as the senior strategist and lays out the major strategic directions for the coming year. More importantly, the annual forecast will provide the underlying assumptions for making day-to-day management decisions. Hospitals do manage their future, but they do so by means of the many tactical and operational decisions that are made routinely. These decisions drive and shape the future of the organization. Ideally, they will be informed by a forecast of where the local health care market is going in the year ahead so that the hospital can avoid the threats and capitalize on the opportunities the future will bring. Start this next year!

Part II

The New Medicine

Chapter 2

Medicine's New Economics

As an economic good, health care is fundamentally a commodity product and is affected by some simple economics: extent of availability, number of buyers, and therefore, a competitive market. Attempts to overcome these economic realities have led to the commercialization of health care.
    —John H. Moxley III, *The Changing Health Care Market*

Throw the old textbooks of medical economics away. These are changing times. The health care industry is in transition from a regulated to a free market economy. As a result, a social good—medical care—has clearly become an economic commodity, even a commercial product. This creates complex problems, both for the economics of medical care and for social policy and the health care profession it affects. Change—continuous, sometimes jolting shifts in every aspect of health care—will be common for the next 10–15 years. Not until the turn of the 21st century will the industry be restabilized (Coile 1986).

The trendlines of change point in all directions. New patterns are forming, but which will dominate? Economists are in disarray. There are many possible futures and scenarios. The future of medicine arrives daily and it impacts every health service provider. But although the future is near, it is far from clear.

What will the future bring? For some health care providers, the years ahead are threatening. Doomsday forecasts suggest hundreds of hospitals could be swept into bankruptcy and thousands of physicians into early retirement by payer pressure and vicious market competition. For others, the future will bring opportunity by creating new products, new markets, and redefining their base business as health, not illness. Their futures will only be limited by their imagination. The starting point for managing the future is awareness of the driving forces that will transform the industry in the next 5–15 years.

THE NEW ECONOMICS OF MEDICAL CARE

First the good news: Health care is expanding—and at double-digit rates. Hospital expenditures rose at a rate of 11.6 percent in the first half of 1988 and expenditures for physician services at a rate of 9.3 percent, according to the medical care component of the CPI. Health care's share of the gross national product (GNP) soared to 11.1 percent by the end of 1988. HCFA predicts health spending will continue to rise in the 1990s, reaching 15 percent of the GNP by the year 2000.

Now the bad news: Physicians and hospitals are making less money than ever, despite record-level revenues, as their costs rise faster than reimbursement. The problem is simple. Per-unit reimbursement for health services is not keeping pace with health cost inflation. Half of all U.S. hospitals lost money in 1988; as few as one in four institutions may be profitable in 1989, according to predictions by the Healthcare Financial Management Association. Physician incomes rose by 3.2 percent in 1987, according to *Medical Economics'* annual survey. But the gain in practice earnings was more than offset by the 4.4 percent hike in the overall cost of living, so physicians lost buying power (Owens 1988).

National Health Expenditures

Dramatic changes in health care reimbursement have not resulted in lower health costs, only in shifting the pattern of health care spending from inpatient to ambulatory. That conclusion is becoming clear from an analysis of trends in national medical care expenditures since the mid-1980s. The overall trend in health spending continues upward.

In 1988, national health expenditures reached $541 billion, up from $500 billion in 1987. On average, almost $2,000 was spent on health care for every person in the United States. Health spending continued to outpace the cost of living in 1987, as national health costs rose by 9.8 percent, compared to a 4.4 percent climb in the CPI. The distribution of health spending in 1987 is illustrated in Figure 2-1.

In 1987, expenditures for hospital services reached $195 billion, or 39 percent of all national health care spending. Hospital inflation has been steadily moving upward since 1984. The 1987 inflation rate of 9.1 percent was the steepest since 1982, the year prior to implementation of prospective payment systems (PPSs).

Hospital costs appear to be caught in a new upward spiral of double-digit inflation. One of the driving factors is the nursing shortage, which has resulted in many hospitals boosting nurse wages by 7–15 percent in 1987–1988. Better wages for nurses are helping reduce the shortage, but the nurse vacancy rate fell only from 13.6 percent in 1987 to 11.3 percent in 1988. This has come at a high cost in terms of hospital overhead, since more than 50 percent of most

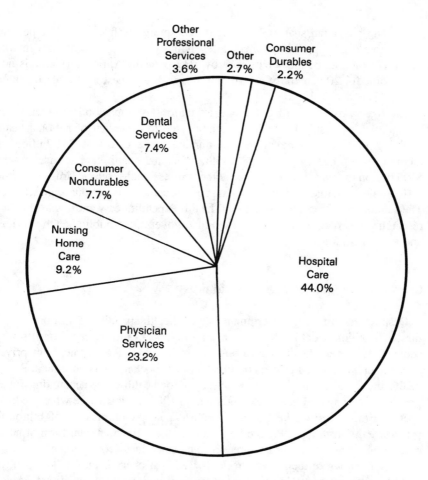

Figure 2-1 Distribution of the Personal Health Care Dollar in the United States (1987)

hospital budgets goes for personnel. Wage inflation is predicted to fall to 5–8 percent in the next three years, but the cost structure of hospitals has been permanently inflated at a time when per-unit reimbursement is falling and will continue to fall, at least in the near future.

Hospital expenditures are a shrinking piece of the health care pie. In 1987, hospitals had a 39 percent share of the pie, down from almost 41 percent five years earlier. The impact of PPSs has been to shift demand from inpatient to ambulatory care.

Spending for physician services increased twice as fast as community hospital inpatient revenues in 1983–1987 (Owens 1988). National expenditures for physician services topped $100 billion for the first time, reaching $103 billion in

1987. The physician share of the health care pie grew from 19 to 21 percent, and double-digit increases in medical spending pushed up the doctors' market share. Hospital ambulatory care rose by 16.7 percent. Ambulatory care is now responsible for 20 percent of community hospital revenues, a gain of 50 percent in only five years.

The age wave has still not made an enormous impact on long-term care expenditures. Nursing home services amounted to 8 percent of national health spending in 1987. The total cost of nursing home care was $41 billion, an increase of 8.6 percent over 1986. Other personal health care services totaled $105 billion in 1987, for dental care, other professional services, drugs and other nondurables, durable medical products, and miscellaneous personal care services. The remaining 12 percent of national health expenditures went toward medical research, construction of medical facilities, government public health services, and administration.

Sources of National Health Expenditures

Despite fears of "big government," most health spending is still private. Of the $500 billion spent on health care in 1987, $293 billion came from private sources. For every health care dollar spent in 1987, $.59 came from private pockets, either from employers or directly out of pocket from consumers. Private health insurance is the largest single payer for health care, accounting for 32 percent of all national health expenditures in 1987, almost twice what Medicare spends. Employers, workers, and individuals paid premiums of $158 billion for private health insurance. Private health insurance is the dominant form of health care reimbursement, covering three in four Americans (76.6 percent).

Consumers wrote their own checks for $.25 of every health dollar spent. In 1987, consumers spent $123 billion from their own pockets, for direct services as well as insurance copayments. The more expensive the service, the more insurance covered. Only 10 percent of hospital care costs were paid by consumers themselves. For small-ticket items, such as drugs and nondurable medical products, consumers covered 75 percent of the expenditures.

Government covers 41 percent of all health costs: Medicare, 17 percent, Medicaid, 10 percent; and other government programs, 17 percent. Medicare is the largest publicly funded health program. In 1988 Medicare expenditures were more than $87 billion, and spending will top $97 billion in 1989. Medicaid spent $52 billion for health services provided to 23.2 million of the nation's poor. Special entitlements and targeted programs funded by tax dollars account for another 17 percent of all health costs. Other governmental health spending covered groups such as the military and their dependents, veterans, injured workers, Native Americans, and those who do not qualify for Medicaid.

Soaring Medicare costs are partially a myth. The rate of increase of government spending for health care is not higher than the rate for other payers. Indeed, health spending by all payers—private health insurance, Medicare, Medicaid, and consumers—has been going up at about the same rate for the past five years (at an average of 9.1 percent).

MEDICAL ECONOMICS: TRENDS IN PHYSICIAN INCOMES

While hospital revenues fell, doctor earnings slowly climbed at a rate of 5.6 percent for the five years prior to 1987. Hikes in physician fees in 1986, in response to payer pressures, resulted in a 10 percent gain in medical revenues in 1986. Double-digit increases in earnings did not last long. Rising practice costs and declining reimbursement quickly reversed the trend in 1987.

Physicians have reason to worry about their incomes. For more than five years, medical practice costs have been climbing faster than fees or revenues. Doctors are still among the most highly compensated professional groups, but their real incomes have been declining for most of the 1980s. Rising fees have not covered costs. Physician fees advanced 6.3 percent in 1987, moderating after an average rise of 7.1 percent over the previous five years. Professional expenses rose sharply, with practice cost inflation averaging 10.4 percent in the same five-year period. Rapidly growing practice costs outpaced physician revenues for most of the 1980s. Even in 1987, when doctors managed to hold their practice expenses down to a 6 percent boost, mounting costs were almost double their net practice incomes.

Is this trend of lower net physician incomes permanent? The reality is that medical fee increases cannot cover rising costs. In the future, physicians can only improve their net incomes by cutting overhead costs or increasing service volume. The alternatives are just that simple.

Income Variations

All doctors are not equal when it comes to revenues or profits. The typical cardiovascular surgeon earned more than twice the 1987 norm for all physicians, whereas the typical G.P. fell nearly one-third short. In terms of dollar medians, cardiovascular surgeons, the highest earners according to *Medical Economics* annual survey, netted $191,640 more per doctor than G.P.s (Owens 1988). The net incomes comparison: $271,550 for the cardiovascular surgeons versus $79,910 for G.P.s. The average doctor's net income in 1987 was $116,440 on gross revenues of $210,480.

Physicians in groups do better than solos, and the gap is widening. Those who share both income and expenses in groups netted $38,070 more than their counterparts in solo practice, a difference of 35 percent in 1987. Only two years before, the gap was 25 percent. The reasons are lower office expenses per doctor (efficiency) and, primarily, higher volume. Doctors in groups see more patients: Multispecialty groups average 17 percent more patients and single-specialty groups pull in almost 25 percent more.

Location is a factor in physician earnings. Urban physicians netted 5.4 percent more than colleagues in the suburbs, and they made $14,060 (13.1 percent) more than rural doctors. The mid-South was the best place to practice from an earnings standpoint. Among the best-paid physicians, regardless of specialty, were doctors located in Alabama, Kentucky, Mississippi, and Tennessee. They averaged a net income of $135,000—16 percent above the national median and 35 percent more than New Englanders, the lowest earners among U.S. physicians.

PHYSICIAN FEES: TARGETS OF INCREASED REGULATION

Physician fees are becoming the number one target of America's health care payers. Doctors can expect reimbursement reform, and soon. Congress and HCFA are pointing to doctors as the source of the problems facing Medicare. An 18 percent jump in Medicare Part B costs for physician services in 1987 triggered the mounting criticism of physician fees and earnings. Medicare spending for Part B physician services may be capped by Congress, putting an arbitrary limit on medical payments.

Physician Fee Freeze

Washington's experiments with regulating physician reimbursement have not always produced the results that policy makers and Congress desired. A physician fee freeze was imposed in July 1984 and continued through April 1986 for "participating" physicians and through December 1986 for "nonparticipating" physicians. Even while the freeze was in effect, Medicare expenditures per beneficiary increased by 26 percent.

Physicians figured out how to "game" the new system by increasing volume and substituting more expensive services for less expensive ones. This accounted for two-thirds of the increase in Medicare's physician costs during the three-year freeze. Surgery, radiology, and special tests had the highest growth rates. For example, the number of hip replacement operations per 1,000 Medicare beneficiaries increased only slightly, but the volume of coronary artery bypass surgery grew 19 percent, the volume of knee replacements grew 39 percent, and the volume of lens procedures surged upward 50 percent.

General surgeons increased volume by 9 percent during the freeze, and internists saw their Medicare visits rise 17 percent. Most of the growth occurred in the specialties: thoracic surgery, up 42 percent; cardiology, up 49 percent; ophthalmology, up 57 percent; and gastroenterology, up 73 percent.

Harvard RVS Study

The long-awaited study by Harvard's William Hsiao (1988) was delivered to HCFA in the late fall of 1988. Many expect the study to provide the basis for setting national price controls on physician fees in the 1990s. Medicare, state Medicaid programs, and many private insurers are expected to utilize the Harvard RVS scale to set payment for physician services. Moving to a single standard of payment would eliminate most of the regional differences in physician charges and service patterns.

The Harvard study developed a resource-based relative value scale (RBRVS) as an index of the relative levels of resource input expended when physicians provide services or perform procedures. The RBRVS is divided into nonmonetary units. When used as a conversion scale, the RBRVS is multiplied by a monetary conversion factor (dollars per unit). The scale was developed using three factors: (1) the work expended on a particular service, which is determined by the amount of time before, during, and after the service and the intensity of activity during that time; (2) the practice costs of providing the service; and (3) the opportunity costs of specialty training.

The Harvard RVS study was conducted for HCFA in order to help devise a new and standardized approach for physician payment. The researchers assumed that the new scale would not change the overall volume of services and procedures and that it would be "budget neutral" (i.e., it would not increase Medicare spending for physician services).

Implicit in the new scale are biases intended to reduce fees for specialized procedures and increase compensation for the "cognitive medicine" of G.P.s, family practitioners, and internists, who typically diagnose and treat patients without using high-cost procedures. The most sharply affected specialists would be cardiovascular surgeons and ophthalmologists ("losers") and family practitioners and allergists ("winners"), as graphically illustrated in Figure 2-2. An average family practitioner could receive 60–70 percent more in revenues from Medicare if the RBRVS schedule were adopted, whereas cardiovascular surgeons could earn 40–50 percent less from Medicare.

Doctors should brace themselves for a national fee schedule. Although the RVS study is widely controversial, the American Medical Association (AMA)

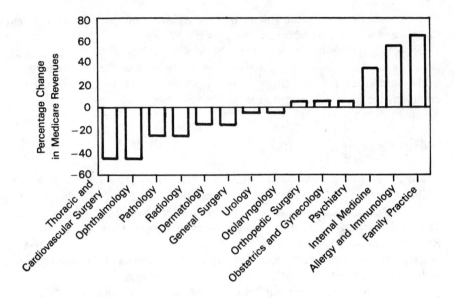

Figure 2-2 Results of simulation of the impact of an RBRVS-based fee schedule on 1986 Medicare payments, according to specialty. *Source*: Reprinted from *Medical Benefits*, Vol. 5, No. 20, p. 2, with permission of Kelly Communications, © October 1988. (Data obtained from a study by William C. Hsiao, Harvard School of Public Health.)

has already endorsed it in principle (their assumption is that some fine-tuning will be done before implementation). The RVS scale is likely to be adopted by federal regulators and widely used by private insurers and third party payers.

HOSPITALS IN TRANSITION

The coming changes in health care will be painful, especially for hospitals. The state of America's hospital economy can be described in a word: *recession*. For the five-year period from 1983 to 1987, the economic signals were flat or declining and the downward trend accelerated (see Figure 2-3). Hospital inpatient admissions reached a plateau in 1981. By 1982 the decline in patient days had begun, and by 1984 the downturn had become precipitous. Further erosion continued until 1987, and only in 1988 did the hospital industry begin to recover.

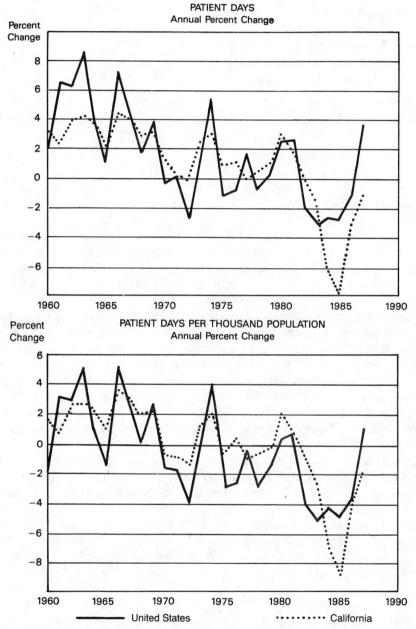

Figure 2-3 The Rate of Hospital Use 1960–1987. *Source*: Data from *Hospital Statistics: 1985 Edition*, American Hospital Association, Chicago, IL.

Hospitals want to know the following:

- Is the recession permanent?
- How soon (if ever) will growth resume?
- Where will recession hit hardest?
- Who will get hurt? Or benefit?
- Will the overall *health* market continue to grow even as the hospital market declines?
- How can hospitals participate in that growth?

Profile of the Downturn

All hospitals lost ground in 1983–1987. Whereas admissions registered 36 million in 1984, about the same as 1983, the length of hospital stay decreased from 7.6 days to 7.3 days, and the national average daily census decreased by 6.3 percent in 1984. The trend continued in 1985, with a further decline in length of stay to 6.7 days (Morse 1988).

The nation's 5,800 short-stay community hospitals have experienced a decline of 5–15 percent in patient days over the past two years, depending on location and case mix. Some regions have been hit harder. The midwest and the Mountain States, with traditionally longer lengths of hospital stay, experienced the sharpest decline in patient days in 1984. According to the American Hospital Association, (AHA), average daily census fell between 7.6 and 9.6 percent in the Midwest and 6.7 percent in the Rocky Mountain area. Every region experienced downturn: New England, 3.5 percent; Middle Atlantic, 2.0 percent; Southeast, 7.2 percent; and Pacific, 3.7 percent.

Small hospitals were more vulnerable to declining census. Facilities under 25 beds lost 13.1 percent of their patient days, and those with 25–49 beds saw their patient days erode by 10.7 percent. Larger hospitals have been somewhat more recession resistant thus far: Facilities of 300–399 beds lost 6.5 percent of their daily census, and very large hospitals (over 500 beds) slipped only 5.4 percent. Midsize hospitals (200–299 beds) were least affected by the downward trend, losing only 4.6 percent compared with the national decline in average daily census of 6.3 percent.

The Hospital Economy under the "New Medicine"

Hospitals are adjusting to the realities of the new medicine. Despite the Doomsday forecasts, there has been no widespread failure of American hospitals. After the introduction of PPSs, 24 U.S. short-stay community hospitals were closed or consolidated in 1984, consistent with the ten-year trend toward a less numerous industry base of larger hospitals. In 1985, 56 hospitals were closed; in 1986, 71; and in 1987, another 79. The trend continues but is not accelerating at a doomsday rate. In 1988, 81 hospitals were closed (Burda 1989).

In this transition, the average hospital size grew from 158 beds in 1974 to 177 beds in 1984, whereas the number of hospitals shrank gradually from 5,875 to 5,759. At the end of 1988, America had experienced a net loss of nearly 500 hospitals in the 1980s.

For-Profit Hospital Companies

Many hospitals continue to prosper under prospective payment and case reimbursement, although profit margins have slipped from double to single-digit levels (Cahan, Deveny, and Hamilton 1986). Shrinking profits have had their most visible impact on investor-owned health care companies. Hospital Corporation of America had flat earnings growth for 1986, and projected earnings by other major investor-owned health care management companies were well below the 15–25 percent levels of the past. In response, Wall Street took a $3 billion bite out of the market value of the biggest publicly traded health care issues in late 1985, and the stocks were slow to bounce back, despite the upward surge of the stock market to record highs in 1987 (Hull 1985). The October 1987 stock market crash wiped out up to 40 percent of the gains of the for-profits, but the largest companies have generally recovered their ground. Hospital Corporation of America, National Medical Enterprises, and Humana again are achieving strong earnings records and high per-share prices.

All of the investor-owned systems went through painful downsizings, reducing overhead, eliminating or selling off unprofitable divisions, and divesting nonperforming hospitals. Companies like Republic, NuMed, Summit, and Paracelsus, which specialized in smaller, low-margin facilities, have been hit harder and are taking longer to recover. Several of the investor-owned hospital companies have taken a lesson from the private sector in boosting stock value by spinning off less profitable facilities into new companies financed by employee stock ownership plans. The result of decreasing the drag on earnings of low-margin facilities has been improved balance sheets and better net income.

It now seems unlikely that investor-owned hospitals will achieve the market share once forecast for them: double-digit growth and 30 percent of the hospital market. Investor-owned hospitals have remained stable at 15 percent of U.S. hospitals, with their growth coming primarily in specialty facilities (e.g., acute psychiatric and rehabilitation units).

Future Threats to U.S. Hospitals

Under the economics of the new medicine, the greatest threats to hospitals may lie ahead: growth of HMOs and selective contracting by major buyers (insurance companies and employers). Contracts will be the lifeblood of tomorrow's hospitals, and physicians will account for 60–75 percent of all patients by 1995. One Los Angeles hospital has more than 150 contracts; many have 50–60 HMO or PPO agreements. Those hospitals which are not "preferred providers" or part of an HMO network will lose a significant share of the market.

Development of a Seige Mentality

Confidence in the future health care economy among senior hospital executives and physician leadership is guarded. In a 1987 Delphi survey on the health industry in the 1990s conducted by the accounting firm of Arthur Andersen and Company in conjunction with the American College of Hospital Administrators, the majority of health care executives and medical society leaders surveyed believed that hospital failures would increase, especially in small, free-standing nonprofit hospitals (*Health Care* 1987). The panelists predicted that 700 U.S. hospitals would close. The trauma would be greatest in the near future, with 84 hospitals closing per year until 1990. From 1990 to 1995, the number of hospital failures was predicted to be 75 per year.

Chief financial officers show even more caution about economic prospects for hospitals. The January 1986 issue of *Healthcare Financial Management* carried articles with titles like "Filing for Bankruptcy: A Sign of Failure or Hope for the Hospital," "Organizational Downsizing: Streamlining the Healthcare Organization," and "Hospital Closure: Who Will Be at Risk in the Upcoming Decade."

The decline in patient days had been foreseen by the Institute for the Future in a 1988 study entitled *Healthcare Services Environment: Hospital Utilization to 1995*, which was prepared for the Robert Wood Johnson Foundation of Princeton, New Jersey. The Menlo Park–based futurists predicted the boom in hospital admissions would end in the 1980s, and they forecast an 8 percent decline by 1995. If current trends continue, their analysis may have underestimated how rapidly the reduction in length of stay would cut into total hospital patient days.

Blame the Buyers for Hospital Slump

The damage to America's hospital industry has multiple causes, which are summarized in Table 2-1. The decline is primarily attributable to the cost-containment initiatives of the major purchasers (government, employers, and

Table 2-1 Role of Major Buyers in the Hospital Economy

Major Buyers	Trigger Factors	Cost-Containment Strategies
Government	Medicare cost rise, federal deficits, Social Security bankruptcy	Shift to prospective pay, freeze on physician fees, reductions in Medicaid dollars
Business	1981–1983 recession, health cost rise of 15% to 30% per year	Greater use of HMOs and PPOs, employer health coalitions, reinstallment of employee front-end deductibles and coinsurance
Insurance companies	Hospital cost rise of 15% to 30% per year, no effective controls over hospital or M.D. use	Develop HMOs, PPO contracts, concentrate on administrative services to employers, 2nd opinions
Consumers	Increasing out-of-pocket costs, rising coinsurance, malpractice	HMO enrollment, fitness and wellness, consumer activism
Integrated health plans	Fee-for-service system not cost competitive, rising HMO enrollment, physician surplus creates labor pool	National HMOs and PPOs forming, new alliances between providers and insurance companies, mainstream M.D.s join HMOs and PPOs

insurance companies) and secondarily to increasing competition from HMOs and ambulatory services.

For the long term, the decline signals a profound shift in consumption patterns that will reshape the hospital industry over the next 5–15 years. The downturn began in 1984 when hospital revenues rose only 5.4 percent, the first time hospitals failed to achieve a double-digit growth rate in the past ten years. In response, U.S. hospitals took nearly 11,000 beds off line in 1984, the first time there was no increase in acute hospital capacity in almost 40 years. The hospital work force lost over 600,000 jobs. Losses at the nation's hospitals more than doubled between 1980 and 1984, when they totaled $5.7 billion.

FUTURE MACROTRENDS IN THE HOSPITAL INDUSTRY

Although the demand for hospital services and beds appears to be restabilizing, more changes lie ahead. The hospital industry is in the midst of a fundamental restructuring of supply and demand, moving rapidly away from a predictable pattern of cost-based payment to the rough and tumble of competitive market forces.

The main trends are summarized in Exhibit 2-1. As these trends gain momentum, they will reshape the face of the American health care industry. All are evident today, but the new patterns are not fully established. The question each physician and hospital must ask is, If this is the shape of the future, how do we participate?

Recession

On the product life cycle curve, the hospital industry is mature and declining. Like any producer whose product has reached the mature phase, each hospital is faced with three strategic choices:

1. *Sell* while the product still has potential market value.
2. *Hold* operating costs down and defer capital investment while taking maximum profit out, then pursue one of the other two strategies.
3. *Innovate* to break through the life cycle curve by creating new markets for the existing product or by recycling through product extension, enhancement, or renewal.

Expanding Boundaries

Although the nation's hospitals are heading into a recessionary trough, the health industry is continuing to grow and the health component of the GNP is rising. By 1990, health care may account for more than 12 percent of the GNP, up from 10.5 percent in 1984. Consumer spending constitutes more than two-thirds of the GNP, and consumer surveys show health is still a high priority.

Exhibit 2-1 Hospital Industry in Transition

1. Recession
2. Expanding Boundaries
3. Market Warfare
4. Merchandising
5. Global Market
6. Integrated Health Plans
7. Diversification
8. New Managers
9. Technopush
10. Spirit of Enterprise

The health market could account for 13 percent of national expenditures by 1995 and 15 percent by 2000. At current rates, national spending on health will easily reach one trillion dollars in the mid-1990s.

Market Warfare

As the traditional base business of hospitals—inpatient care—stabilizes, competition for market share will become intense. In the past ten years, a number of other industries have experienced sharply rising competition and economic destabilization, often prompted by deregulation. Hospitals can learn how to beat the life cycle curve from the "ABCs": airlines, banking, and communications. Competition and deregulation shook those industries to the core. If their history is any guide to the future of the hospital industry, these strategic responses can be predicted:

- marketing
- price competition
- new competitors
- niche seeking
- diversification
- consolidation

Take the airlines industry, for example. Price competition is rampant, and fare wars have become a permanent facet of the market. America West, Southwest Air, and other new competitors overcame barriers to entry and created new niches in the marketplace. Consumer choice regarding price, service, and amenities increased substantially. Air miles and passengers are up, but not without side effects. Low airline margins cut service to many small communities. Not all carriers will survive. Braniff went to the brink of collapse, then came back, while Continental, Pan Am, and Eastern have been driven to the financial wall. Airline mergers are rampant. Industry consolidation is predicted to reduce the major carriers (those having one billion dollars in annual revenues) from twelve to eight, or even six, by 1995. In the same marketplace, American, United, and U.S. Air have flourished. Hospitals can expect their future to follow much the same pattern.

Merchandising

In the fiercely competitive watch industry, the Japanese watchmaker Casio calculates it has a three-month lead from the time it introduces a new product to the time competitors copy its move. Merchandising is making health care buyers more fashion conscious, and health care product life cycles are shortening. Thanks to advertising, the American consumer believes there is an epidemic of disorders: stress, anorexia and bulimia, sexual dysfunction—even baldness is being treated as a health problem. Advertising and promotional expenditures are projected to double in the next 2–3 years. From the private sector, hospitals are importing concepts such as product line management and customer relations. Pricing will become a primary merchandising weapon. Already, popular products such as cataract surgery are being discounted heavily. HMO price wars became rampant and the tactic of discounting spread, badly bruising the HMO industry. The national battle for brand-name leadership is taking shape now. American Medical International (AMI) and Humana have put their corporate brands on all products, and other investor-owned companies are following suit, followed more tentatively by nonprofit ''supergroups'' like Voluntary Hospitals of America.

Global Market

With their surplus of physicians and hospital managers, American health care firms will develop new markets overseas. A preferred target will be the countries of the Triad (United States, Europe, and Japan), which contain 600 million customers with similar values, attitudes, and consumption patterns. In Triad countries, as well as in newly industrialized countries, U.S.-style health care is the standard that is aimed at. Overseas expansion will follow the global strategies of industries like electronics, automotives, and computers. Joint ventures, consortia, and innovative arrangements will create market entry points for U.S. health care products and expand opportunities for foreign investment in American companies. The influx of foreign capital into the U.S. health system could be significant. Direct foreign investment in American companies and assets has swelled from $30.6 billion in 1978 to $174 billion in late 1985.

Integrated Health Plans

The distinction between health care providers and payers is disappearing rapidly. Tomorrow's very large health care companies will, as integrated health plans (IHPs), combine insurance, financing, and service delivery. The health industry is entering a period of rapid change and experimentation. Capitation and prepayment will come to dominate the industry. HMOs will enter a new growth phase as employer satisfaction with lightly controlled PPOs fades. HMOs in the 1990s can anticipate a quickening pace of consumer and Medicare acceptance. They can look for annual enrollment gains of 15–25 percent, giving them a 30–40 percent market share by 1995. HMOs are one type of IHP, but PPOs will also contend strongly, as will "OWAs" (Other Weird Arrangements), the new experimental organizational forms that are now taking shape. Large hospital companies are acquiring insurance companies or developing joint ventures with the carriers. Watch the turnabout strategy, as major insurance companies buy hospital chains or merge with them. Several investor-owned health care companies could become candidates for this scenario.

Diversification

With increasing pressure on traditional inpatient lines of business, a number of hospitals have set themselves the goal of getting 25–40% of their revenues from noninpatient sources by 1995. This goal may be ambitious. Even companies whose hallmark is innovation, like 3M and General Electric, do well to get 20–25 percent of their revenues from new (one- to five-year-old) product lines. The experience of the private sector is clear: Diversify only into related businesses and capitalize on the organization's strengths. Alternatively, hospitals may develop new business alliances with other firms whose strengths facilitate market entry into desired new fields. Joint ventures with medical staff fall in this category of business development. Acquisition as a market entry strategy is gaining popularity, and not just among investor-owned health care firms. Acquisition of physician office practices became one of hottest recent market trends and is now commonplace. To develop new products and business ventures, hospitals are increasing their R & D investment. Companies like the Lutheran Hospital Society of Southern California (now UniHealth America), Hospital Corporation of America, and American Medical International's Presbyterian/St. Lukes Medical Center established R & D units to foster innovation.

New Managers

As the heart of the Baby Boom generation reaches age 40 in the 1990s, the glut of middle managers will become more apparent. Health care will follow the lead of insurance, retail, communications, and manufacturing companies by downsizing middle management ranks and "flattening" the organization, removing redundant tiers in corporate offices and operational units. An estimated 15–25 percent of today's middle managers may be affected. Reduction of the middle ranks may actually increase administrative opportunities for front-line supervisors as part of the "worksite democracy" movement to decentralize authority and distribute it to the operating units. Women are rising rapidly in health care management. Incoming students in health administration programs are now more likely to be women. Carol McCarthy's selection to head the AHA heralded the arrival of the woman health care executive. The next newcomers are likely to be physicians. Medical directors will take on increasing levels of administrative responsibility and, soon, line authority, with titles such as Vice-President for Patient Care Services. A small but growing number of hospitals, such as Pasadena's Huntington Memorial, are hiring physician CEOs.

Technopush

The pace and force of technology is increasing. The technology capital investment in "knowledge workers" like health care professionals is less than $5,000 per employee, compared with $25,000 in the manufacturing sector. Think of the hospital as the factory of the future. All efforts will be made to speed up the "throughput" by using a case management approach, reducing the length of stay, and increasing the efficiency of resources utilization. Computer-aided diagnosis and computer-assisted medicine will move beyond the prototype phase into early market entry before 1990. The new software of medicine will link hospitals, physicians, and payers and provide common data bases via computer local area networks. Genetically engineered diagnostics and therapeutics are just coming to market. Laser and microsurgery have enormous potential. Linking new imaging technologies with robotic surgery will become common by 1990. Technology-rich hospitals can differentiate themselves from competitors and charge premium prices.

Spirit of Enterprise

If Peter Drucker (1985) and George Guilder (1985) are right, health care will be galvanized by innovation and entrepreneurship in the decade ahead. Corporate restructuring among hospitals has created new vehicles like B.E.D.S. (Business Enterprise Development Services of Santa Monica Hospital Medical Center, California) to pursue diversified business development. Use of financial incentives for health care managers is rising. An estimated 25 percent of nonprofit hospitals have incentive programs, and the practice is virtually universal in the investor-owned sector. Hospitals such as Good Samaritan of San Jose, California, and Port Huron Hospital in Michigan are experimenting with "intrapreneurship" initiatives to foster employee entrepreneurship. A recent study by Illinois-based Witt Associates of hospital CEOs revealed a new executive type, the "sociopreneur," who can maintain the social values of an organization while pursuing complicated, risky business ventures. These farsighted managers are changing the shape of the hospital industry by making it innovative and competitive.

THE END OF THE HOSPITAL SLUMP

If the health market is expanding while the hospital market is retracting, this paradox leaves hospitals with two questions: How long will the hospital recession persist? And what health products and services will gain most in the next 5–15 years?

The current slump in patient days already eased in 1988, and the recovery should be national by the end of the decade—although some pockets of decline may persist, especially in rural regions with depressed economies. The average length of stay for those over 65 is now stabilizing at around 7 days; the average length for those under 65 will bottom out at between 4 and 5 days by 1990. Admission rates will be the next trend to recover. Hospitals should anticipate that admissions will follow length of stay trends in the next five years. The growing number of elderly will constitute the rising tide that lifts all boats, as admission rates rise again by 1990. Regional differences will disappear. The overall result in the 1990s will be a national level of acute hospitalization averaging 400–500 patient days per 1,000 population—much like the most efficient HMOs today.

In the midrange future, beyond 1990, hospital stays will be longer and cheaper, leading to a new boom in the construction of small, low-cost, and highly efficient hospitals. These "quick-stay" hospitals will replace today's 300- to 500-bed white elephants, which are overbuilt for tomorrow's noninvasive, low-acuity care.

These changes will not result in a "fire sale" of U.S. hospital facilities, however. Most hospitals will diversify into related businesses and develop new high-margin products. Hospitals with good locations will be sold for their real estate value or to foreign investors as health care becomes a global business. By the 1990s, the hospital asset base will be significantly depreciated, opening the door to recapitalization for a variety of health and nonrelated businesses at a lower square-foot price.

Many community hospitals may step down their base level of care, giving 50 percent or more of their beds over to subacute or long-term care, or they may specialize only in limited lines of inpatient business. A smaller number of exclusive medical centers will provide the highest levels of service and amenities and become the dominant centers of new technology. Public hospitals will find it increasingly difficult to compete, and at least 25 percent of teaching medical centers will align with other community hospitals to develop their own feeder systems.

Hospitals will be like computers. Today's $1,500 microcomputer has the computing power of a $250,000 room-sized mainframe of a decade ago. Similarly as technology such as lasers, magnetic resonance imaging, and the new medical software becomes cheaper and more widely available, even a 50-bed hospital can be a "medical center."

INNOVATION, COMPETITION, AND INTEGRATION

There is no secret path to future success. In health care, as in other industries, the high-performance organizations will be masters of the strategic triangle: innovation, competition, and integration (Figure 2-4).

Innovation

Innovation provides the "attacker's advantage." That is the message of the management best seller by Richard Foster (1986) of McKinsey and Company. From his studies of American industry, Foster learned that businesses that are on the cutting edge achieve above-average returns. Sustaining high-level performance depends on how successfully a company can maintain its innovative stance. If it coasts, more innovative competitors will take away its markets and its margins. When breakthrough technology is introduced, the market share of defending producers can erode as much as one share point per month.

There is a lesson here for health care. Take the experience of computed tomography (CT). Introduced barely 20 years ago, CT has already evolved

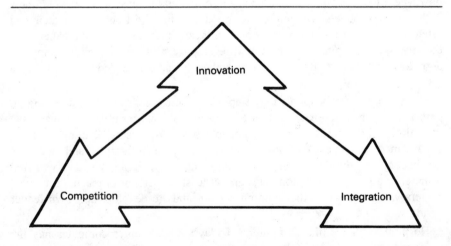

Figure 2-4 The Strategic Triangle

through four "generations" of technological innovation. The next innovation—an imaging speed increase from 10 seconds to 50 milliseconds per scan—gives cine CT the potential to dynamically image the heart in real time, heartbeat by heartbeat.

Change has already taken its toll. EMI, the British company that introduced CT, could not sustain its advantage and exited the imaging market after five years. Hospitals that bought the first million-dollar brain scanners are now writing them off as obsolete. CT is moving out of the hospital into free-standing diagnostic imaging centers, often owned by entrepreneurs. What's next? CT is rapidly being displaced by magnetic resonance imaging, a superior technology that has both imaging and biochemical analysis capacities. As the CT experience graphically illustrates, innovation is a continuing necessity in a dynamic marketplace.

Competition

Competition now provides the central dynamic for the health care industry. Competition is taking place at three levels:

1. among *major buyers* of health care—government, employers, insurance companies—who foment price wars of competitive bidding between hospitals and providers
2. among *integrated health plans*—the HMOs, PPOs, and health insurance plans that also provide direct care—competing to entice the 85 percent of Americans who use fee-for-service medicine into capitated plans
3. among *hospitals and physicians* who are battling for a share of the fastest-growing market in health care: ambulatory services

Competition in health care is still in its adolescence. Many providers still know very little about their competitors, but they are learning. Competitor intelligence will become a critical piece of every strategic decision. Marketing is more than a management hula hoop. It is a central preoccupation of all levels of health care management, and it affects every provider and every management decision.

The future of the health care industry will be shaped in the marketplace, not in Washington, D.C., or in state capitals. Today, consumers make 30–70 percent of the choices to purchase health care services (Jensen 1986). The health care purchase still involves a complex decision, one significantly influenced by physician opinion but no longer doctor dominated. In this new market-driven environment, every health care program, product, and service must meet the test of the market: Does it sell?

Integration

Integration is the key to future success. The many and varied health care services offered under a wide range of sponsorships are converging. Old boundaries are breaking down. As fee-for-service medicine declines and more consumers are covered by integrated health plans, case management will integrate the clinical and financial decisions of health care. In a managed care environment, the distinctions between a physician's office and hospital practice are rapidly disappearing. So are the differences between health insurance, financing, and service delivery. Often, these are coordinated by or combined within a single entity—an HMO, PPO, or services broker.

The *continuum of health care* is becoming a marketplace reality. Both consumers and providers accept the concept, and the market shift is gaining speed. More comprehensive health care benefit plans are being offered in the marketplace, and more integrated provider organizations are making coordinated services and settings available. This trend aligns well with the future. It has considerable power to reshape health care for the 21st century.

LOOKING FORWARD

Despite the current economic crunch for physicians and hospitals, the outlook is far from bleak. Health care providers today can be divided into three groups. The first group—perhaps 50 percent of today's physicians and hospitals—are well positioned, have a sound market strategy, and are pursuing their future with vigor. A second group—estimated at 25 percent of physicians and hospitals—are searching for a strategic path and will probably find it. The final 25 percent are just awakening to market realities and could be in real peril. Office location, hospital size, and payer mix are not the critical factors—it will be the quality of farsighted leadership that will determine success or failure in this era of new economics for medicine.

For now, medicine and health care are very much in transition. Old patterns are eroding rapidly and new forces are beginning to make a noticeable impact. The experience of other recently deregulated and more competitive industries— airlines, banking, brokerage, communications—is instructive. In every case, the industry was underprepared for the magnitude and speed of the transition. Managers of top companies like United Airlines, Continental Illinois, and AT&T underestimated how quickly and powerfully their markets would shift. Companies that saw opportunities in the transition and moved swiftly to capitalize on them, such as Security Pacific, Compaq, and MCI, have become some of America's most successful and high-growth corporations.

As physicians and hospitals look to the future, they may take heart from the experience of stock brokerage. More than 15 years ago, on May 1, 1975, brokerage was deregulated. Forecasters predicted widespread calamity: More than 20–25 percent of the 500 Wall Street firms were expected to fail. The surviving brokerage houses would cater only to the big institutional buyers, abandoning individual investors. The reality was quite different: Wall Street flourished! Competition unleashed innovation. Options, no-load, and specialty funds of all sorts developed, and consumer choice multiplied. Major buyers did get discounts averaging 30–40 percent of fees, but Charles Schwab appeared to give individuals the same price break. On Wall Street, only 38 firms consolidated or disappeared. Today, more than 640 brokerage houses exist, and Wall Street has broken through the "Dow Jones $1,500" and every other limit, surviving the "crash" of October 1987 and pushing outward the boundaries of its market again.

There should be a lesson for physicians and hospital executives here.

BIBLIOGRAPHY

Burda, David. 1989. "Why Hospitals Close." *Modern Healthcare*, 24 March, 24–35.

Cahan, Vicky, Kathleen Deveny, and Joan O. Hamilton. 1986. "Health Care Costs: The Fever Breaks." *Business Week*, 21 October, 41–42.

Coile, Russell C., Jr. 1986. *The New Hospital: Future Strategies for a Changing Industry*. Rockville, Md.: Aspen Publishers.

Drucker, Peter F. 1985. *Innovation and Entrepreneurship: Practice and Principles*. New York: Harper & Row.

Feldman, Roger, and Frank Sloan. 1988. "Competition among Physicians, Revisited." *Journal of Health Politics, Policy and Law*. 13 (Summer): 239–61.

Foster, Richard. 1986. *Innovation: The Attacker's Advantage*. New York: Basic Books.

Guilder, George. 1985. *The Spirit of Enterprise*. New York: Doubleday.

Health Care in the 1990s: Trends and Strategies. 1987. Chicago, Ill.: Arthur Andersen & Co. and American College of Hospital Administrators.

Hevesi, Dennis. 1989. "Polls Show Discontent with Health Care." *New York Times*, 15 February, A8.

Holoweiko, Mark. 1988. "Which Practice Expenses Are Biting Deepest into Earnings?" *Medical Economics*, 7 November, 162–85.

Hsiao, William. 1988. "Results and Policy Implications of the Resource-based Relative Value Study." *New England Journal of Medicine*, 29 September.

Hull, Jennifer B. 1985. "Four Hospital Chains, Facing Lower Profits, Adopt New Strategies." *Wall Street Journal*, 10 October, A-1.

Jensen, Joyce. 1986. "Women Pick the Providers Who Treat Their Illnesses, Those of Their Children." *Modern Healthcare*, 9 May, 66–67.

Jolly, Paul. 1988. "Medical Education in the United States, 1960–1987." *Health Affairs* (Supplement): 144–56.

Kirchner, Merian. 1988. "Fee Hikes: Who's Rocking the Boat?" *Medical Economics*, 3 October, 126–62.

Levit, Katharine R., and Mark S. Freeland. 1988. "National Medical Care Spending." *Health Affairs* (Winter): 124–36.

Madison, Donald L., and Thomas R. Konrad. 1988. "Large Medical Group-Practice Organizations and Employed Physicians: A Relationship in Transition." *The Milbank Quarterly* 66:240–82.

Marder, William D., et al. 1988. "Physician Employment Patterns: Challenging Conventional Wisdom." *Health Affairs* (Winter): 137–45.

Morse, Larkina. 1988. *1988 Hospital Fact Book*. 13th ed. Sacramento, Calif.: California Association of Hospitals and Health Systems.

Owens, Arthur. 1988. "How Much Did Your Earnings Grow Last Year?" *Medical Economics*, 5 September, 159–80.

Paxton, Harry T. 1988. "Could You Make it in Private Practice Today?" *Medical Economics*, 21 November, 157–74.

Stevens, Carol. 1988. "Are You Ready for the Doctor Rating Game?" *Medical Economics*, 19 September, 58–67.

Chapter 3

The New Consumer

"Today's healthcare consumer is a sleeping giant—one who is awakening to his power. Fully awakened, he will be the master and healthcare providers will be the servants. For the patient is a customer."
— Leland R. Kaiser, *"Healthcare's Sleeping Giant"*

The American social mosaic is changing rapidly. By the turn of the century—only eleven years away—new demographic patterns will be causing profound changes in health care. The trends will affect every sector of the health industry and every provider, insurer, and payer. For physicians, hospitals, and health systems, tomorrow's consumers will provide both an opportunity and a challenge. The demographic changes of the next five to ten years will provide health care with a continuously moving target for service development in a competitive marketplace. The future will also challenge the ability of health providers to meet the problems of new immigrants, the medically uninsured, the elderly poor, and special needs groups.

HIGHLIGHTS OF THE CHANGES AHEAD

America's *growth* is slowing. Although the United States will grow by more than one million residents each year for the next 20 years, the rate of growth is slowing, continuing a trend set in the 1960s.

The *aging of America*, the subject of chapter 4, is the most important trend in American demographics for health care.

Social and population *mobility* is stabilizing. Although the United States continues its general tilt towards the South and West, the rate of internal migration is slowing. Some regions are enjoying a renaissance. New England is prospering, with new high-tech industry and 3–4 percent unemployment. California will continue to flourish. Florida will age faster than any state.

43

Farm states will keep on emptying. Economic downturns in the energy-dependent Southwest and Rocky Mountain region will continue to dampen their growth into the 1990s. Fewer Americans are moving to urban areas. Indeed, fewer are moving, period.

The *income gap* between richest and poorest is widening. The problem of the *homeless* is national and worsening. Fewer than a third of young Americans can afford to buy a home. The rate of savings is low and not improving. As sociologists observe the decline of the middle class, a growing number of the U.S. households are "two paychecks and a crisis" away from the poverty line.

The *Baby Boom generation* will continue to set the trends. As the nation's largest population segment moves through the years ahead, it will define market trends and consumption patterns. Upper-income yuppies will mature through child rearing and become "empty nesters" by the mid-1990s. The Echo Boom— consisting of the children of the Baby Boom—has already peaked and will now make its impact in day-care shortages, overfilled schools, and swelling college enrollments for the next 15 years.

A problem for the 1990s, *labor shortages,* is arriving ahead of schedule. Behind the Baby Boom is the *Baby Bust generation.* The nursing shortage is the tip of an iceberg that will affect all employers, from Burger King to high-tech companies. There will not be enough workers to fill jobs of any kind. For U.S. employers, 80 percent of the work force for the next 20 years is already working. Unemployment may fall below 6 percent, which economists have considered the minimum possible in an industrialized country. In response, the U.S. may expand immigration and recruit worldwide for skilled professionals such as nurses, engineers, and scientists and for workers to staff low-skill entry jobs.

America will rapidly become a *multicultural society.* In the 1990s, many of the top 20 U.S. cities will lack any population majority and instead will contain a new multiracial blend of many groups. Although the number of *new immigrants* will likely continue at present levels, their higher birth rates are propelling high growth. Their numbers may increase further if Congress raises immigration quotas to help solve the problem of the labor shortage.

The *American family*, feared to be an endangered species in the early 1980s, is restabilizing. Divorce rates are slowing and marriage rates rising. Still, the fastest-growing type of household consists of a single person.

No group will be affected as much as *women* in the decade ahead. Their role in society and the economy shifted dramatically in the 1970s and 1980s, and the changes seem permanent. The prevalence of *women in the work force* has changed the American family in the past decade. The number of women heading households continues to rise. If employment inequality and wage inequality for women persist, the *feminization of poverty* will be a growing problem in the 1990s for health and human service agencies. As age discrepancies widen among aging Americans, older women living alone on marginal incomes will compose an underrecognized pocket of poverty and social need.

The *AIDS epidemic* is growing rapidly. The number of AIDS cases will reach 100,000 in 1990, and the Centers for Disease Control forecast 270,000 by 1991 (Pascal 1987). Every state has AIDS patients. New York City hospitals are experiencing a bed shortage that is exacerbated by the AIDS crisis. AIDS will tax the moral reserves of America's health care providers, calling for quality, competent, compassionate, and ethical care. Ethical issues faced by providers include testing, confidentiality, and refusal to treat. AIDS will put financial and staffing pressure on hospitals in a growing number of metropolitan areas as the disease spreads, new cases emerge, and new therapies like AZT postpone death. Already the case mix is shifting from gay males (as the primary vector) to drug abusers. In New York City more than half the AIDS cases are drug related, and the disease is spreading through the ghettos via needle sharing and heterosexual transmission. AIDS could spread to inner-city heterosexuals if no cure is discovered, and this would place enormous burdens on inner-city hospitals. Case management, out-of-hospital care, and new drugs offer promise in treating people with AIDS.

The *poor and homeless* are a perennial challenge to mission-oriented health institutions. Their numbers are increasing, despite a relatively healthy economic growth of 3–4 percent and shrinking unemployment, now below 6 percent. The percentage of Americans below the federal poverty line has remained relatively stable, around 15 percent, but the numbers of the medically disadvantaged are growing, since state-level Medicaid programs have restricted benefits and eligibility to limit budget outlays. Religious and nonprofit hospitals are carrying an increasing burden, as indicated in the Catholic Hospital Association's widely read report *No Room in the Marketplace: The Health Care of the Poor*. The conditions spotlighted by the report persist today and may be worsening. State legislatures are giving high priority to health care for the poor, but few states will be able to increase funding. Public hospitals are being overwhelmed by high demand and inadequate funding.

Medical uninsurance is an emerging problem now gaining recognition, and perhaps a solution. There is a growing underclass of Americans without health insurance, estimated at 37 million by the Employee Benefit Research Institute, based in Washington, D.C. Perhaps as many as 75 percent are employed, at least part-time. Washington, Florida, Minnesota, and other states have created self-insurance pools for the medically uninsured, but state-level solutions so far have made little impact on the problem. Congress is considering legislation which would mandate all employers to provide at least minimum employee health benefits. The bill is given limited chances for passage before 1992 and faces stiff opposition from small business. The proposal may be ultimately attractive to Congress despite the opposition of the Bush administration, since the cost would be borne by employers, not government.

SHIFTING DEMOGRAPHICS: TOMORROW'S CONSUMERS

In the final decade of the 20th century, America's population will experience changes at an accelerating rate. Aging, the rise in ethnic diversity, and labor shortages are only a few of the demographic forces that will affect health care institutions in the near and midrange future. The central factors in this demographic phenomenon are

- aging
- life extension
- racial diversity
- immigration
- fewer children
- low unemployment
- the changing definition of *household*
- a population growth of 40 million
- 37 million medically uninsured people
- the AIDS epidemic

The demographic changes ahead will alter many assumptions about the "average American." Futurist Hank Koehn (1986) anticipates a "mosaic society" of many subgroupings that differ by race, sex, income, education, region, age, life style, values, and attitudes. Understanding market shifts is the key to future strategic planning by hospitals and health plans.

Population Forecasts

Recent estimates by the federal government's National Center for Health Statistics forecast a national population of between 271.6 and 279.9 million by the 21st century, a gain of 40 million (Exter 1986). The lower projection assumes constant mortality. The higher estimate is based on a continuation of the declining mortality rate, an already evident trend that may play an increasingly important role in health care utilization and marketing (see Chapter 4).

Although the population is growing, the rate of increase is slowing. U.S. population growth is predicted to slow further between now and the turn of the century, even if there should be medical breakthroughs or major changes in immigration policy. Since the Baby Boom of the 1950s, when America grew yearly at a rate of 17.1 per 1,000 population, the trend has been downwards. The average annual growth rate between 1980 and 1987 was 9.9 per 1,000, according to the Bureau of the Census. This growth rate was below the pace of 10.5 per 1,000 of the 1970s and well below the 12.6 rate of the 1960s.

Family Structure

As population growth has slowed, more substantial changes are taking place in the underlying structure of American society. Only 27 percent of American families today fit the stereotype of 20 years ago—husband, wife, and children. Couples with no children, unmarried couples who cohabit, and people who live alone make up 57 percent of all households today. The single-parent family is the fastest-growing type of household today. Many such families are headed by women.

Families are shrinking. The average number of people per household in the United States plunged to 2.67 in 1986, the least ever recorded by the Census Bureau. The aging of the population and the decrease in children per family are responsible for this dramatic shift in household size. The trend toward smaller families dates back to the 1970s. Family size fell from 3.14 in 1970 to 2.76 in 1980, and it declined to 2.69 three years ago, in 1985. Could the typical American "family" of the 21st century be a couple?

Don't mistake the shrinking size of households for the decline of the family. New family formation outpaces population growth. The number of households mushroomed 10.5 percent from the 1980 census to 1986. The term *household* masks a growing diversity of living arrangements among related and unrelated persons, trends driven by changing life styles, the soaring cost of housing, and the return of adult children to live at home with older parents. More than 8 million new households have been formed in the 1980s, boosting total households from 80.4 million to 88.8 million (in 1986). At this rate, there will be 90 million households in 1990 and more than 100 million by the year 2000.

Marriage is regaining prestige as a social institution, and social observers see traditional values making a renaissance. Fear of AIDS may be a contributing factor. The number of marriages had declined consistently in the 1980s, from 10.6 per 1,000 population in 1980 to only 10.0 in 1986. Married couples numbered 51.7 million in 1986. Don't bet on the decline of this traditional institution. The number of married couples increased by nearly 2 million in the 1980s. More importantly, divorces are declining, after reaching an all-time high of 5.4 per 1,000 population in 1980. By 1986, divorces had fallen to a rate of 4.8 per 1,000 population.

The rise of *single-parent families* has been widely recognized as one of the results of changing life styles and welfare policies. More than 10.2 million women head households and maintain them alone. One-quarter are black, one-third are under 35, and another 15 percent are over 65. The forecasts are gloomy. The single-parent family headed by women increased 17.3 percent in the 1980s. At this rate, nearly one-quarter of all families may be headed by single women in the year 2000. Single-parent households headed by women have household incomes significantly below those headed by men. Two out of three divorced women receive no child support. As a result, women heading households find it difficult to purchase health care, copay health insurance deductibles, or afford health insurance (unless provided by their employers).

Many new households consist of a *single* person living alone. More than 21.1 million Americans live the single life, and over 60 percent are women. The number of singles has tripled since 1960, from 7 million, when women held a 2:1 edge among those living alone.

Fewer Children

The *Echo Boom* of the 1980s will be over by the early 1990s. The number of live births shrank by 18,000 in 1986. The birth rate declined in 1986 to 15.5 per 1,000 population from the decade-high rate of 15.7 in 1985. Even that was well below the rate for 1970 (18.4) and a far cry from the 25.3 recorded in 1954 at the height of the Baby Boom.

As women delayed marriage and childbirth in the 1970s, a new birthing boomlet began in 1977 and is now peaking. At this point, the Baby Boomers are moving into their post-40 middle years. As fewer women enter childbearing years in the future, the birth rate may fall further in the 1990s. America need not yet fear zero population growth before the 21st century. Live births continue to outnumber deaths almost 2:1 (e.g., 3.7 million births versus 2.1 million deaths in 1986).

Employment

In the small print of the index in the December 28, 1987, issue of *Business Week*, the turnaround of America's unemployment situation was visibly demonstrated. Only 291,000 initial claims for unemployment were filed, down from 350,000 a year before. The *Wall Street Journal* reported that unemployment fell to 5.8 percent at the end of 1988, below the 6 percent "full employment" rate that some economists consider the lower limit because of the hard core of unemployables present in all Western industrial economies (Gutfeld 1988). This economic success comes only seven years after unemployment jumped to double-digit levels at the outset of the Reagan administration.

Not all the improvement can be credited to supply-side economics. America's resurgent economy is the result of national economic policy initiatives, changes in the global economy, and surging growth in small businesses and entrepreneurship. Lower unemployment is likely for the future, even if economic growth falls below 3 percent annually. The reason is demographics: There will not be enough young workers to replace retirees and also fill the new jobs resulting from normal economic growth.

Middle-class satisfaction has not grown with the economy. Despite economic and employment growth, fewer middle-class Americans rate themselves satisfied with their economic circumstances in 1986 than in 1956. Pay raises have come at a slower rate than in the 1950s and 1960s, whereas prices have nearly quadrupled. The typical American family's income in 1986 dollars rose from $19,500 to $29,548. The 50 percent improvement in family income has been achieved in the 1980s by the widespread entry of women into the workplace. The aggregate gains have not been equally shared between rich and poor. From 1960 to 1986, the share of total income earned by the top two-fifths of families grew, but the share earned by others declined.

Behind the Baby Boom generation is the Baby Bust cohort, the 20-year result of declining birth rates and fewer children. More than 80 percent of those who will be in the American work force during the next 20 years are already in it. The problem of labor shortages is here today. McDonald's and Burger King are paying premium wages and busing teenagers from inner cities to the suburbs, but jobs still go begging. There are only as many 17-year-old teenagers today as there were in 1970. As a result, unemployment among teenagers looking for work was only 16.1 percent in December 1987, down 0.5 percent from a year before. One possible strategy is to recruit older workers back into the work force. For example, McDonald's "McMasters" program provides flexible hours and work opportunities for retirees.

Labor Shortages

Low unemployment is likely for the decade ahead. Labor shortages will become widespread, affecting all industries from fast-food chains to farms and factories. The problem will hit labor-dependent services hard, including hospital, nursing, and health-related technical services. In 1986 the nursing shortage gained national attention when hospitals reported their nursing vacancies rose from 6 percent to 13 percent. Some hospitals are covering 25–33 percent of their nursing positions by using registry personnel and contract employees. Shortages in hospital intensive care units and emergency departments are now being reported in many regions. The problem is widespread, affecting health care providers in all regions, urban and rural. Nursing school enrollments are down 5–10 percent. A national panel responding to a recent Delphi survey for *Healthcare Forum* predicted the nursing shortage is "permanent" and will not yield to short-term financial incentives (Coile and Grossman 1988).

This trend will affect high-tech manufacturing, low-tech services, government, finance, education, and all types of employers. The nursing shortage presages the limited supply of workers in every field that will vex U.S. employers and hospitals for the next decade. Labor shortages and wage inflation are inevitable unless there is a substantial return of the elderly to the work force or the United States revises immigration policies to increase the importing of labor from foreign countries.

Immigration

America is still a beacon for emigrants throughout the world. To cope with the problem of illegal aliens, an amnesty program enacted in 1987 qualified nearly two million aliens for U.S. citizenship. By some estimates, seven to ten million aliens may be in the United States, but they either did not fit the new amnesty criteria or feared any contact with authorities. The immigration amnesty program yielded fewer than two million new citizens before it expired in 1988, but could be renewed in the 1990s if labor shortages worsen.

If the past is any guide to the future, America is unlikely to loosen the immigration floodgates in the next decade. Once the beacon for emigrants, America has maintained close controls over entry since the 1920s. In the 1980s, new legal immigrants have averaged 550,000 to 600,000 per year. The number could be doubled or tripled easily, but any increase would face stiff political opposition.

Congress is unlikely to increase immigration quotas unless the problem of labor shortages becomes acute. In the life cycle of public issues, most policy changes take 6–10 years. Awareness of labor shortages is just beginning. For legislation to be enacted by Congress, American business and elected officials must recognize the problem, see immigration as a solution, and overcome objections from groups whose status might be threatened. Political forecasting is difficult, but experience suggests that major national legislation to further ease immigration restrictions is unlikely before 1995.

Racial Diversity

America is moving rapidly from a white society of European origin to a multiracial and multicultural mixing pot without a clear ethnic majority. The trend is still spotty and inconsistent, but it is rippling out from urban centers to suburban and rural settings. Major metropolitan areas like Los Angeles, Miami, Detroit, Atlanta, and others have nonwhite majorities, and dozens more cities and towns will follow in the decade ahead. The bellwether states of California and Texas may experience nonwhite majorities by the year 2000. The trend will be evident in their public school enrollments by the mid-1990s.

Asians and Hispanics are the fastest-growing immigrant groups. America's immigrants are increasingly from Asia and Latin America. In 1970, Asians constituted 25 percent of foreign immigrants. By 1986, nearly 45 percent of all newly immigrated Americans came from Asian nations. Another 38 percent is new arrivals from the Americas, principally the West Indies and Latin America. The Census Bureau estimates that 500,000 illegal immigrants cross American borders each year, principally from Latin America. European immigrants now constitute only 10 percent of new Americans, with a trickle from Africa, Australia, and the Pacific Islands. Further expansion of the immigrant quotas is highly uncertain—a "wild card" for the future. Immigration is a highly political issue. There may be more temporary immigration programs, such as the extraordinary granting of entry to Southeast Asian boat people in the 1970s and similiar programs for Haitian refugees and Cuban exiles in the 1980s. To cope with shortages of skilled labor such as nurses and pharmacists, Congress may expand quotas for workers with needed expertise while changing the current policy of automatically accepting as immigrants the family members of U.S. citizens.

Population growth patterns are impacted by immigration as an underlying factor in the polyethnic cultural shift that is changing America. Immigration now accounts for 28 percent of national population growth and will provide 40–50 percent of U.S. population expansion by the turn of the century if the current low birth rate of 1.8 births per woman continues. Health care providers will respond to the shifting demographics with multilingual staff and culturally sensitive health programs.

Persistent Poverty

Despite lower unemployment and an economy that has recovered strongly from the 1981–1982 recession, a large underclass of Americans continues to live in poverty. The underlying reason is the prevalence of certain deeply rooted socioeconomic conditions, not a lack of jobs. Despite rising labor shortages, the culture of poverty may limit participation or income gains by the poor. In 1985, the Census Bureau estimated that 33 million people, or 14.0 percent of U.S. residents, have incomes below the poverty line, which is currently set at $11,203 in annual cash income for a family of four. Whereas 11.4 percent of whites are poor, a disproportionate number are minorities: 31.3 percent of blacks and 29.0 percent of Hispanics live in poverty. These percentages are similar to those of a decade ago and seem unlikely to change soon—unless labor shortages become so acute that employers reach out and train these marginal workers.

Children in poverty are a special needs population. As many as one-third of black children live in poverty. A new generation of "hotel children" are growing up in welfare hotels in America's inner cities. Some are offspring of third- and fourth-generation welfare families. Rural poverty, less seen and recognized, is also a serious problem. Unless these children can break the cycle of poverty with education and employment, they will drop out of school. With limited literacy, their employment opportunities will be limited. High rates of unemployment continue to frustrate minority teenagers and create new cycles of poverty.

Of those Americans living in poverty, an estimated 9–10 million are *working poor*, who were profiled in a January 11, 1988, *U.S. News and World Report* cover story (Whitman 1988). The working poor include members of households in which the wage earners work full- or part-time but still have incomes below the poverty line. Many of these families are white, and the majority are two-parent families. They are divided about evenly between center cities, suburbs, and rural areas. Their numbers have grown 52 percent from 1978 to 1986 (rising to 7 million), whereas the number of Americans on welfare and public assistance grew only 14 percent (to 4 million).

One common factor that links the working poor is lack of health insurance. According to one estimate, two out of three working poor have no employer-provided or union-subsidized health insurance (Whitman 1988). The Employee Benefits Research Council estimates the number of medically uninsured at 37 million today, up almost 10 million in the past three years. This increase is the dysfunctional result of an economy in transition. Whereas the Fortune 500 companies have shed 2.5 million workers in the past decade, small businesses have created 8 million new jobs. Many of these small employers are in service industries, are nonunion, and pay no fringe benefits or health insurance.

The *medically uninsured* are the target of new programs, such as Massachusetts' requirement that small employers with five or more employees be mandated to provide health insurance. Another dozen and a half states have programs to help the uninsured, such as Washington State's recently enacted self-insurance pool. Congress is considering legislation to require employers to provide a minimum level of health insurance benefits to all workers. The goal is commendable, but the national cost could be sizeable. The Institute for Research on the Economics of Taxation estimates the potential cost of such universal health insurance coverage at $37 billion per year in direct costs, plus another $16.3 billion in increased insurance costs for workers with existing coverage.

Regional Differences

The notion of America as the "melting pot" is obsolete. There are nine "Americas." Social observer Joel Garreau (1981) identified nine distinct regions based on sociocultural and economic differences. Garreau's regions are New England, the Foundry (the Central Northeast), Dixie (the Southeast), the Islands (Puerto Rico and the West Indies), Breadbasket (the Midwest), the Empty Quarter (the Rocky Mountains and Western Canada), Mexamerica (the Southwest, Mexico, and Southern California), Ecotopia (the Northern California and the Northwest), and Quebec.

Despite the leveling influence of television on American culture, strong *regional differences* persist. Take Garreau's Empty Quarter, which comprises many states of the old West. This region has only 6–100 persons per square mile. Distances are great, the climate harsh, and work is hard. A 1987 study of mortality data for Utah showed that modern residents of this "frontier" region suffered high rates of working years lost due to suicide, auto accidents, work-related accidents, and infant diseases. The rural figures were 33.5 percent higher than urban figures.

Mortality rates vary by region. Washington, D.C., led the nation with 13.0 deaths per 1,000 population in 1985. Arkansas, Florida, Missouri, Pennsylvania, and Rhode Island all had double-digit death rates. Alaska had the nation's lowest death rate (3.9), followed by Hawaii (5.8) and Utah (5.7). Dr. John Wennberg's studies of regional patterns in health care utilization in New England over the past 20 years have demonstrated that local and regional differences in medical practice have very different outcomes.

Differences in mortality are not all attributable to variations in medical practice or physician distribution. Arizona, Nevada, New Mexico, and Utah have the highest adolescent mortality rates in the United States, according to a report by Frank Popper, chair of the urban studies program at Rutgers (Applebombe 1987). Western states ranked highest and Northwestern states lowest in death rates for youths 15–24. The West's high death rates are the result of more dangerous occupations and the high number of fatal auto accidents, which reflects widespread drinking, dangerous roads, and the difficulties in providing emergency care in rural areas.

AIDS

The AIDS epidemic is no longer a wild card for the health industry. By the end of 1989, some 100,000 AIDS cases will have been diagnosed in the United States, and more than half of these cases will have resulted in death. The American AIDS caseload broke 50,000 in 1988. The Centers for Disease Control

(CDC) estimates that 270,000 Americans will have contracted AIDS by 1991 and that perhaps 1 to 1.5 million people are carrying the HIV virus. Of these, researchers estimate that 3 in 10 will get full-blown AIDS or AIDS-related complex (ARC) and that most will eventually develop some form of immune deficiency.

On a global basis, the AIDS problem may already be much worse. World health experts now estimate that 100 to 150 million may get AIDS, although "official" estimates are much lower, reflecting a combination of underreporting and national pride. Africa could be hard hit, possibly losing 25 percent or more of its population. Every country in the world now has reported AIDS cases.

The future magnitude of the AIDS epidemic in America is unknown. Data for precise estimates do not exist. The CDC is currently launching three epidemiologic studies to identify how many people in the general population may be HIV-positive. The homosexual community may already have achieved some control over the disease. Fewer new cases involving gays are being reported in San Francisco and New York, but the disease is spreading among intravenous (IV) drug abusers and into the ghettos of New York City, Washington, D.C., and other urban centers. More than 700 infants have been diagnosed with AIDS, most the offspring of IV drug abusers. The fear among epidemiologists tracking the spread of AIDS is that the disease, through heterosexual transmission, could reach epidemic proportions in low-income areas, for example, among ghetto teenagers, who seldom use safe sex practices.

Health care workers fear occupational exposure. Nine health workers have contracted AIDS through occupational injuries—needle sticks or blood contact. Worse yet, a lab worker has been stricken with the AIDS virus through an "inapparent exposure," that is, where there was no obvious blood spill or needle stick prior to infection. Until a cure is discovered, AIDS will be one of America's most serious public health problems.

SPECIAL FOCUS: WOMEN AS HEALTH CONSUMERS

Women are among the "prime customers" of the health industry. They consume health care at a higher rate than men and are more often the family decision makers when health services are needed. Further, women outnumber men, and they have a significantly higher life expectancy.

The "women's market" for health care is currently undergoing a number of important shifts that have strategic implications for health providers.

Life Span

Women have traditionally outlived men, and the gap is widening. According to a 25-year forecast of life expectancy by the National Center for Health Statistics, in the year 2003 women will outlive men by 10 years (84.2 years for women versus 74.2 years for men) if current patterns of declining mortality hold (Verbrugge and Wingard 1986). By comparison, the gap was only 4 years in 1953 and 7.9 years in 1978.

A generation ago there were approximately an equal number of men and women in the United States. Today there are 6.4 percent more women than men, and this numerical advantage is predicted to persist well into the next century. For the foreseeable future, Peter Francese (1986), the publisher of *American Demographics*, predicts that a clear majority of the adult population as well as a majority of patients in virtually every hospital will be women. Experts believe that two-thirds of women's higher longevity is due to environmental exposure, health habits, and life style rather than genetically determined physical differences.

Since women die later than men, they suffer more chronic illnesses and disabilities before death. Whereas older men spend more days in the hospital, older women are more likely to be institutionalized in a nursing home or need home care services. About 75 percent of nursing home residents are women. Over half of nursing home residents have serious organic brain syndrome (senility), and more women suffer this condition because of their longevity and numbers.

Older Women

The graying of American women will be especially important for health care strategists and marketers. In 1982, women represented 59 percent of those over age 65, and they incurred 63 percent of medical care expenses. The problem is intensified for older single women, who spend a greater share of their income for out-of-pocket health expenses and insurance premiums. This percentage rises from 10.2 percent for 70-year-olds to 42 percent for women over age 85.

Medically Uninsured Women

More women are becoming medically uninsured. Among the estimated 37 million Americans without health insurance, women between the ages of 45 and 64 may constitute one of the most overlooked groups. Largely invisible, this group consists of dependent homemakers and part-time workers. Married women may be eligible for health insurance under their husbands' employment coverage. However, more than one-third of American women do not fit this traditional pattern. Single, divorced, and widowed women who have not earned their own health benefits through a consistent career in the labor market are most likely to be uninsured.

Access to medical care before age 65 is almost entirely tied to employer-sponsored health insurance programs for full-time workers, a policy which discriminates against women. More than one quarter of women in the work force are part-time. The problem is compounded for women entering and exiting the work force to raise children or accommodate a spouse's job shifts. Thus women are more likely to lose health coverage due to interrupted work patterns.

Baby Boomers

The median age of women in 1985 was 33. As Baby Boomers move into their middle years in the coming decade, their health needs and utilization will increase, which could lead to a boom market for health care.

With more disposable income, women are making a major impression in the health marketplace. Many hospitals are organizing women's health centers to cater to their specialized needs. Nationally, 40 free-standing women's centers had been established by 1987, but most women's health programs were hospital-based. Most centers focus on ambulatory care, offering diagnostic services, urgent care, and preventive services such as mammography and bone scans. Hospitals benefit from increased ambulatory revenues as well as inpatient referrals.

Many women in this age group have postponed childbearing and are becoming mothers at an older age. The fastest-growing age group for childbearing consists of women 30–34 years old. This trend roughly parallels the increased rate of Cesarean sections that has caused growing concern in the medical profession. In the past 15 years, this rate has tripled. Since deliveries by section require an average of 3.1 extra days of hospital care, this has significant economic consequences. Physicians also note with alarm the increased health risk from a delivery by C-section, which has lead to a call by the National Institute of Child Health and Human Development to reverse this trend (Gleicher 1984).

Working Women and Changing Households

In 1960, only one of every three women aged 25–34 was in the paid work force. After their childbearing years, labor force participation increased, but even among women aged 45–54 fewer than half worked out of the home. In the last 15 years this pattern has changed dramatically. Nearly three-quarters of women aged 25–34 and 35–44 are working. The shape of the curve of labor force participation is now essentially identical to the one for men. This change is most probably permanent.

As women moved into the work force, the "family" underwent major changes. In the past 15 years the only type of household to decline was the traditional family of husband, wife, and children. In 1985 there were 300,000 fewer such families than in 1970. The number of single-parent households grew 125 percent and the number of people living alone grew 90 percent. By 1985 over one-quarter of all households were single-parent (mostly single-woman) households.

Women in Poverty

Whereas about 15 percent of the elderly have incomes below the poverty line, a disproportionate share of those in poverty are women living alone or households headed by women. About 16 percent of all Medicaid recipients are women above age 65, and nearly three-quarters of them are women. Even this bleak statistic masks a worsening situation. Over the last decade, according to the University of California's Institute for Health and Aging, the percentage of the poor and near poor covered by Medicaid declined from 63 percent in 1975 to 46 percent in 1985 (Estes, Gerard, and Stone 1986). The proportion of aged poor who are eligible for Medicaid also declined between 1976 and 1982.

Women as Health Care Decision Makers

Traditionally, women have played a lead role in health care decision making. That tradition persists, despite alterations in their working status and the changing American household. Women choose 63 percent of regular physicians. They are more likely to have regular physical exams (83 percent of women versus 72 percent of men). A national survey done by the National Research Corporation of Lincoln, Nebraska, for *Modern Healthcare* found that men are more likely to consult their wives on the selection of a doctor than vice versa. The importance of women as decision makers is even made clearer by the following facts: Only 4 percent of consumers relied on a hospital's referral in selecting a doctor, and only 3 percent let their HMO select a doctor for them.

STRATEGIC IMPLICATIONS FOR PHYSICIANS

1. *Physician practices will change as the population changes.* Physicians who saw their practices erode in the 1980s know they cannot take their patient base for granted. Important demographic shifts such as women in the workplace have significantly altered family health-seeking behavior and physician office hours. A number of medical specialties will be significantly impacted by demographic changes such as the aging of the Baby Boom generation.
2. *Medical uninsurance will remain an important issue.* Organized medicine needs to be actively involved in the debate on how best to make health

insurance available to employees of small companies, the self-employed, and the working poor.

3. *Labor shortages will increasingly impact physician offices.* Physicians have been buffered in part from the worst effects of the labor shortage, since nurses and other health professionals have tended to shift from the hospital into ambulatory care. Hospitals have been left short-handed, but physician offices were largely unaffected. Physician offices will be hard-pressed in the 1990s, as the large wage hikes hospitals granted in 1987–1990 make hospital work more attractive. The salary discrepancies between hospitals and ambulatory settings will drive up labor costs by at least 10 percent in physician practices and other nonhospital sites, such as independent laboratories and nursing homes.

STRATEGIC IMPLICATIONS FOR HOSPITALS

1. *Hospitals and health systems will need to closely track current shifts and future trends in consumer demographics to develop market-based strategies.* America's demographics have changed dramatically in the past 15 years and continue to change. Strategic planning needs to anticipate changing community needs. Programs must be continuously matched to shifting markets and tested using focus groups and other research approaches. Large health systems should consider hiring a research director to continuously assess demographics, consumption patterns, and consumer needs. For mission-oriented health care providers, future plans and strategies must be sensitive to the changing socioeconomic needs of their communities and must reflect their values and preferences.

2. *Regional differences will tend to disappear.* Anticipate that national health standards will eliminate many regional differences in medical practice and hospital care. The Harvard RVS study will accelerate this leveling trend. As hospitals and health systems plan ahead, scenarios for the near and midrange future should reflect the impact of national trends and norms. Rural hospitals and physicians can expect their differences to persist, but these too will be gradually eroded in the coming decade.

3. *The continuum of care must include the poor.* The strategic challenge for health care providers in the future will be to develop a comprehensive array of health programs and related support services. In the current competitive environment, there is a danger that hospitals will neglect special needs populations: the poor, the elderly, women, minorities, and the medically uninsured. It will be important to take a comprehensive and holistic approach when planning for future community health needs, combining

wellness and health promotion, home care, and self-care with traditional institutional and ambulatory care.

4. *Strategy will focus on high-profit niches.* In the "31 flavors" health marketplace of the future, every mini–market segment will be the target of specialized health programs and market strategies. Future health care competition will be in the niches: cardiac care, oncology, stroke therapy, and others. Programs will be customized by disease and population group.

5. *Labor shortages will plague health care and many American industries.* Shortages will not be limited to nursing but will be experienced by many health professions. They will have a significant impact on health care operations, cost of care, and service availability. Wages may rise 5–15 percent in the year ahead, and wage inflation is likely for the next 2–5 years. Labor shortages should be anticipated, monitored, and factored into the strategic plans of hospitals and health systems.

6. *In the future, every hospital will have AIDS patients.* In the grimmest scenario, AIDS scorches America's inner cities and breaks into the middle class. Blood recipients constitute a special problem. Hospitals should contact blood recipients and alert them to the potential danger. Health workers should step up their vigilance against accidental contact with HIV-infected blood. AIDS education campaigns for staff and communities should be ongoing. Hopefully, research will find a cure, but few believe it will be discovered in the next 2–3 years.

BIBLIOGRAPHY

Abrums, Mary. 1986. "Health Care for Women." *Journal of Obstetric, Gynecologic, and Neonatal Nursing* (May-June): 250–55.

Adamache, Killard W., and Louis F. Rossiter. 1986. "The Entry of HMOs into the Medicare Market: Implications for TEFRA's Mandate." *Inquiry* 23 (Winter): 349–64.

Applebombe, Peter. 1987. "Some Say Frontier Is There, and Still Different." *New York Times*, 12 December, 11.

Arnett, Ross H., III, and Gordon R. Trapnell. 1984. "Private Health Insurance: New Measures of a Complex and Changing Industry." *Health Care Financing Review* 6 (Winter): 31–42.

Arnould, Richard J., Lawrence W. Debrock, and John W. Pollard. 1984. "Do HMOs Produce Specific Services More Efficiently?" *Inquiry* 21 (Fall): 243–53.

"As California Goes. . ." 1986. *American Demographics*, 26 November, 66.

"As HMOs Grow, Acquisitions, Mergers Thrive." 1985. *Group Health News* (September): 3–6.

"Baby Bust Incomes." 1987. *American Demographics* (October): 70.

Blendon, Robert J., and Drew E. Altman. 1984. "Public Attitudes about Health-Care Costs: A Lesson in National Schizophrenia." *New England Journal of Medicine* 311:616–24.

Blume, Sheila B. 1986. "Women and Alcohol." *JAMA* 256:1467–69.

Buchanan, Joan L., and Shan Cretin. 1986. "Risk Selection of Families Electing HMO Membership." *Medical Care* 24 (January): 39–51.

Burda, David. 1987. "The Nation Looks for New Ways to Finance Care for the Aged." *Hospitals*, 20 September: 48–54.

Coile, Russell C., Jr., and Randolph M. Grossman. 1988. "Macrotrends." *Healthcare Forum* (November-December): 50–53.

Daily-Melville, Cheri. 1986. "Women's Primary Care Clinics: Addressing the Women's Market." *Group Practice Journal* (July-August): 22–28.

Dalton, John J. 1987. "HMOs and PPOs: Similarities and Differences." *Topics in Health Care Financing* 13 (Spring): 8–18.

"Data on Nursing Homes Reflect Population." 1988. *New York Times*, 30 March, 9.

Davidson, Ezra C., Jr., and Teiichiro Fukushima. 1985. "The Age Extremes for Reproduction: Current Implications for Policy Change." *American Journal of Obstetric Gynecology*, 15 June, 467–71.

Dearing, Ruthie H. 1987. "Marketing to Attract Women." *Health Progress* (January-February): 26–28.

Deigh, Robb. 1987. "Population on the Road Again: Relocating American Dreams." *Insight*, 25 May, 18–20.

de Lissovoy, Gregory, et al. 1987. "Preferred Provider Organizations One Year Later." *Inquiry* 24 (Summer): 127–35.

de Lissovoy, Gregory, et al. 1986. "Preferred Provider Organizations: Today's Models and Tomorrow's Prospects." *Inquiry* 23 (Spring): 7–15.

Dutton, Diana B., Deanna Gomby, and Jinnet Fowles. 1985. "Satisfaction with Children's Medical Care in Six Different Ambulatory Settings." *Medical Care* 23:894–11.

Epstein, Arnold M., Colin B. Begg, and Barbara J. McNeil. 1986. "The Use of Ambulatory Testing in Prepaid and Fee-for-Service Group Practices." *New England Journal of Medicine* 314:1089–94.

Estes, Carroll L., Lenore Gerard, and Robyn Stone. 1986. "The Policy Implications of Caring for Older Women." *Business and Health* (March): 38–40.

Exter, Thomas. 1986. "Census Bureau's Household Projections." *American Demographics* (October): 44–47.

————. 1987. "How Many Hispanics?" *American Demographics* (May): 36–67.

Francese, Peter K. 1986. "Women as Healthcare Consumers." *Healthcare Forum* (January-February): 22–24.

Friedman, Emily. 1986. "The Health Lifeline: Out of the Reach of Women and Children?" *Hospitals*, 20 October, 46–51.

Fuchs, Victor R., and Leslie Perreault. 1986. "Expenditures for Reproduction-related Health Care." *JAMA* 255:76–81.

Gabel, Jon, and Dan Ermann. 1985. "Preferred Provider Organizations: Performance, Problems, and Promise." *Health Affairs* 4 (Spring): 24–40.

Garreau, Joel. 1981. *The Nine Nations of North America*. New York: Avon Books.

Gilman, Thomas A., and Cynthia K. Bucco. 1987. "Alternative Delivery Systems: An Overview." *Topics in Health Care Financing* 13:114–20.

Gleicher, Norbert. 1984. "Cesarean Section Rates in the United States." *JAMA* 252:3273–76.

Greenberg, Jay N., Walter N. Leutz, and Stanley S. Wallack. 1984. "A Vertically Integrated, Prepaid Care System for the Elderly." *Healthcare Financial Management* (October): 76–86.

Gutfeld, Rose. 1988. "Jobless Rate Dropped to 5.8% in December." *Wall Street Journal*, 11 January, A-2.

Hibbard, Judith H., and Clyde R. Pope. 1986. "Another Look at Sex Differences in the Use of Medical Care: Illness Orientation and the Types of Morbidities for Which Services Are Used." *Women and Health* 11 (Summer): 21–36.

Hughey, Michael John. "Routine Prenatal and Gynecologic Care in Prepaid Group Practice." *JAMA* 256: 1775–77.

Inglehart, John K. 1984. "HMOs (For-Profit and Not-for-Profit) on the Move." *New England Journal of Medicine* 310:1203–8.

———. 1984. "Opinion Polls on Health Care." *New England Journal of Medicine* 310: 1616–20.

———. 1985. "Medicare Turns to HMOs." *New England Journal of Medicine* 312:132–36.

Jensen, Joyce. 1986. "Women Generally Select Their Family's Physicians." *Modern Healthcare*, 31 January, 60–61.

———. 1986. "Women Pick the Providers Who Treat Their Illnesses, Those of Their Children." *Modern Healthcare*, 9 May, 66–67.

Kenkel, Paul J. 1987. "More Hospitals Enter Long-Term Care Business." *Modern Healthcare*, 20 November, 30–34.

Koehn, Hank. 1986. "The Social Mosaic of the '90s." *Healthscan* 1 (May): 1–11.

Langwell, Kathryn, et al. 1987. "Early Experience of Health Maintenance Organizations under Medicare Competition Demonstrations." *Health Care Financing Review* 8 (Spring): 37–55.

Lesser, Arthur J. 1985. "The Origin and Development of Maternal and Child Health Programs in the United States." *American Journal of Public Health* 75: 590–96.

Levin, Bruce Lubotsky, and Jules D. Levin. 1986. "Differential HMO Organizational Structures." *Group Health Association of America Journal* (Spring): 43–48.

Lewis, Myrna. "Older Women and Health: An Overview." *Health Needs of Women as They Change*, 1–15.

Luft, Harold S. 1978. "How Do Health Maintenance Organizations Achieve Their 'Savings?' " *New England Journal of Medicine* 208:1336–42.

Lutz, Sandy. 1987. "Hospitals Develop Satellite Clinics to Tap Emerging Women's Market." *Modern Healthcare*, 2 January, 76.

McMillan, Alma, James Lubitz, and Delores Russell. 1987. "Medicare Enrollment in Health Maintenance Organizations." *Health Care Financing Review* 8 (Spring): 87–93.

Manning, Willard G., et al. 1984. "A Controlled Trial of the Effect of a Prepaid Group Practice on Use of Services." *New England Journal of Medicine* 310:1505–10.

"Maternity Services Shift in Response to Consumer Demand." 1985. *Hospitals*, 16 April, 82–88.

Mechanic, David, Norma Weiss, and Paul D. Cleary. 1983. "The Growth of HMOs: Issues of Enrollment and Disenrollment." *Medical Care* 21:338–47.

"Men on Their Own." 1987. *American Demographics* (July): 62.

"Money and the Single Mother." 1987. *American Demographics* (June): 70.

Moran, Donald W., and Theresa E. Savela. 1986. "HMOs, Finance, and the Hereafter." *Health Affairs* (Spring): 51–65.

Morrisey, Michael A. 1984. "The Nature of Hospital-HMO Affiliations." *Health Care Management Review* (Spring): 51–60.

Naeye, Richard L. 1983. "Maternal Age, Obstetric Complications, and the Outcome of Pregnancy." *Obstetrics and Gynecology* 61 (February): 210–15.

Newhouse, Joseph P., William B. Schwartz, Albert Williams, and Christina Witzberger. 1985. "Are Fee-for-Service Costs Increasing Faster than HMO Costs?" *Medical Care* 23:960–66.

O'Hare, William. 1986. "The Eight Myths of Poverty." *American Demographics* (May): 22–25.

Pascal, Anthony. 1987. *The Costs of Treating AIDS under Medicaid: 1986–1991*. Santa Monica, Calif.: The Rand Corporation.

Powills, Suzanne. 1987a. "Segment Marketing: Less Costly, More Efficient." *Hospitals*, 20 January, 38.

_____. 1987b. "Diversity Key to Targeting Women's Market." *Hospitals*, 5 February, 38–41.

_____. 1987c. "Women's Health Care Market: Here to Stay?" *Hospitals*, 5 July, 38–40.

Rappaport, Anna M. 1986. "Flexible Compensation for Effective Benefit Management." *Topics in Health Care Financing* 12(4): 74–83.

Rasky, Susan F. 1988. "Senate, 88 to 4, Passes Bill Setting Immigration Limits." *New York Times*, 16 March, 10.

Reinhold, Robert. 1988. "Church and Immigration Officials Coaxing Aliens." *New York Times*, 8 March, A23.

Rice, Thomas, et al. 1985. "The State of PPOs: Results from a National Survey." *Health Affairs* 4 (Winter): 25–40.

Richman, Dan. 1986. "Enrollment Soars 291% in HMOs Sponsored by Hospitals Chains." *Modern Healthcare*, 6 June, 132–34.

_____. 1986. "Number of PPOs Rises at Fast Pace." *Modern Healthcare*, 6 June, 138–40.

Robey, Bryant. 1987. "Locking up Heaven's Door." *American Demographics* (February): 24–55.

Rosenberg, Lynn. 1985. "Myocardial Infarction and Cigarette Smoking in Women Younger than 50 Years of Age." *JAMA* 253:2965–69.

Rundle, Rhonda. 1987. "Doctors Who Oppose the Spread of HMOs Are Losing Their Fight." *Wall Street Journal*, 6 October, 1.

Russell, Cheryl, and Thomas G. Exter. 1986. "America at Mid-Decade." *American Demographics* (January): 22–29.

Schlesinger, Mark M. Blumenthal, and Eric Schlesinger. 1986. "Profits under Pressure: The Economic Performance of Investor-owned and Nonprofit Health Maintenance Organizations." *Medical Care* 24:615–27.

Siu, Albert L., et al. 1986. "Inappropriate Use of Hospitals in a Randomized Trial of Health Insurance Plans." *New England Journal of Medicine* 315:1259–66.

Steinwachs, Donald M., et al. 1986. "A Comparison of the Requirements for Primary Care Physicians in HMOs with Projections Made by the GMENAC." *New England Journal of Medicine* 314:217–22.

Super, Kari E. 1987. "Women Slow to Respond to Bone Scanning Services, While Arthritis Units Show Promise." *Modern Healthcare*, 31 July, 40–42.

Supple, Terry Stevenson. 1986. "The Labor Shortage." *American Demographics* (September): 32–35.

U.S. Department of Labor, Bureau of Labor Statistics. 1986. *Employee Benefits in Medium and Large Firms, 1985*. Bulletin 2262. Hyattsville, Md.: U.S. Department of Labor.

Verbrugge, Lois M., and Deborah L. Wingard. 1986. "Sex Differentials in Health and Mortality." *Women and Health* 12(2): 103–43.

Wagner, Lynn. 1987. "Nursing Homes Develop Special Alzheimer's Units." *Modern Healthcare*, 24 April, 40–46.

Waldrop, Judith W. 1987. "The Demographics of Diabetes." *American Demographics* (April): 45–47.

Ware, John E., Jr., et al. 1986. "Comparison of Health Outcomes at a Health Maintenance Organization with Those of Fee-for-Service Care." *The Lancet*, 3 May, 1017–22.

Welch, W.P., and Richard G. Frank. 1986. "The Predictors of HMO Enrollee Populations: Results from a National Sample." *Inquiry* 23 (Spring): 16–22.

Whitman, David. 1988. "America's Hidden Poor." *U.S. News and World Report*, 11 January, 18–24.

Wilensky, Gail R., and Louis F. Rossiter. 1986. "Patient Self-Selection in HMOs." *Health Affairs* (Spring): 66–79.

Wilner, Susan, Stephen C. Schoenbaum, Richard Monson, and Richard Winickoff. 1981. "A Comparison of the Quality of Maternity Care between a Health Maintenance Organization and Fee-for-Service Practices." *New England Journal of Medicine* 304:784–87.

"Who's Having Babies?" 1987. *American Demographics* (September): 62.

"Women: Target of New Marketing Efforts." 1985. *Hospitals*, 16 April, 82.

Zillmer, Theodore. 1986. "Stop-Loss Insurance Can Reduce Employers' Risks." *Topics in Health Care Financing* 12(4): 68–73.

Chapter 4

The Age Wave

When a physician makes a prognosis, it usually is based on years of experience with similar cases. Today, when eldercare futurists make prognoses, there are no analogous experiences upon which to base predictions. Never before have we seen the confluence of so many unprecedented social trends in America.

—Ken Dychtwald and Mark Zitter,
The Role of the Hospital in an Aging Society

The aging of society, the most powerful trend affecting tomorrow's health care, will impact every facet of the health system, from ambulatory to extended care. Rising costs of care for the elderly are placing real financial burdens on hospitals, and talk of rationing is getting louder. To manage the coming demographic shift toward the elderly, physicians and all health providers will need a coordinated continuum of elderly services network so that they can implement their social commitment to care for the aged sick and poor (see Chapter 5).

For health care, the aging of American society is the most profound demographic change in the 20th century. Its effects will be felt well beyond the year 2000. In simple terms, in 1980, one in nine Americans was over age 65; in another 30 years, the ratio will be almost one in five. The crest of the aging trend will be in the year 2010, when those born during the peak of the Baby Boom reach age 65. Then more than one million citizens will reach age 65 each year for 20 years.

Today's health system is still acute care focused; tomorrow's health needs will be chronic and the care holistic. As the percentage of the population enrolled in managed care plans rises to 50 percent and more in the 1990s, physicians and hospitals will have a long-term contractual responsibility for maintaining high health levels among their older patients—and Americans will live a long time, gaining another two years of life expectancy before the year 2000.

Don't think of the aging of society only as a future trend. In many ways it is arriving now. Aging will be one of the leading forces for change for tomorrow's health system. Older adults are health care's most frequent customers and the largest segment of the health care market. Diseases of old age will dominate hospital care and medicine. Medicare will pay for more than half the nation's hospital and medical bills in the years ahead. Older voters are becoming America's most potent political bloc, and health care is their number one issue. The needs, values, and attitudes of older adults will set the trends in health care access, costs, and service.

THE AGING OF AMERICA

The following are key trends that may influence health needs and services in the near and midrange future.

Coming of the Gerontocracy

Since 1960 the population aged 65 and over has grown more than twice as fast as the younger population. The elderly increased from 16.7 million in 1960 to 24.9 million in 1980 (a 55 percent increase, while those under 65 increased by 24 percent). From 8.1 percent of the population, the elderly increased to 11.2 percent in 20 years. By the year 2000, their numbers will exceed 12 percent and will reach 15 percent before the year 2020.

The older the age segment, the more the numbers are increasing. In the 1960–1980 period, the "Golden Years" segment (age 75–84) rose by 65 percent while the "oldest old" (over 85) grew an astonishing 174 percent. Population forecasts from the Census Bureau predict that at the turn of the century 10.4 million more Americans will reach age 65, an increase of 40 percent (Table 4-1). Those aged 75–84 will increase in number by almost 5 million, and those over 85 will double in number, reaching 1.5 million. Most impressive, the "Centenarians" (over age 100) are forecasted to increase from 25,000 in 1980 to 75,000 in the year 2000.

America's health system is only beginning to understand the magnitude of this population trend. Planning should begin with the assumption that older adults will be the number one patients of America's hospitals, doctors, and health plans. Every hospital and health system should have a long-range strategic development plan for the health care services and facilities the older population will need. Think chronic care (not acute care) and long-range development when planning for the elderly. Creating a continuum of care for the elderly will be at least a ten-year process.

Table 4-1 Forecast of the over-65 Population (1950–2030)

Year	Population over Age 65	Percentage of US. Population
1950	12,397,000	8.1%
1970	20,087,000	9.9
1980	24,927,000	11.2
2000	31,822,000	12.2
2010	34,837,000	12.7
2020	45,102,000	15.5
2030	55,024,000	18.3

Source: U.S. Bureau of the Census

Declining Mortality and Rising Life Expectancy

Not only is the nation's population aging, people are also healthier and living longer. Consider these forecasts developed by Dr. Dorothy Rice, former director of the National Center for Health Statistics. They indicate the trends for the 25 years between 1978 and 2003 (Rice and Feldman 1983):

- The national death rate per 100,000 population will decline almost 50 percent for males and 40 percent for women.
- Deaths due to heart disease will decline 50 percent for men and nearly 60 percent for women.
- Cancer deaths will rise 25 percent for men and 20 percent for women.
- Vascular diseases will decline more than 200 percent for men and 300 percent for women.
- Deaths due to respiratory diseases will drop more than 33 percent for men but less than 10 percent for women.

The fastest growing age group in the nation is the same one on which the federal government spends the most money. The number of people aged 80 and over is growing five times faster than the total population, and this age group will double in size in 20 years. The primary reason for this rapid growth is rising life expectancy. According to a recent study by the Census Bureau, the United States spent $51 billion on health and social services in 1984, which came to $8,500 per person. The expenditure per person will exceed $10,000 before 1990 (Rice and Feldman 1983).

Physicians, hospitals and health plans should track the trends closely for shifts in mortality and morbidity among their older adults. Looking ahead, cardiac care will decline and cancer care will grow. Respiratory disease is generally declining, but that is less true for women. As Americans age, the main causes of death will be different in the decade ahead. Older adults are living longer and will suffer higher rates of stroke and Alzheimer's disease.

Longer Lives and Shifts in Morbidity Patterns

Some demographers believe that changes in life style and improved medical technology will reduce death by chronic disease and restrict high levels of morbidity to the older age groups. Instead of fading away gradually, the elderly are surviving spells of acute illness—heart attacks, strokes, breast cancer—and returning quickly to health. These experts forecast a continued decline in premature death and the emergence of a pattern of natural death at the end of a natural life span.

This shifting pattern of morbidity in the survival curve is seen today in factors such as

- higher survival rates for breast cancer treated by mastectomy
- improving recovery rates for stroke victims
- higher life expectancy post–heart attack (a number of bypass surgery patients survive long enough to need a second bypass procedure)

Elderly people recovering from the acute phases of chronic illness are now returning to high levels of function and productivity. They are surviving to lead independent, quality lives, many well into their 80s and above. The "squaring of the demographic curve" is contributing to a rising need for home care, both health care and support services, in order to keep these relatively healthy elders functioning at home and out of institutions. It is more than health status that makes the elderly "frail." At older age levels, it is their increasing need for maintenance and assistance with daily living that determines whether older Americans can live independently or require institutional care. Physicians, hospitals, and health systems will need to take a lead role in coordinating health care with social support services, working with public agencies, local charities, and community programs.

Growing Dependency Ratio

A major concern in the shifting ground of American demographics are the *dependency ratios*. These are crude indexes of the total burden on the working population as a result of its support of old and young dependents. Since the future of the Social Security trust fund for Medicare depends on the ratio of retirees to workers, dependency ratios serve as useful indexes of the burden on society of the aging of the population. The *aged dependency ratio* is defined as the number of people aged 65 and over divided by the number of people aged 20–64. This ratio was .174 in 1960 and .195 in 1980. It is expected to increase to .215 in 1990 and to .226 in 2000.

Health care providers should anticipate that Social Security and Medicare funding may be inadequate to provide income and health care for the elderly in the future. Assuming present trends, the Medicare trust fund could be bankrupt by the turn of the century. To compound the problem, Congress may stop indexing Social Security benefits in the early 1990s in an attempt to balance the federal budget. This situation may come before 1995 if federal budget deficits cannot be managed, forcing Congress to make massive cuts in Medicare and Social Security. The charitable capacity of physicians and hospitals would be a "safety net" for the elderly in such a scenario.

Gender Gap

Women have traditionally outlived men, and the gap is widening. In a 25-year forecast of life expectancy by the National Center for Health Statistics, women will outlive men by 10 years (84.2 years for women versus 74.2 years for men) in the year 2003 if current patterns of declining mortality hold (Verbrugge and Wingard 1987). By comparison, the gap was only 4 years in 1953, spreading to 7.9 years in 1978.

A generation ago there was approximately an equal number of men and women in the United States. Today there are 6.4 percent more women than men, and this numerical advantage is predicted to persist well into the next century. Peter Francese (1986), the publisher of *American Demographics*, predicts that for the forseeable future a clear majority of the adult population as well as a majority of patients in virtually every hospital will be women. Experts believe that women's higher longevity is two-thirds explained by environmental exposure, health habits and life style rather than by genetic physical differences.

The gender gap and the aging of American women will be especially important for health care strategists and marketers. In 1982, women constituted 59 percent of those over age 65 and incurred 63 percent of medical care costs. The problem is intensified for older single women, who will spend a greater share of their income for out-of-pocket health expenses and insurance premiums. For single-woman households, this percentage rises from 10.2 percent for those aged 70 to 42 percent for those aged 85 and over.

Since women die later than men, they will suffer from more chronic illnesses and disabilities before death. Whereas older men spend more days in the hospital, older women are more likely to be institutionalized in a nursing home or need home care services. About 75 percent of nursing home residents are women. Over half of nursing home residents have serious organic brain syndrome (senility), and more women than men suffer this condition—because of their longevity and numbers. Environmental, genetic, and life style differences combine to make older women living alone extremely vulnerable. Hospitals and health systems can develop outreach and support systems particularly targeted to older women living alone, including Lifeline, daily telephone calls by volunteers, friendly visiting, pastoral care, transportation, and home health or homemaker services. Support for caregivers—family, friends, or neighbors—may make the difference between independent living and institutionalization. Holy Cross Hospital of Detroit is illustrative of community providers who have created caregiver support groups. Few of these outreach services are reimbursable, but they offer many opportunities for volunteerism. Doctors and hospitals should coordinate joint efforts with local charities, churches, volunteers, and community agencies on behalf of their elderly patients.

Income and Old Age

There is a persistent myth that to be old is to be impoverished. Old age poverty has largely been remedied in the past 20 years through the indexing of Social Security benefits, improvements in Medicare benefits, and better private pension plans. Today only 15 percent of those over age 65 have incomes below the poverty line, which is roughly the percentage for the general population (Kirchner 1985).

For the past decade, the money income of households headed by an elderly person has increased faster than the rate of consumer inflation. Data from the Bureau of Labor Statistics for 1977–1983 show the median income of those over 65 rose 74 percent. This increase substantially exceeded the 49 percent rise in median income of all households as well as the 59 percent hike in the CPI. The "young elders" (ages 55–64) have the highest per capita disposable incomes of any age category. These income trends show considerable strength and are forecasted to continue for the next decade.

The elderly have among the highest levels of disposable income of any adults, but they also spend more of it on health care than other age groups. Older Americans are actually divided into many minisegments. Developing and marketing health services for the elderly must deal with a broad range of needs, from the affluent with discretionary income to the poor on subsistence incomes.

Older Workers

One reason for their economic health is that many older adults are still working. More than half of those over age 60 are working at least part time. A third of the working elders hold down a full-time job. As the nation's labor shortage grows, hospitals and health organizations may look to the elderly and retirees as a new labor pool. McDonald's, one of the few U.S. companies with a full-time futurist, began to recruit "McMasters" older workers in response to labor shortages in 1985.

As the population ages, the proportion of retirees to workers continues to shrink. Currently, an estimated two-thirds of workers in medium and large firms will receive postretirement health coverage, as will 71 percent of those taking early retirement. All this may change in the future if the Financial Accounting Standards Board (FASB) requires employers to disclose their unfunded liability for postemployment health and welfare benefits. For American business, that unfunded health insurance liability is estimated at one to two trillion dollars. The cost of funding the liability would be more than five thousand dollars per employee per year, by one estimate. Employers may abandon supplementing Medicare coverage for retirees altogether if the FASB standard is imposed.

Older workers are underrecognized as a target for health care services and marketing. For many older Americans, the problems of chronic disease and health limitations begin while employed and prior to retirement. Few doctors, hospitals, or health plans have targeted these older workers as a priority for specialized programs or attention, yet business has a substantial obligation in terms of health benefits for these workers after retirement.

Older workers and retirees may also help solve health care's labor shortage. They have invaluable experience and wisdom, as well as loyalty and a strong work ethic. They may help hospitals cope with shortages by working part time, flextime, or "minishifts" of less than eight hours. A hospital's older workers and "recycled retirees" may need continuing education to maintain skill levels, and it will need to make scheduling and compensation policies more flexible to accommodate older workers.

Social Problems of Older Americans

For many older Americans, old age and retirement do not resemble the situation of Fonda and Hepburn in *On Golden Pond*. Poverty, crime, loneliness, drug abuse, and suicide are growing problems among the elderly. Rising numbers of the elderly are moving in with adult children for reasons of economics or failing health, signaling the return of the multigenerational family. The strains of living with aging parents are reflected in the increase in elder abuse, an underreported problem. Poverty rates among elderly blacks are triple those for whites, and twice as many elderly Hispanics are poor than elderly non-Hispanic whites. These trends persist, despite overall gains in income achieved by the elderly over the past 20 years.

Those involved in protecting and promoting the health of older adults must recognize the social factors that contribute to health and disease. As the nation ages, the social problems of the elderly are growing. Doctors, hospitals, churches, and charities should coordinate their efforts to combat alienation, elder abuse, alcohol and drug use, and suicide among the elderly.

MARKET PROFILE: OLDER AMERICANS TODAY

A landmark event in American demographics occurred in July 1983. For the first time in U.S. history, the number of older adults (over age 65) surpassed the number of teenagers. America is gradually becoming less youth-oriented, and its vision and values are increasingly those of a maturing society. Every 18 months more people reach age 65 than made up the total elderly population in 1900.

The aging of America is picking up speed. Today there are over 30 million older adults, and they constitute more than 12 percent of the population. The Census Bureau predicts that the number of seniors will rise to 32 million by 1990 and to 35 million by the turn of the century. At this point, 1 in 7 Americans will be over age 65. The growth curve of aging will continue to rise as the Baby Boom generation reaches old age. By the year 2020, 1 in 5 Americans will be over 65, and the trends push upwards.

RISING LIFE EXPECTANCY: AGING WILL DOMINATE THE 21ST CENTURY

What demographic factors are driving the age wave? Rising life expectancy and a declining birth rate are the primary ones. A newborn today has a life expectancy of 75 years. There is a real gender discrepancy, and the gap is widening. Men will live 71.2 years, whereas women can expect a life span of 78.2 years. Not surprisingly, women constitute 60 percent of the elderly. Among those over age 85, more than seven in ten are women.

The aging of the population is complemented by a declining birth rate, which shifts the age curve toward older age cohorts. Since its high point in the late 1950s, the birth rate has dropped from 106 live births per 1000 to less than 64.9 in 1986, an all-time low. The outlook for fertility in the 1990s is for a continued low birth rate. Demographers estimate that perhaps 20 percent of the Baby Boom generation will not have children, and another 25 percent may have one child per couple. Thus the elderly will make up an increasing share of the population, and the median age will continue to rise.

INCOME, WEALTH, AND SPENDING

Forget what you may have thought about aging. The older generation is the most diverse of all age groups. The popular perception of the elderly as poor, lonely, and failing is simply not accurate. Economic well-being varies widely, but the elderly are not generally poor. Older adults have lower financial resources and average incomes than younger adults, but they have fewer financial demands. As a result, older adults have the highest level of discretionary income of any age group.

Not all the elderly are affluent, by far. Black and Hispanic elders have far lower cash incomes than their non-Hispanic white counterparts. This is true for both sexes and all ages. More of the elderly fall below the poverty line, but the difference is small. About 12.4 percent of older adults fell below the 1984 poverty level, compared with 11.7 of those 18–64 years old. Many more of the elderly live near the poverty level. The Census Bureau reported that 16.7 percent of older adults lived in near poverty (between 100 and 150 percent of the poverty level), compared with only 9.6 percent of younger adults (Dychtwald and Zitter 1986).

At the other end of the spectrum, a growing number of seniors live comfortably on high incomes. An estimated 30 percent of all households with incomes above $55,000 are headed by persons over age 55. These households account for 28 percent of all discretionary spending, buy half of the luxury automobiles, and are heavy users of travel and entertainment credit cards.

Spending patterns vary by age. Compared with younger households, elders spend more of their pretax income—at rates between 90 and 105 percent. Four-fifths of personal spending by seniors goes for food, transportation, housing, and health care, compared with less than 75 percent for those aged 25–64. People over age 55 account for about half of all health care expenditures.

LOCATION, DISTRIBUTION, AND MIGRATION

Many of the popular perceptions about older Americans are far from accurate. For example, not all seniors have migrated to the Sunbelt. Far from it. Half of those over age 65 are concentrated in eight states: California, New York, Florida, Pennsylvania, Texas, Illinois, Ohio, and Michigan. This is no surprise, for these are also the most populous states in the nation. Only Florida and Pennsylvania have proportions of the elderly significantly above the national average. Florida is a bellwether state: Its 17.7 percent share of elders is similiar to what the nation can expect in the year 2020.

Most states with high percentages of the elderly are in the Midwest and Northeast. At least 10 states had proportions of elder residents above 13.5 percent (the national average is 12.1 percent): Florida, Pennsylvania, Rhode Island, Arkansas, Iowa, South Dakota, Missouri, Massachusetts, Nebraska, and West Virginia. The high percentages in these states resulted from a net emigration of younger residents from the Midwest, low fertility rates in the North Atlantic states, and continuing immigration of seniors to Florida.

Other myths about the elderly likewise miss the mark. Not all seniors have retired to rural areas or are huddled in inner cities. Although many older adults are located in cities, more live in suburbs. In 1980, more than 10 million seniors lived in suburban areas and 8.1 million were city dwellers. Another 7.3 million were located in rural areas.

HEALTH STATUS: HEALTHIER THAN MANY BELIEVE

Older adults are in better health than is commonly realized. The majority of seniors are relatively healthy and far less limited in physical and mental activity than might be imagined.

The elderly do consume more health care than any other age group, especially in the eighth and ninth decades of life. But they feel healthy. Various studies report that between 66 and 85 percent of seniors rate their own health as "excellent," "very good," or "good" in comparison with others their age. Fewer than one in 10 report their own health as relatively poor (Kirchner 1985). A recent study of 237 retirees in the *American Journal of Public Health* reported that 40 percent enjoyed an improvement in their health after retirement and that 37 percent maintained the same health levels (Zitter 1988).

Money helps! A direct relationship exists between perceived health status and income. More than 40 percent of seniors with incomes above $25,000 rated their health "excellent," whereas less than 25 percent of those with incomes below $7,000 gave their health this rating. Older adults in the lowest income group are more than twice as likely to report poor health as those in the next income bracket up.

Besides income, there are other factors that correlate with better health among older adults. Education may be the most important. Public health experts speculate that more educated people may heed messages about health promotion and plan for the future. Other indicators for longevity and happiness include job satisfaction, strong family and social support, and a history of satisfying sexual relationships.

Better health perceptions are related to less use of health services. In a 1982 study, persons over age 65 who reported themselves in excellent health averaged only 3.3 days in bed as the result of an illness or injury per year, compared with 62.2 bed days for those who reported poor health. The same discrepancy held for physician utilization: Elders claiming excellent health made 2.5 doctor visits per year, whereas those reporting poor health visited the doctor an average of 15.3 times. Data on health perceptions may be an important marketing tool for eldercare services.

HEALTH AND DISABILITY

Relatively few elders are severely limited by some type of disability. Seniors may be rated on their ability regarding six activities of daily living (ADLs): eating, bathing, dressing, toileting, continence, and mobility (Figure 4-1). Disability is rated by determining how many of these activities require some assistance. One in five seniors has at least a mild amount of disability or is limited in one or two ADLs. Only 3.5 percent of those over age 65 suffer from severe disability (limitations in five or more ADLs).

Disabled seniors are more likely to be women (20.9 percent) than men (16.0 percent). The proportion of those who are limited in ADLs rises dramatically with age. Nearly half of those over age 85 are limited in at least one ADL. Not all limitations require special assistance. Although 18 percent of people over 65 suffer some degree of limitation in mobility, less than two-thirds of those need special help to get around and only one in three is housebound.

MENTAL HEALTH

In terms of mental health, the elderly may be the healthiest of all population segments. Studies by the National Institute of Mental Health and the Office of Technology Assessment estimate that 15–25 percent of noninstitutionalized older adults suffer some symptoms of mental illness, with 5–15 percent of these suffering from Alzheimer's disease (Zitter 1988).

Institutionalized elders have more mental illness. Among nursing home residents, more than half suffer from a chronic mental condition or some form of mental impairment. Over 20 percent of those in nursing homes have a mental disorder or senility without psychosis as their primary diagnosis.

Some experts fear that mental disorders may be more easily overlooked or misdiagnosed among the elderly. Symptoms of mental problems may be wrongfully assumed to be the natural consequences of aging. Depression is a major problem for older adults. Between 2 and 7 percent of those over 65 have clinically

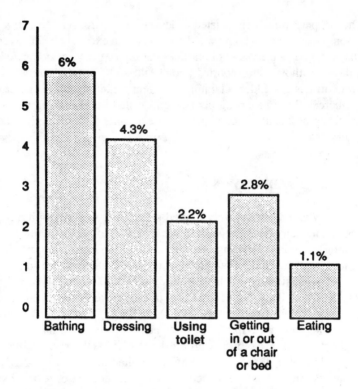

Figure 4-1 Dependency in Selected Activities of Daily Living. *Source*: Reprinted from *Marketing Healthcare to Older Adults* by M. Zitter with permission of Age Wave Publications, © 1988.

diagnosed depression. The problem is most likely to occur among older women who have suffered a loss of spouse, health, or home.

Loss of mental functioning is often acute and can be reversed with appropriate diagnosis. Half of all cognitive impairment problems are due to drugs, illness, or environmental factors (e.g., confusion due to new surroundings). Other health-related factors such as heart disease, hyperthyroidism, kidney disease, infection, sensory loss, hypothermia, or malnutrition can contribute to the appearance of irreversible mental illness.

NATURE OF HEALTH PROBLEMS AMONG THE ELDERLY

The health needs of older Americans are different from and more frequent than those of younger adults. Hospitals developing eldercare programs must begin with a fundamental understanding that eldercare is different. The diseases of young and middle-aged adults are acute, involve short hospitalizations, and seldom require more than a few days or weeks for complete recovery. The diseases of older adults are chronic and degenerative. Hospital stays are longer, and the conditions require continuing medical follow-up and treatment, in many cases for a lifetime.

Despite the heavy preponderance of older health care users, health care plans orient reimbursement toward cure rather than care; yet the chronically ill need the latter, not the former. Medical science's successes in curtailing acute diseases has allowed people to live longer, thereby contributing to the increasing prevalence of chronic diseases. More than 80 percent of the older population suffer from at least one chronic health condition. According to the U.S. Federal Commission on Chronic Disease, older adults average 4.4 chronic conditions per person, although many of these are minor. Most visits to hospitals or physicians are related to chronic health conditions, which account for 75 percent of restricted-activity days among the elderly (Waldo and Lazenby 1984).

The leading causes of death among older persons are heart disease, cancer, and stroke. These illnesses account for more than 75 percent of all deaths for people over age 65. Heart disease is responsible for 45 percent of deaths among seniors, more than twice the percentage of those dying from cancer, the second leading cause of death. Stroke accounts for one in nine deaths among elders.

HOSPITAL UTILIZATION

Seniors need acute care, too. Acute problems such as injuries and digestive and genitourinary conditions are currently the leading causes of hospitalization for older adults.

Older adults are hospitalized twice as frequently as younger people, stay nearly twice as long, and spend three times as many days in the hospital. Based on the 1986 National Hospital Discharge Survey, the National Center for Health Statistics reported the following:

- Older adults constitute 12 percent of the population but account for more than 31 percent of hospital discharges.
- Short-stay hospitals reported 367.3 discharges per 1,000 for those over age 65, compared with 162.2 for the 45–64 age group and only 143.1 for the population as a whole.
- Hospital stays in 1986 averaged 8.5 days for those over 65 and 6.8 for the 45–64 age group.

- Average hospital stays for those over 85 were 61 percent longer than for the population as a whole and 21 percent longer than for younger elders aged 65–74.
- Older adults spent 3,574.8 days in the hospital per 1,000 population, twice the number of days (2,318.5) used by those aged 45–64 and three times the number of days (1,033.7) used by the entire population.

PHYSICIAN SERVICES

Older adults are more frequent visitors to physician offices and heavier users of services. Those over age 65 averaged 4.8 doctor visits in 1985, compared with 3.1 visits for those aged 45–64 and 2.7 for all age groups. These figures do not include visits by physicians to the elderly in hospitals, which seniors use more often and for longer periods of time, as noted above.

Older adults use services more intensely than other age groups. Those over 65 tend to see doctors at their offices rather than visiting an ambulatory care center or calling by phone. Most seniors (81.4 percent) see a doctor at least once a year, compared with less than two-thirds of those aged 18–64.

NURSING HOMES, HOME CARE, AND PHARMACEUTICALS

The demand for nursing homes and institutional care continues to expand, primarily driven by the expansion of the older population ("Data on Nursing Homes" 1988). The use rate for nursing homes and other institutional care facilities is holding constant at about 5 percent of the over 65 population. Long-term care experts predict there will eventually be more demand for personal care facilities and continuing care retirement communities that contain assisted-living units.

Most of the growth of home care has already occurred, due to reimbursement shifts. Home care could expand at a rate of 12–20 percent, but home care use will be restrained unless there are significant changes in Medicare and health plan benefit policies (Anderson 1986). About 80 percent of the 5 million non-institutionalized elderly receive unpaid home care from family or friends, experts estimate. About 20 percent use a combination of paid and unpaid home health services, and only 5 percent rely on paid home care services. The burden of home care primarily falls on adult children, who on average support their aging parents for an estimated 17 years beyond age 65.

The aging of the population has sent pharmaceutical use soaring. More than 75 percent of seniors have at least one prescription annually, compared with less than 60 percent of the total population. Elders use twice as many prescription drugs as all other age groups. More than 30 percent of drugs prescribed in America are used by people over age 65.

Health care entrepreneurs don't need to be demographers to see the trends. The implications of the changing demographics are clear. As America shifts towards an older population, the need for eldercare services of all types and in all settings is growing.

STRATEGIC IMPLICATIONS FOR PHYSICIANS

1. *The elderly are physicians' most important patients.* The elderly now exceed 11 percent of the population and will be the source of 40–50 percent or more of physician revenues. Some physicians, primarily from internal medicine, are taking examinations to become board-certified gerontologists.
2. *The patterns of disease are shifting.* Growing numbers of the elderly are affecting traditional American patterns of morbidity and mortality. Death rates for older men and women are declining, life expectancy is rising, and patterns of disease are shifting. Cardiac mortality will decrease and cancer incidence will grow. As adults live longer they will suffer higher rates of stroke and Alzheimer's.
3. *The income gap among seniors is widening.* First the good news: The income levels of the elderly are rising. Now the bad news: Income is "bimodal" among the elderly. That is, the rich are getting richer and the poor are growing poorer. Physicians should consider older adults as prime markets for discretionary health care, including health promotion, wellness, and cosmetic surgery. At the same time, the elderly poor may need special efforts from physicians and hospitals in collaboration with community agencies. Physician charity may be the safety net if public spending cannot keep pace with rising costs and the needs of the elderly.
4. *As the number of older adults grows, meeting the health needs of the elderly will become one of America's top legislative priorities—in the U.S. Congress, state legislatures, and local government.* Physicians, hospitals, and health systems need to be a strong voice in support of senior health needs. They also must form an alliance with the American Association of Retired Persons (AARP) and other concerned organizations. Equal attention should be given to emerging social problems in our aging society, especially poverty, crime, loneliness, drug abuse, and suicide.

STRATEGIC IMPLICATIONS FOR HOSPITALS

1. *Older adults will be the largest market for hospital services in the 1990s.* More than half of all community hospital inpatients will be over age 65

by the year 1995. This is the most important customer segment hospitals will serve. The survival of individual hospitals will be determined by how effectively they respond to the needs and expectations of the elders.

2. *Shifting patterns of disease will affect hospital use.* Changing patterns of disease will be driven by demographic trends of the "age wave." Cardiology is already established as a major service. In the future, oncology, orthopedics, and urology will become more important, while obstetrics declines. As adults live longer, they will suffer higher rates of stroke and Alzheimer's disease.

3. *Prepare for a fundamental paradigm shift from acute to chronic care.* The decade of the 1990s will be a transition period for the health industry, moving away from a focus on acute curative medicine and toward long-term chronic care that will be punctuated by periodic flareups of acute illness. This mindshift will drive a gradual transformation of the entire health system.

BIBLIOGRAPHY

American Hospital Association. 1988. "Key Trends through Third Quarter." *Economic Trends* (Winter): (reported in *Medical Benefits*, 15 March, 1988, 1–2.)

Anderson, Howard J. 1986. "Home Care Providers Business Expanded Rapidly during 1985." *Modern Healthcare*, 6 June, 168–69.

Arnett, Ross H., III, David R. McKusick, Sally T. Sonnefeld, and Carol S. Cowell. 1986. "Projections of Health Care Spending to 1990." *Health Care Financing Review* 7 (Spring): 1–63.

"Blue Shield First to Add Wellness Benefit to Individual Health Plans" 1987. (press release). San Francisco: Blue Shield of California, 23 November.

Changing Mortality Patterns, Health Services Utilization, and Health Care Expenditures: United States, 1978–2003. 1983. Hyattsville, Md.: U.S. Department of Health and Human Services. PHS 83-1407.

Chollet, Deborah J., and Robert B. Friedland. 1987. "Employee-Paid Retiree Health Insurance." In *The Changing Health Care Market*. Edited by Frank B. McArdle. Washington, D.C.: Employee Benefit Research Institute.

Coile, Russell C., Jr. 1987. "Overview: Environmental Forces and Trends in Long Term Care." In *Managing the Continuum of Care*. Edited by Connie J. Evashwick and Lawrence J. Weiss. Rockville, Md.: Aspen Publishers.

"Data on Nursing Homes Reflect Population." 1988. *New York Times*, 30 March, 9.

Doty, Pamela, Korbin Liu, and Joshua Weiner. 1985. "An Overview of Long-Term Care." *Health Care Financing Review* 6 (Spring): 69–78.

Dwight, Maria B. 1985. "Affluent Elderly Want to Live Where Quality Care's Available." *Modern Healthcare*, 26 April, 74–76.

Dychtwald, Ken, and Mark Zitter. 1986. *The Role of the Hospital in an Aging Society.* San Francisco: Age Wave.

―――――. 1988. "Looking Beyond the Myths of Aging America." *Healthcare Financial Management* (February): 40–43.

Estes, Carroll L., Lenore Gerard, and Adele Clarke. 1984. "Women and the Economics of Aging." *International Journal of Health Services* 14(1): 55–67.

Evashwick, Connie, Thomas Rundall, and Betty Goldiamond. 1985. "Hospital Services for Older Adults." *The Gerontologist* 25:631–37.

Francese, Peter K. 1986. "Women as Healthcare Consumers." *Healthcare Forum* (January-February): 22–24.

Graham, Judith. 1987. "Declines in Bed Prices at Nursing Homes Expected by Year-End, Industry Experts Say." *Modern Healthcare*, 22 May, 94–96.

Halpert, Burton P., and Mary K. Zimmerman. 1986. "The Health Status of the 'Old-Old': A Reconsideration." *Social Scientist Medicince* 22:893–99.

Harel, Zev, Linda Noelker, and Brian F. Blake. 1985. "Comprehensive Services for the Aged: Theoretical and Empirical Perspectives." *The Gerontologist* 25:644–49.

"Hospitals Reserving Nursing Home Beds." 1985. *Modern Healthcare*, 26 April, 68.

Jensen, Joyce. 1986. "Women Pick the Providers Who Treat Their Illnesses, Those of Their Children." *Modern Healthcare*, 9 May, 66–67.

Kaiser, Leland R. 1988. "Healthcare's Sleeping Giant." *Healthcare Forum Journal* (March-April): 35–37.

Kirchner, Merian. 1985. "Sifting Fact from Myth." *Medical Economics*, 29 April, 35–43.

Koch, Hugo, and Richard J. Havlik. 1987. "Use of Health Care–Ambulatory Medical Care." In *Health Statistics on Older Persons: United States, 1986*. Hyattsville, Md.: U.S. Department of Health and Human Services. DHHS Pub. no. PHS 87-1409.

Lazer, William, and Eric H. Shaw. 1987. "How Older Americans Spend Their Money." *American Demographics* (September): 36–41.

Leutz, Walter. 1986. "Long-Term Care for the Elderly: Public Dreams and Private Realities." *Inquiry* 23 (Summer): 134–40.

Lewis, Mary Ann, Shan Cretin, and Robert L. Kane. 1985. "The Natural History of Nursing Home Patients." *The Gerontologist* 25:382–88.

Linden, Fabian. 1986. "The $800 Billion Market: Economic Profile of the Mature Market: 1984." *American Demographics* (February): 4–6.

Lubitz, James, and Ronald Prihoda. 1984. "The Use and Costs of Medicare Services in the Last Two Years of Life." *Health Care Financing Review* 5 (Spring): 117–30.

McDonald, Stephen. 1988. "Designs for the Elderly but Not 'Geriatric.' " *Wall Street Journal*, 31 March, 27.

Magill, Judith R., and Janet L. Scheuermann. 1985. " 'Baby Boomers' a Ripe Market for Healthcare Providers: Study." *Modern Healthcare*, 29 March, 128–32.

Manton, Kenneth G. 1985. "Future Patterns of Chronic Disease Incidence, Disability, and Mortality among the Elderly." *New York State Journal of Medicine* (November): 623–33.

National Center for Health Statistics. 1987. *Health Statistics on Older Persons: United States, 1986*. Hyattsville, Md.: Department of Health and Human Services.

Olshansky, S. Jay, and A. Brian Ault. 1986. "The Fourth Stage of the Epidemiologic Transition: The Age of Delayed Degenerative Diseases." *Health and Society* 64:355–91.

Powills, Suzanne. 1986. "The Elderly: A Health Marketer's Challenge." *Hospitals*, 20 March, 70–74.

Punch, Linda. 1985. "Long-Term Care Industry Develops Alternatives to Meet Needs of Elderly." *Modern Healthcare* 26 April, 59.

Rice, Dorothy P., and Jacob J. Feldman. 1983. "Living Longer in the United States: Demographic Changes and Health Needs of the Elderly." *Health and Society* 61:362–96.

Roos, Noralou P., Evelyn Shapiro, and Leslie L. Roos, Jr. 1984. "Aging and the Demand for Health Services: Which Aged and Whose Demand?" *The Gerontologist* 24:31–36.

Smallegan, Marian. 1985. "There Was Nothing Else to Do: Needs for Care before Nursing Home Admission." *The Gerontologist* 25:364–69.

Super, Kari E. 1986. "Hospitals Are Beginning to Focus on Services for Older Patients." *Modern Healthcare*, 11 April, 80–82.

"Surgicenter Firm Has Geriatric Care." 1985. *Modern Healthcare*, 29 April, 68.

Tatge, Mark. 1985. "Providers Will Offer Care in New Settings." *Modern Healthcare*, 26 April, 70.

U.S. Congress. Senate. Special Committee on Aging. 1986. *The Health Status and Health Care Needs of Older Americans*. 99th Cong., 2nd sess., Senate Report 99–200.

Verbrugge, Lois M., and Deborah Wingard. 1987. "Sex Differentials in Health and Mortality." *Women and Health* 12(2): 103–43.

Wagner, Lynn. 1987a. "Seattle HMO, Insurer Offer Long-Term Care Option." *Modern Healthcare*, 10 April, 92.

_____. 1987b. "Measures to Bolster Nursing Home Quality Considered." *Modern Healthcare*, 14 August, 72–74.

_____. 1988. "States Exerting More Control over HMOs." *Modern Healthcare*, 5 February, 22–24.

Waldo, Daniel R., and Helen C. Lazenby. 1984. "Demographic Characteristics and Health Care Use and Expenditures by the Aged in the United States: 1977–1984." *Health Care Financing Review* 6 (Fall): 1–27.

White, Elizabeth C. 1985. "Competition for Healthcare Markets Spurs Race for Demographic Data." *Modern Healthcare*, 27 September, 79–80.

Zitter, Mark. 1988. *Marketing Healthcare to Older Adults*. Emeryville, Calif.: Age Wave.

Chapter 5

Continuum of Care

Imagine this scenario for elderly services in the year 1995—the "de-institu-tionalization of long term care." More than half of the nation's nursing homes have been closed or converted to other uses. More are closing daily; the trend is like the de-institutionalization of mental health 20 years before. . . . A com-bination of advanced medical science and progressive social thinking is reducing the need for institutional care for elderly. Health benefit policy has radically shifted from acute and institutional to ambulatory and home care. Long term care insurance never did catch on in the 1980s; health plans and HMOs altered their benefit mix to favor non-institutional services. The goal is the maintenance of high health levels among the elderly, now more than 15% of the population; by 1995, more than 50% of Medicare beneficiaries have enrolled in an HMO or Medicare Preferred Provider Organization. . . . Housing for older adults is a high-growth market. Builders and bankers are responding with innovative financing and new housing alternatives for older Americans. Continuing Care Retirement Centers (CCRCs) have doubled since 1987, numbering more than 1,800 in 1995, and growing at a rate of 200 projects per year. Lifecare, condominium ownership, leasing, rental, and time-share provide older Amer-icans with a wide array of housing choices in projects designed for their needs and lifestyle. CCRC housing for the elderly includes assisted living, congregate care, mobile services, and on-site health services in larger CCRC projects. . . . Every hospital has a continuum of elderly services, from inpatient subacute, skilled nursing to limited care; many hospitals have on-site senior health centers and medical hotels which are used for the residential component of acute care.

—Russell C. Coile, Jr.

CONTINUUM OF CARE: JUST WHAT THE ELDERLY NEED

Does the above scenario sound far-fetched? With growing numbers of the elderly impacting the U.S. health industry, physicians, hospitals, and health systems will need an overarching elderly services strategy for providing services

and establishing a network for older adults. The rising acuity—and age levels—
of today's health care patients signal that the time to begin developing tomorrow's
elderly services system is now.

Many experts on aging and health recommend development of a "continuum
of care" containing a broad array of health and health-related support services.
Connie Evashwick and Lawrence Weiss (1987) identify the following categories
of care and assistance as constituting the continuum of care for the elderly:
extended, acute, ambulatory, home, outreach, wellness, and housing (Figure
5-1).

Comprehensive eldercare systems will be developed by many hospitals and
multihospital systems to meet the needs of tomorrow's elders. Religious-spon-

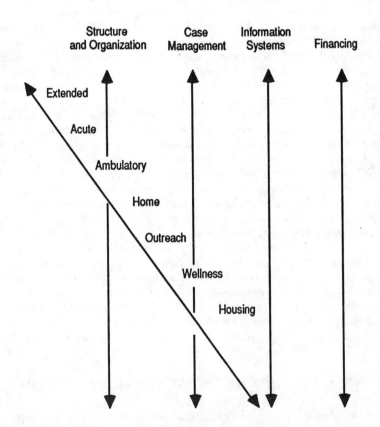

Figure 5-1 Continuum of Care Services and Integrating Mechanisms. *Source*: Reprinted from
Managing the Continuum of Care by C.J. Evashwick and L.J. Weiss (Eds.), p. 25, Aspen Publishers,
Inc., © 1987.

sored health systems have been creating multilevel continuums of health care for 100 years. For example, Providence Systems of Springfield, Massachusetts, has developed a multilevel system of care over decades. The system currently includes three acute hospitals, a 121-bed skilled nursing home, two personal care homes, a 153-bed skilled nursing facility and congregate care center, a home health agency, and a spiritual life center. New refinements include the recent merger of a non-Catholic community hospital into the system, the creation of an Alzheimer's unit, and the extension of pastoral counseling to local nursing homes. Providence is an example of a "multihealth corporation" that has anticipated the aging of the community it serves.

BUILDING BLOCKS: CONSTRUCTING THE CONTINUUM OF CARE

The continuum of care is essentially a set of building blocks for providing health and health-related services to older Americans. The coordinating mechanisms that facilitate the referral of patients across the service spectrum are as important as the services and facilities that make up the continuum. The continuum concept revisualizes the hospital as the hub and focal point of a coordinated service network for the elderly. Alternatively, a social service agency such as San Francisco's On Lok program may provide the point of coordination. Following are the major components of the continuum of care.

Long-Term Care

Long-term or extended health care for older Americans is supported by more than 80 federal programs. These programs directly and indirectly support people with long-term care problems through cash assistance, in-kind transfers, and the provision of services. Federal spending for the elderly climbed 250 percent between 1977 and 1984. Nursing-home care costs for older Americans increased 13 percent annually in that period, but the yearly increases have fallen below 10 percent since 1985 (Figure 5-2).

There will be little change in sources of payment for long-term care in the near to midrange future, even if long-term care insurance begins to sell in quantity. About half of the costs are now privately paid by patients and families, and government expenditures cover most of the rest. Medicaid is the largest long-term care payer, covering 42 percent of the costs. Medicare offers limited nursing home coverage, paying only 2 percent of the costs of long-term care for the elderly. State governments make limited nursing home expenditures, if any. Long-term care insurance is now offered by more than two dozen insurers, but high premiums, eligibility restrictions and limited benefits have dampened en-

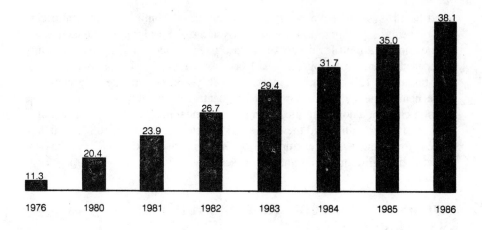

Figure 5-2 Nursing Home Expenditures 1976–1986 (in Billions of Dollars). *Source*: "Trends in Medical Care Costs," *Statistical Bulletin*, Jan-Mar., 1987, p. 5.

rollment. The number of long-term care policies sold to date is disappointingly low.

Although the nursing home population is growing steadily, the growth is due to population increases, not increases in the incidence of ill health. The percentage of people institutionalized in nursing homes is remaining stable as the population ages, according to a study by the National Center for Health Statistics (1987). About one percent of Americans between ages 65–74 are confined to institutions. For those 85 years and older, the number rises to 22 percent. Driven by the growth of the older population, nursing home population grew 50 percent between 1970-80, growing in size from 4 percent of the population to 4.8 in 1980.

That could pale in comparison with future demand for nursing home services. From the National Center for Health Statistics comes the forecast that the nursing home population could grow by more than 75 percent by the turn of century, from 1.3 million in 1980 to 2.3 million in the year 2000 (National Center for Health Statistics 1987). The "oldest old" over age 85 would generate the greatest increase, from 562,000 to 1.2 million nursing home residents in the 20-year period. It is clear that the aging of America is going to have a great impact on nursing homes.

Acute Hospital Care

As Americans age, hospital care becomes a more frequent and more important component of personal health care. As previously noted, 23 percent of males and 17 percent of women age 65–74 were hospitalized yearly, according to the national health survey. For those age 75 and over, about 25 percent of both sexes were hospitalized.

A much greater impact on hospitals is predicted for the future. The number of short-stay hospital days used by the elderly may increase 50 percent from 1980 to the year 2000. The greatest increase would be in hospital days used by those aged 75 and over, almost doubling from 56.1 million days in 1980 to 102.1 million days in the year 2000.

Hospital costs are a substantial share of all health expenditures, especially for the elderly. Hospital expenditures are slowly declining as a percentage of national health expenditures, from 46.0 percent in 1983 to 44.4 percent in 1986. If the trend continues, hospital costs will account for only 40 percent of the health care dollar in the mid-1990s. Two of every three Medicare dollars (65.5 percent) went for hospital services in 1986. Hospital costs for the elderly grew at a rate of 16.2 percent between 1977 and 1984, but the increases fell below double digits in the mid-1980s. Now hospital costs are rising again, from 7.7 percent in 1987 to 9.1 percent for 1988 according to the U.S. Department of Commerce (Francis 1988). With increasing nursing and other wage costs, hospital costs for the elderly could again achieve double-digit increases in the 1990s, unless there is a major shift in federal Medicare policy. Policy makers fear the federal Medicare trust fund may be broke by the late 1990s.

After more than five years of shrinkage in the supply of hospital beds, the United States is beginning to experience bed shortages. This trend is now driven by the aging of the population. U.S. hospitals and health systems will need to build more hospitals and beds in the 1990s. Tomorrow's building boom will focus on two kinds of facilities: (1) small "institutes" (50–100 beds) that specialize in specific diseases and are built as towers of existing hospitals, and (2) "minihospitals" (100–200 beds) in growth areas, with a complementary nursing home and retirement center built on the same campus. As the acuity and complexity of inpatient care rise, med-surg units are becoming intensive care units for older patients in the average hospital. Plan to put at least 50 percent of med-surg beds on telemonitoring or boost staffing levels to cope with sicker patients by the early 1990s.

Ambulatory Care

How will the aging of the population affect the use of health services? Regarding physician services, those over age 65 will visit their doctors over 230 million times per year in the year 2000, up 40 percent from the 165 million visits in 1980, according to the forecast of the National Center for Health Statistics (1987). Only 6 percent of the soaring demand for physician services in the future will be due to a higher use rate; most of the increase will reflect the rapidly growing numbers of the elderly population.

Only 10 to 20 percent of the elderly do not see a physician at least once annually. Most older Americans get their care the old-fashioned way, namely, in the doctors' office; 60.4 percent of visits by those over age 65 to a physician occurred in the office. The hospital is an important source of ambulatory care for the elderly; 12.1 percent were treated in hospital emergency rooms or hospital clinics. Despite the mushrooming growth of urgent-care centers, only 8 percent of the elderly sought treatment there. A surprising 6.8 percent were seen by physicians at home, and another 12.5 percent contacted their doctors by telephone.

The elderly can be divided into three groups of users for ambulatory care: low, intermediate, and high. The average number of annual physician visits recorded in the most recent National Health Interview Survey was between 6.2 and 9.2, depending on age, race, and sex (Koch and Havlik 1987). Health status is a major factor. For those whose health was considered "fair or poor," 10.2–12.9 visits per year were needed. In contrast, those whose health was "good or excellent" needed only 4.1–6.1 visits per year. A small proportion of the elderly are considered high users, with 20 or more physician visits per year. Data from the National Medical Care Utilization Survey show that 3.8–6.7 percent of men over age 55 were high users, as were 7.7–12.5 percent of women in this age group.

What are the most frequent diagnoses of the ambulatory elderly? Chronic ischemic heart disease is ranked first, followed by hypertension, diabetes mellitus, and osteoarthritis. Cataracts are another high-frequency disorder, especially for the oldest old. For those over age 85, cataracts are the fourth largest diagnosis for ambulatory care, with 68 visits per 1,000 (compared with 29 visits for those aged 65–74).

Many ambulatory visits of the elderly result in drug prescriptions. More than 70 percent of those over age 65 seen by a doctor receive at least one prescription drug; 80 percent of those over 75 do so. The most frequently prescribed or provided drugs for persons age 55 and older are diuretics, cardiovascular drugs, and analgesics. Aspirin is also among the top drugs for the elderly. Hydrochlorothiazide, propranolol, digoxin, and triamterene are among the most frequently prescribed generic drugs. Surprisingly, vitamin B12 is still widely prescribed for older Americans.

For the elderly, the shift continues from inpatient to ambulatory care. Since 1983, Medicare has changed more than 200 procedures from inpatient to outpatient. Medicare policies encourage provision of services in free-standing ambulatory facilities. Rising Part B Medicare costs for physician services may force the federal government to impose "ambulatory visit groups" before 1995. Physicians can anticipate national payment standards for all ambulatory care, regardless of whether it is provided in doctors' offices, free-standing centers, or hospital-based programs.

Home Care

In-home health and support services constitute a rapidly expanding component of the continuum of care. Between 1980 and 1985, the number of hospitals having formal home-health programs increased from 12 percent to more than 20 percent, according to a national survey by the AHA (Evashwick, Rundall, and Goldiamond 1985). Home care has expanded at annual rates of 10–15 percent for the past five years, and it will continue to grow at this high level, a national expert panel recently predicted for *Healthcare Forum* magazine (Coile and Grossman 1988).

Home care today is an intensely competitive industry segment with many small providers. Consolidation is already taking place (Anderson 1986), and the trend in the 1990s will be toward regional and national home health firms. There are now five companies with more than 100 local home health operations. Tender Loving Care acquired Staff Builders in 1986, and it now has 140 offices in 26 states. Lifetime Corporation, which is owned by a British holding company, purchased Kimberly Services and now operates more than 100 offices in 32 states. These national firms join Upjohn (300 offices), Medical Personnel Pool (250), and Quality Care (200). National firms will compete for large insurance company accounts, major HMOs and PPOs, and EPAs with major employers.

High-tech services will be increasingly delivered in home settings, including parenteral feeding, antibiotic therapy, and intravenous chemotherapy. AIDS patients are being successfully treated at home for cancers and pneumonia. This is a high-growth market for the future, as medical services and technology are modified for home delivery.

Social factors compound the problems of home care for the elderly. For a growing number of older adults, there is no spouse or companion caregiver. Some older persons will have to be institutionalized who might otherwise have maintained their independence. Holy Cross Hospital of Detroit, Michigan, a member of Franciscan Services Corporation sponsored by the Sisters of St. Francis in Sylvania, Ohio, has developed a caregivers counseling program for the many individuals who are providing care for their aging relatives or friends. A caregivers support group meets monthly at the hospital to make available social and health-related counseling.

Outreach

Many hospitals are developing new programs to reach the senior market. The definition of "seniors" has been broadened to include ages 50–55 in order to reach a broader audience of older Americans who are beginning to experience chronic illnesses.

Aging resource centers combine a consumer health library with information and referral services. Resource centers provide comprehensive collections of information on issues and organizations relevant to health, wellness, care needs, and life style. Centers include books, magazines, films, and videos relating to the health and well-being of older adults, as well as professional journals and books in geriatric medicine. Most aging resource centers are located outside of acute hospital facilities, with some based on and others off the hospital campus. Age Wave of Emeryville, California, has assisted more than 50 hospitals in establishing aging resource centers.

The Planetree program, which pioneered the resource center concept at Pacific Presbyterian Medical Center in San Francisco, was so successful that it has developed a 13-bed "model unit" in the hospital based on an informed consumer philosophy. Staffing of the resource centers by trained librarians provides expert information and referral assistance. The program is now being implanted in half a dozen other hospitals nationally to provide models of consumer-centered care in different types of facilities. Planetree's resource centers are oriented to the broad public and not limited to the elderly. Some resource centers market memberships to physicians, dentists, and other local providers, with annual fees of $100 to $500 in order to subsidize free services to their patients.

Senior membership plans are growing rapidly. St. Francis Hospital of the Daughters of Charity system was a pioneer of the senior membership plan concept. Its Senior Circle program provides assistance in coordinating benefits, which eliminates much of the paperwork burden seniors face when using Medicare. Consultant Peter Yedidia of Geriatric Health Systems estimates that 40 percent of U.S. hospitals now offer the senior plans; more than two-thirds of all hospitals may have senior plans by the early 1990s (Yedidia 1988). Costs to establish and operate the programs range between $15,000 and $100,000, depending on staffing and marketing. Baylor's 55-Plus program has been highly successful, with more than 25,000 members drawn from a multistate region in the Southwest. A key 55-Plus service is physician referral; 25 percent of the 55-Plus members indicated they would like to be connected to a Baylor physician. Most membership plans offer discounts on hospital services, and some waive Medicare deductibles for inpatient care.

As the senior market expands, many hospitals will use outreach programs to effectively bond older consumers to the hospital and its medical staff. When many hospitals have such programs in the future, then more benefits must be added to senior membership plans to keep the plans competitive so they can remain effective as marketing tools. Such benefits might include medical credit cards, preferred VIP treatment, and even bonus plans with health-related premiums for good customers.

Health Promotion and Wellness

A recent survey by the AHA reported more than 60 percent of U.S. hospitals offered some type of elder health promotion program (Longe 1986). Just 3.3 percent of these programs are specifically designed for older adults. Dychtwald and Zitter (1986) identify a continuum of health promotion and wellness programs for seniors: (1) health education classes, (2) self-care instruction, (3) accident prevention, (4) life style education, (5) behavior change programs, (6) peer support groups, (7) emergency medical training, (8) physical fitness and exercise, (9) life enhancement or socialization programs, and (10) spiritual or pastoral counseling.

The reimbursement factor will continue to limit health promotion and wellness efforts until insurers come to recognize their value. Medicare and "medi-gap" insurance policies cover few health promotion services that are not directly related to illness. Blue Shield of California is one of the first insurance plans to offer a personal health management program as an integral part of its medi-gap policy. The Healthtrac program was initiated in January 1988. Developed at Stanford University, Healthtrac is an ongoing health risk assessment and reinforcement program that uses individualized health plans for Blue Shield–covered members (each plan is updated every six months). Participants receive a copy of *Take Care of Yourself*, a 400-page self-health manual, and risk reduction kits tailored to the health plan goals.

Health promotion services are rarely sponsored to earn a profit. Health promotion activities for seniors may function as loss leaders for other services and as feeders for other hospital services. Excellent hospital-based health promotion programs can be established for under $20,000 per year. These programs emphasize self-health instruction and life style education and often use volunteers and medical staff to minimize overhead expenses. Few hospitals have realized profits on substantial capital investments in health clubs and fitness centers. Some hospitals run their health promotion programs through the hospital foundation. Education programs are one of the principal benefits of enrollment in senior health membership plans.

Health promotion activities often include health screening for physical conditions, mental disorders, nutritional problems, and drugs and drug interactions. Some hospitals have found that 25–50 percent of the older persons tested have significant health problems and often require treatment and referral. Costs of special screening programs can run $500 to $2,500 per day, depending on tests administered and whether staff are paid or volunteers. Although most hospitals test at no charge, some tests are chargeable at rates of $35 to $50 per procedure (or possibly charged at a discount). Ongoing screening programs for conditions such as osteoporosis may process 100–150 patients per month at test prices of $25 to $50 per screening. Companies such as ElderMED, a subsidiary of non-profit Unihealth in Chatsworth, California, sell prepackaged health screening programs.

The long-range future of health care will see a shift from acute care to holistic health care. Health care providers need to know more about the biology of aging. Doctors, hospitals, and health systems should educate their staff about the psychosocial needs of their older patients. Under managed care, maintaining high health levels among older Americans will be a contractual as well as a social responsibility. Most hospitals will provide health promotion, wellness, and screening programs to older adults as part of their community service. Senior health promotion programs should be part of an integrated eldercare strategy. As part of a holistic approach, health promotion and screening should be coordinated with ambulatory, acute, and home care services. Senior health membership plans may provide the coordinating nexus for older adults reached through health testing or wellness activities.

Housing and Congregate Care

The housing needs of tomorrow's elders will predictably change in four phases, as illustrated in Table 5-1.

Housing the nation's dependent elderly will require a mosaic of private and public efforts. A growing response to the wave of older Americans is congregate housing with services for the elderly (CHSE). CHSE communities provide an array of health and support services in the context of congregate housing. (These communities are also referred to as continuing care retirement communities [CCRCs].) The CHSE concept is elaborated in *Elderly Housing Options*, by Terrence J. Scott and Robert F. Maziarka (1987), of Elderly Management Corporation, a subsidiary of Consolidated Catholic Health Care in Westchester, Illinois. CHSE communities meet a growing need, and many of the sponsors of these communities are hospitals or health systems. Most of the CHSE communities built or planned involve rent or leases; a few are based on the "life care" concept of meeting total health service needs for an all-inclusive fee.

Demand for life care and retirement housing with services is expected to grow at a dramatic rate. Already, the nation needs 1,800 CHSE communities (there are 600 today) according to Laventhol and Horwath (personal communication 1989). Another 83 communities will be needed in the future for each additional

Table 5-1 Four Phases of Elder Housing Needs

Phase	Age Period	Housing Needs
The empty nest	50–65	Preretirement households sell home; downsize to smaller (2–3 bedroom) house, condo, or apartment; may buy second home; full health, mobility, and independence
The golden years	55–75	Retirement (Phase 1) households based in small house or apartment; may travel (motor home) or split time between first and second home; some chronic health and activity limitations
Dependence	70–90+	Retirement (Phase 2) households may downsize further to condo or apartment; death of spouse triggers move to congregate housing or into home of adult child; may need increasing levels of in-home health and chore services (or a companion)
Institutionalization	85+	Declining health and mobility levels compel move to congregate care facilities, then eventually to intermediate care and nursing homes

million people over age 65. Life care, including CHSE, is a $725 million segment of the health care market and is growing at an annual rate of 15 percent.

Capital will be the key factor in the future development of CHSE communities. In today's market, only 40 percent of the communities are estimated to be profitable, and capital is beginning to dry up. One hospital had its bonds downgraded by Standard and Poor for using part of its funding for a CHSE project. Access to capital will need innovative approaches, such as joint ventures, general limited partnerships, and capital pooling. If private funding slows, the "senior lobby" may push the federal government to expand its role in subsidizing senior housing construction.

Meeting elder housing needs is a strategic market opportunity for diversification and development by hospitals and health systems. CHSE communities can return substantial return on equity plus appreciation, and they can be refinanced or sold over time, yielding additional return. Many communities are joint ventures and require limited capital from their sponsors.

Managed Care

Eldercare could be much affected by the growing popularity of managed care. The outlook for managed care and the continuum of care is still unclear. So far, the elderly have shown only limited interest in signing up with HMOs. HCFA has set a goal of having 20 percent of Medicare beneficiaries enrolled in an HMO or "competitive medical plan" by 1990. To date, Medicare enrollment has been well below expectations; at current enrollment rates, only 10 percent of Medicare enrollees may belong to HMOs by 1990.

HMOs with Medicare contracts are publicly unhappy with rates and restrictions, according to a study by InterStudy that was widely circulated throughout the industry (Baldwin 1987). In response, two dozen Medicare HMO contractors dropped out of the program in 1987; most had few or no enrollees. The well-publicized withdrawal of four Minnesota HMOs from Medicare contracting left more than 25,000 enrollees scrambling for coverage. These events have had a chilling effect on the program. Medicare HMO enrollment will only expand in the near future if payment is increased. Expanding Medicare HMO enrollment to meet HCFA's goal will take a significant boost in rates to draw in new contractors and get existing HMOs to expand their Medicare membership.

Medicare PPOs may help fill the gap and provide a new opportunity for hospitals and health systems. HCFA is experimenting with five Medicare PPOs to determine their popularity, effectiveness, and efficiency. A much broader opportunity exists to restructure medi-gap policies now held by an estimated 80 percent of Medicare beneficiaries. ElderMED, a subsidiary of UniHealth America (formerly HealthWest) in Los Angeles, has recently introduced a Medicare supplemental program with lower premiums than traditional medi-gap policies. Hospitals participate in the PPO program by accepting a negotiated Part A reimbursement, whereas physicians agree to accept the plan benefit as payment in full. The Medicare PPO concept offers a way to "lock in" senior citizens as customers.

Another innovative approach is the "long-term care HMO," such as the plan offered by Group Health Cooperative of Puget Sound in a joint venture with Metropolitan Life Insurance Company. Group Health will provide the services and Metropolitan will price and market the long-term care product to Group Health members age 65–80. In the future the program will be marketed to all members over age 55. Cost will range from $25 to $200 per month, depending on age and coverage. A low-option plan will cover nursing home services, whereas the high-option plan covers a broad range of extended care services.

Over the long term, managed care will dominate the health industry. Medicare beneficiaries may be the most difficult market segment for managed care to penetrate. High costs and utilization levels, coupled with low rates and risk sharing, make the Medicare managed-care market highly risky for providers now. Don't think just of Medicare HMOs. There will be Medicare PPOs and other innovations, like Group Health's long-term care HMO option. This is the time for physicians, hospitals, and health systems with HMOs to explore and pilot Medicare managed-care plans. Most hospitals and many physicians depend on Medicare to provide their "bread and butter." Their market share could dwindle or evaporate as Medicare HMOs channel patients only to a select number of hospitals and doctors. Medicare HMOs are still experimental. Ground rules and reimbursement may be changed in the next one to three years, but ultimately the federal government will seek to shift its responsibility for Medicare to a few exclusive health plans. Get in on the ground floor of this trend, take leadership, and reach for that preferred leadership position in the market consisting of America's most frequent health care customers, the elderly.

Marketing the Continuum of Care

Marketing the continuum of care will be a challenge for physicians, hospitals, and health plans. The multifaceted elder market is actually many minimarkets whose health needs vary by age, sex, household status, and income. The elderly are America's most frequent users of health services. Strategic planning for marketing health services to the elderly must take account of their diverse needs and abilities.

In recognition of the growing significance of the elderly in the health care market, hospitals will create advisory groups and focus groups and place seniors in responsible positions in the health care organization. Far from tokenism, such strategies will assist health providers to stay close to their most important consumers.

Service Line Management

Since the elderly are the most frequent users of health services, hospitals and health systems should refocus services for them using a service line management approach. Baptist Medical Center's Third Age Life Center is a well-developed model that has produced good results in Oklahoma City, and the program is being franchised nationally. Another experiment with this approach by St. Mary's Hospital and Medical Center in San Francisco includes case management; results are modest, but the program is still developmental. Programs that coordinate Medicare benefits, such as Senior Circle, can help provide a more focused market approach. Such programs could be critical for maintaining and expanding Medicare market share.

There are multiple segments of the older population, each with its own demographics, needs, preferences, and health problems. The young elders (age 55–70) are biologically younger, healthier, and may not need as many institutional services they have traditionally used. The frail elders (over age 85) will need higher levels of home health and support services to maintain independence. Many of these home care services are inadequately funded, with the result that wealthier seniors are able to maintain home-based independence whereas poor older adults are often forced into nursing homes if tax-supported home health services are inadequate.

READY, AIM, FIRE AT THE ELDERCARE MARKET

Health care executives agree that the future of health care will largely be a matter of serving older Americans. In a recent survey presented in *Healthcare Forum*, 90.0 percent of a national panel predicted that long-term care would be the next "hot spot" for hospital diversification and health care development (Coile and Grossman 1988). It is much less clear which services the elderly will need and how soon the "future of aging" will arrive. Is the concept of the continuum of care a market strategy or a market myth? Some predictions for the continuum of care are highlighted in Table 5-2.

PROVIDER SKEPTICISM: ELDERCARE "DOESN'T PENCIL"

If so many health care executives and industry experts agree that the elderly will constitute the market of the future, why have so few hospitals and health systems made eldercare a top priority? The answer is more than an issue of timing. When it comes to eldercare, America's hospitals and health systems are asking the following questions:

- If Medicare is becoming a below-cost payer, why expand the Medicare market share?
- If current reimbursement policies (mostly Medicare) favor acute care and do not adequately cover nursing home care or home care, why build or expand these services?
- If only one out of three CCRCs are profitable, why build one unless it will clearly "pencil out" profitably?
- If geriatrics is the field of the future, why are fewer than one thousand physicians specializing in gerontology?
- If the elderly constitute the market of the future, where are the new competitors (innovators) who should be entering the field?

Hard questions are being asked about eldercare. America's hospitals want to know *when* the elderly will constitute a viable market and *which* eldercare programs and services will be profitable in the short term. The short answer is that it's early in the process. The window of opportunity is just opening for the continuum of care for elders. There are few models. It is still a time for innovation and experimentation, risks and early rewards, and the inevitable disappointments and losers. On the product life cycle curve, many of the services on the continuum of eldercare are new (e.g., senior membership programs, adult health day care).

Table 5-2 Continuum of Care Trends Forecast 1988–1990

	Agree[a] (%)	Disagree (%)
1. By 1990 hospitals will shift strategic growth from horizontal (mergers or alliances) to vertical (continuum of care).	82.6	8.7
2. Hospitals will invest millions redeveloping their sites into multilevel continuum of care campuses.	69.1	19.5
3. Hospitals will develop assisted living facilities (congregate care homes) and community retirement centers as capital investment priorities.	62.0	24.0
4. Congregate care retirement centers (CCRCs) will become mini-hospitals for the elderly, with ambulatory care centers, pharmacies, lab and rehab facilities.	74.7	13.4
5. HMOs will use more nursing homes without prior hospitalization to avoid hospital costs.	70.7	15.4
6. Nursing homes will increasingly focus on specialized niches such as Alzheimer's or rehabilitation.	80.0	6.0
7. Many—up to 30%—of Medicare patients will be discharged sooner to nursing homes and assisted living facilities by 1990, reducing Medicare inpatient stays by 1–2 days.	75.4	19.3
8. Hospitals will convert 10% to 20% of their inpatient capacity to "step-down," subacute, long-term "swing" beds and self-care units.	90.0	10.0
9. Small and rural hospitals will reposition by moving down the continuum of care: 25% of rural hospitals will convert totally to long-term care and 40% of rural beds will be "swing" by 1990.	75.3	14.0
10. "Life care" will regain popularity as CCRC developers allow buyers to retain or bequeath acquired real estate equity.	56.0	16.7

[a]Data do not include "no opinion" responses.

Source: Healthcare Forum, Association of Western Hospitals, © March/April 1988.

GERIATRIC VENTURES: WHICH WILL BE PROFITABLE?

In a market assessment of eldercare services, the Health Care Advisory Board in Washington, D.C., rated a variety of geriatric ventures as business propositions (see Table 5-3).

The board's surprising finding was that the most popular geriatric innovations are absolutely not the most profitable (Health Care Advisory Board 1986). Its market research suggests that senior citizen membership packages and close

Table 5-3 General Assessment of Geriatric Ventures as Business Propositions

Geriatric Ventures	Near Term	Long Term
Marketing of current services		
Senior membership programs (e.g., Golden Care PLUS, ElderMed)	A	B
Five star quality geriatric assessment	B+	B+
Image advertising for seniors	C+	B
Marketing promotions, VIP services, and high-visibility PR campaigns	C	C
Vertical integration and networking		
Establishment of Medicare HMO	C+	B+
Joint Venture with existing HMOs to pursue Medicare enrollees	A	A
Establishment of "social" HMO	C	C+
Long-term care lines of business		
Life care	C−	A−
Home health care	C+	C+
Adult day care	C−	C−

Source: "Hospital Strategies for Serving the Geriatric: Survey of Most Profitable Ventures," Health Care Advisory Board, Washington, D.C., 1986.

networking with Medicare HMOs bring a rapid and substantial return on investment. Diversification into life care centers, home health agencies, and adult day care are much more risky and, for the present, far less profitable.

Senior Membership Plans

Although some hospital marketers still believe that senior membership plans are "a lot of fluff" which won't result in "cash-register-ringing sales," they are wrong. Twenty-five of 30 hospitals with senior membership programs report that Medicare admissions improved soon after membership introduction. Programs can be started for $25,000 to $50,000. Larger hospitals have experienced marginal profit contributions of two to seven million dollars. Small hospitals and hospitals late in introducing a senior membership plan have reported less success. The membership package offers the potential of recruiting extraordinary numbers of members for each hospital and at a low cost per member.

Medicare HMOs

Like the rest of the population, seniors are moving toward managed care. Physician loyalty is not assured, as the market success of early Medicare HMOs has demonstrated. It is still early in the product life cycle of Medicare HMOs. Low Medicare HMO reimbursement and ignorance about the market have held profitability down (less than 50 percent of Medicare HMOs were profitable in 1987–1988). Few hospitals are direct sponsors of Medicare HMOs. The costs and risks are perceived to be too great. The Health Care Advisory Board (1986) recommends a "superstrategy" of HMO joint venturing and a senior membership package that provides high-volume business for the hospital and high-quality seniors for the HMO.

Life Care and Continuing Care Retirement Centers

The industry consensus clearly is that in the long run health dollars will move away from acute institutional care toward long-term care and home care. There is an emerging industry trend toward long-term care diversification. Unfortunately, these diversification efforts have been generally unsuccessful and there have been few "winners." Hospital experiences with CCRCs and the concept of life care have been high risk and low profitability. Capital investments of $10 million to $25 million are commonplace; so are annual losses of up to $1 million. The Health Care Advisory Board's strong recommendation is to let other hospitals pioneer the retirement centers and wait until profitablity becomes "more formulaic." CCRCs and life care will be better propositions three to five years out. Another market tactic that requires less capital needs is for hospitals to take over failed CCRCs; bankrupt retirement communities have been sold at auction for as little as 25–35 percent of capital investment.

Home Health

The explosive growth of the home care business is no secret. Between 1980 and 1985, the number of home health agencies rose more than 95 percent, and so did revenues. Proprietary chains expanded nearly 100 percent, but hospitals outpaced them, more than doubling the number of hospital-sponsored home care agencies. Today, the future of home health is much less bullish. Volume has peaked and profitability thinned to slim margins. Experts believe the field has too many competitors. Overbuilt, the market is due for a shakeout. Virtually all competitors have been hurt by tightened Medicare policies and claim denials. HMOs could be a future market, but so far they have been disappointing. Barely 1–3 percent of HMO expenditures are for home care. Worse yet, the discounted rates HMOs demand make it barely worth the effort to win HMO business. The best argument for hospital involvement may be strategic. Aggressive discharge planning is essential in a DRG reimbursement system, and hospitals need their own home care agencies to keep patients "in the loop." Home health opens the door for other potential sales: durable medical equipment, pharmaceutical products, private duty nursing, homemaker services, and supplemental insurance. The Health Care Advisory Board recommends focusing on a niche (e.g., home pharmaceuticals) in order to garner home care profits. The growth opportunities in home care will be in high-tech services, where margins of 15–20 percent are still obtainable.

Adult Day Care

Hospitals which have developed an adult day care program have done so primarily for reasons of "mission" rather than "margin." The programs are loss leaders and obtain limited reimbursement from insurance. Medicare will only pay for adult day care in certified outpatient rehabilitation facilities (CORFs), and few state Medicaid programs provide reimbursement. Staff:patient ratios are high (from 1:2 to 1:4). The elderly are inconsistent in their participation, and turnover is high. Few families or patients can afford fees. Most programs offer sliding scale fee schedules and absorb losses or supplement receipts with grants. Alzheimer's patients are not profitable, the Health Care Advisory Board reports. Industry experts predict that demand for adult day care will increase with the aging of the population, but without changes in insurance policies, this service will need subsidizing for the foreseeable future.

TRANSGENERATIONAL DESIGN

The aging of America is beginning to have an impact on product and facility design. As noted in a recent article in the *Wall Street Journal* ("Difficulty in Caring" 1988), designers are striving to accommodate a wider range of users without stigmatizing products as "geriatric." For example, Cuisinart food processors use oversized paddle controls and large black-and-white graphics to help people with limited dexterity and vision. Hospital doors open with paddles, not doorknobs, in deference to the declining grip strength of the elderly. James J. Pirkl, chairman of the design department at Syracuse University, terms these products "transgenerational" because changes in hearing, vision, and movement take place gradually over a lifetime.

In health care, designers are planning the health facilities of the future for older consumers. Phoenix Memorial Hospital has built a 24-bed inpatient skilled nursing unit especially for older adults. Ken Dychtwald and Mark Zitter (1986) cite three key issues for designers:

1. *Mobility limitations*: More than half the residents of nursing homes use wheelchairs; carpeting is a safety factor; bathrooms should have special design features.
2. *Perceptual changes*: Aging of the eyes makes elders sensitive to glare; there should be increased light levels and visual cues for direction.
3. *Patterns of social interaction*: Older adults need individual seating so they can move to hear others better; soft couches are traps for those with limited mobility; chairs should have arms to aid in rising.

Health facilities, both inpatient and ambulatory, should be designed with consideration given to the special needs of the elderly. Older patients may constitute half or more of the caseload of physicians and hospitals in the 1990s. Likewise, the elderly use more ambulatory services than younger adults. Physicians and hospitals should assess their existing offices and facilities from an eldercare perspective. They should retrofit public and patient care spaces wherever possible and incorporate beneficial design features into new facilities. Subtle but significant design features that aid older patients demonstrate the concern of health providers for their needs.

CONCLUSION

Look around! Silver heads are everywhere, wandering shopping malls with golden credit cards, jogging beaches in designer fitness wear, and pictured on the covers of *Time* and *People*. The most important demographic shift of the 1990s is arriving now. Health care's number one consumers are here—older adults. The growing numbers of older Americans in physician waiting rooms and hospital inpatient censuses illustrate one simple truth: The future of health care lies in the aging of society.

STRATEGIC IMPLICATIONS FOR PHYSICIANS

1. *Payers will shift the focus of eldercare onto nonhospital settings*. Physicians can anticipate that insurance plans and HMOs will increasingly encourage doctors to place their patients in nonhospital alternatives. Unfortunately, many communities lack a number of the standard alternatives for the elderly. Nursing homes are often full, especially those of top quality. Home care reimbursement is limited and not all patients have an adequate home setting or family support. The burden of making the best choice among alternatives is placed squarely on the doctor as insurers and third party payers discourage hospital use.

2. *Clinical information systems will need to be linked.* As patient care broadens out past the physician's office and hospital, better linkages between services and settings is essential for quality patient care. Continuity of service is haphazard today, occurring despite the system. Transfer of information is often due to persistent patients and dogged follow-up by providers. Case management offers some promise as a way of dealing with this often chaotic situation.

3. *Physician computer networks will become essential.* In the electronic age, hospital-physician communication is still done through the telephone and paper documentation. Computer networking would provide much needed electronic linkages, at least between the hospital and doctor and between other hospital-sponsored services and facilities in its mini–continuum of care.

STRATEGIC IMPLICATIONS FOR HOSPITALS

1. *Now is the time to invest in the continuum of care.* Every hospital and health system will own, manage, or control long-term care facilities in the future. Small hospitals will use swing beds, whereas larger hospitals may have extended-care units in house, own their own free-standing nursing home facilities, or have nursing home beds available on contract. Growth in long-term care will be primarily in the niches, such as Alzheimer's, mental health, and congregate housing. Increased private spending will support construction of upscale nursing homes and specialized long-term facilities (e.g., an Alzheimer's unit).

2. *Medicare policy is inadequate for long-term care.* Without changes in Medicare policies or more Medicaid funding, few operators will build nursing homes for low- and moderate-income patients. State regulation and certificate-of-need programs have limited the supply of nursing homes in many states, constraining supply further. Some experts believe nursing home use could increase 10–20 percent if supply constraints were lifted and the construction of new nursing homes and long-term care beds was encouraged.

3. *Buying into home care is a reasonable strategy.* Every hospital should own and control a home health agency. Jointly owned home health consortia will be a future trend. Regional "clusters" of hospitals should consolidate their hospital-based home care agencies into regional home health companies to achieve economies of scale, share staff resources, and provide a broader spectrum of services. Hospitals should also explore joint ventures with for-profit firms. In the future, large home health providers will develop

contractual linkages with regional or national hospital companies as these build continuum of care networks.

4. *Money is likely to be lost on continuum of care services.* The reality for today's hospitals and health systems is that many services on the continuum of care do not "pencil" (i.e., lose money or break even at best). An "ethics-economics" dilemma for hospitals and health systems is that if they acquire nursing homes, they will likely raise service and staffing levels above required minimums, making profitability even more questionable. Until reimbursement policies change so as to take adequate account of nonhospital alternatives, the development of the continuum of care will be dampened.

BIBLIOGRAPHY

American Hospital Association. 1988. "Key Trends through Third Quarter." *Economic Trends* (Winter): (Reported in *Medical Benefits*, March 15, 1988, 1–2.)

Anderson, Howard J. 1986. "Two Recent Home Healthcare Mergers May Signal Industry Consolidation." *Modern Healthcare*, 26 September, 118–20.

Baldwin, Mark F. 1987. "Most Medicare HMOs Unhappy with Program." *Modern Healthcare*, 14 August, 26.

"Blue Shield First to Add Wellness Benefit to Individual Health Plans." 1987. (Press release.) San Francisco: Blue Shield of California, 23 November.

Chollet, Deborah J., and Robert B. Friedland. 1987. "Employee-Paid Retiree Health Insurance." In *The Changing Health Care Market*. Edited by Frank B. McArdle. Washington, D.C.: Employee Benefit Research Institute.

Coile, Russell C., Jr. 1987. "Overview: Environmental Forces and Trends in Long Term Care." In *Managing the Continuum of Care*. Edited by Connie J. Evashwick and Lawrence J. Weiss. Rockville, Md.: Aspen Publishers.

Coile, Russell C., Jr., and Randolph M. Grossman. 1988. "FutureTrack: The Continuum of Care." *Healthcare Forum*, March-April, 52–54.

"Difficulty in Caring for the 'Oldest Old.' " 1988. *Wall Street Journal*, 29 March, 31.

Doty, Pamela, Korbin Liu, and Joshua Wiener. 1985. "An Overview of Long-Term Care." *Health Care Financing Review* 6 (Spring): 69–78.

Dwight, Maria B. 1985. "Affluent Elderly Want to Live Where Quality Care's Available." *Modern Healthcare*, 26 April, 74–76.

Dychtwald, Ken, and Mark Zitter. 1986. *The Role of the Hospital in an Aging Society*. San Francisco: Age Wave.

————. 1988. "Looking Beyond the Myths of Aging America." *Healthcare Financial Management* (February): 40–43.

Estes, Carrol L., Lenore Gerard, and Adele Clarke. 1984. "Women and the Economics of Aging." *International Journal of Health Services* 14(1): 55–67.

Evashwick, Connie, Thomas Rundall, and Betty Goldiamond. 1985. "Hospital Services for Older Adults." *The Gerontologist* 25:631–37.

Evashwick, Connie, and Lawrence Weiss, eds. 1987. *Managing the Continuum of Care*. Rockville, Md.: Aspen Publishers.

Francis, Simon. 1988. "U.S. Industrial Outlook, 1988." (Reported in *Medical Benefits*, 15 February, 1–2).

Graham, Judith. 1987. "Declines in Bed Prices at Nursing Homes Expected by Year-End, Industry Experts Say." *Modern Healthcare*, 22 May, 94–96.

Halpert, Burton P., and Mary K. Zimmerman. 1986. "The Health Status of the 'Old-Old:' A Reconsideration." *Social Scientist Medicine* 22:893–99.

Harel, Zev, Linda Noelker, and Brian F. Blake. 1985. "Comprehensive Services for the Aged: Theoretical and Empirical Perspectives." *The Gerontologist* 25:644–49.

Health Care Advisory Board. 1986. *Hospital Strategies for Serving the Geriatric*. Washington, D.C.: Health Care Advisory Board.

"Hospitals Reserving Nursing Home Beds." 1985. *Modern Healthcare*, 26 April, 68.

Jensen, Joyce. 1986. "Women Pick the Providers Who Treat Their Illnesses, Those of Their Children." *Modern Healthcare*, 9 May, 66–67.

Koch, Hugo, and Richard J. Havlik. 1987. "Use of Health Care–Ambulatory Medical Care." In *Health Statistics on Older Persons: United States, 1986*. Hyattsville, Md.: U.S. Department of Health and Human Services. DHHS Pub. no. PHS 87-1409.

Leutz, Walter. 1986. "Long-Term Care for the Elderly: Public Dreams and Private Realities." *Inquiry* 23 (Summer): 134–40.

Lewis, Mary Ann, Shan Cretin, and Robert L. Kane. 1985. "The Natural History of Nursing Home Patients." *The Gerontologist* 25:382–88.

Longe, Mary E. 1986. "Hospital-Based Community Health Promotion: A Status Report. *Family Community Health* (May): 72–78.

Lubitz, James, and Ronald Prihoda. 1984. "The Use and Costs of Medicare Services in the Last Two Years of Life." *Health Care Financing Review* 5 (Spring): 117–30.

McDonald, Stephen. 1988. "Designs for the Elderly but Not 'Geriatric.' " *Wall Street Journal*, 31 March, 27.

Magill, Judith R., and Janet L. Scheuermann. 1985. " 'Baby Boomers' a Ripe Market for Healthcare Providers: Study." *Modern Healthcare*, 29 March, 128–32.

Manton, Kenneth G. 1985. "Future Patterns of Chronic Disease Incidence, Disability, and Mortality among the Elderly." *New York State Journal of Medicine* (November): 623–33.

National Center for Health Statistics. 1987. *Health Statistics on Older Persons: United States, 1986*. Hyattsville, Md.: U.S. Department of Health and Human Services.

Olshansky, S. Jay, and A. Brian Ault. 1986. "The Fourth Stage of the Epidemiologic Transition: The Age of Delayed Degenerative Diseases." *Health and Society* 64:355–91.

Powills, Suzanne. 1986. "The Elderly: A Health Marketer's Challenge." *Hospitals*, 20 March, 70–74.

Punch, Linda. 1985. "Long-Term Care Industry Develops Alternatives to Meet Needs of Elderly." *Modern Healthcare*, 26 April, 59.

Roos, Noralou P., Evelyn Shapiro, and Leslie L. Roos, Jr. 1984. "Aging and the Demand for Health Services: Which Aged and Whose Demand?" *The Gerontologist* 24:31–36.

Scott, Terrence J., and Robert F. Maziarka. 1987. *Elderly Housing Options*. Chicago: Pluribus Press.

Smallegan, Marian. 1985. "There Was Nothing Else to Do: Needs for Care before Nursing Home Admission." *The Gerontologist* 25:364–69.

Super, Kari E. 1986. "Hospitals Are Beginning to Focus on Services for Older Patients." *Modern Healthcare*, 11 April, 80–82.

"Surgicenter Firm Has Geriatric Care." 1985. *Modern Healthcare*, 29 April, 68.

Tatge, Mark. 1985. "Providers Will Offer Care in New Settings." *Modern Healthcare*, 26 April, 70.

"Trends in Medical Care Costs." 1987. *Statistical Bulletin* (January-March): 2–8.

U.S. Congress. Senate. Special Committee on Aging. 1986. *The Health Status and Health Care Needs of Older Americans*. 99th Cong., 2nd sess., Senate Report 99-200.

Wagner, Lynn. 1987a. "Seattle HMO, Insurer Offer Long-Term Care Option." *Modern Healthcare*, 10 April, 92.

————. 1987b. "Measures to Bolster Nursing Home Quality Considered." *Modern Healthcare*, 14 August, 72–74.

————. 1988. "States Exerting More Control over HMOs." *Modern Healthcare*, 5 February, 22–24.

Waldo, Daniel R., and Helen C. Lazenby. 1984. "Demographic Characteristics and Health Care Use and Expenditures by the Aged in the United States: 1977–1984." *Health Care Financing Review* 6 (Fall): 1–27.

White, Elizabeth C. 1985. "Competition for Healthcare Markets Spurs Race for Demographic Data." *Modern Healthcare*, 27 September, 79–80.

Yedidia, Peter. 1988. "Senior Membership Plans—How to Lock In The Elder Market." *Hospital Entrepreneurs Newsletter* (August): 1–5.

Chapter 6

New Technology

"A new dawn may be upon us," states Dr. Michael Bishop, a leading American cancer researcher. Indeed it is. What is really upon us is the culmination of the greatest revolution in the history of medical and biological science, and it will inevitably bring about more profound changes as this century runs out and the next unfolds. Modern medicine is now holding out greater promise of curing illnesses of many kinds, with many different treatments and technologies, in many parts of the world, in ways once inconceivable.
    —Holcomb B. Noble, *Next: The Coming Era in Medicine*

Technology will reshape medical and hospital care. Inpatient care will be increasingly high-tech and focused on acute and complex patients. Ambulatory care will utilize advanced technology to create new services (e.g., arthroscopic surgery) that compete with inpatient services. The use of high technology in both inpatient and ambulatory care will accelerate dramatically.

The pace of technological change is increasing. Some high-tech devices will have life cycles of only 2–3 years, not 10–15. Despite fears that shrinking reimbursement would have a chilling effect on technological development, physicians and hospitals continue to give technology a high priority. Technology will provide new treatment alternatives for physicians and give hospitals a strategic market advantage in the future. New technologies will arrive at a rapid rate in the next decade of the 1990s.

NEW TECHNOLOGY FOR COMMUNITY HOSPITALS

The diffusion of new technology in health care is moving at a quickening pace. The rate of innovation in the biomedical field is rapid. Deregulation in some states has eliminated certificates of need or raised capital expenditure thresholds. This has meant fewer restrictions on hospital acquisition of new equipment and the development of advanced facilities at some hospitals. In all U.S. health care markets, technology is a major strategic factor in hospital competition. At the same time, technology poses difficult ethical issues for physicians and hospitals, which has led to the widespread development of ethics committees and a higher level of concern for the ethical implications of technology.

Following are the diagnostic, therapeutic, and support technologies that will be state of the art for community hospitals in the next five years.

Diagnostic Technologies

Better diagnostic technologies are shortening lengths of stay and providing more precise diagnoses. The effect is to speed the movement of patients through the health care system and to provide treatment at the most appropriate level of care. Hospitals invested an estimated $2.6 billion on diagnostic imaging equipment in 1986, an increase of 13 percent. Computed tomography (CT) scanners, ultrasound scanners, radiographic and fluoroscopy equipment, and mobile diagnostic equipment constituted four of the top five kinds of hospital equipment purchased, and magnetic resonance imaging (MRI) was number 6 on the list.

Computed Tomography

Conventional CT devices are now widespread in community hospitals. Improvements in CT may increase its diagnostic importance. Three-dimensional computed tomography increases the utility of CT imaging, whereas "cine-CT" provides images at four times the speed of conventional CT. Cine-CT has been deployed more slowly than experts predicted in the mid-1980s. Cine-CT is manufactured by Imatron of San Francisco. Enhancement of CT by 3-D or Cine-CT speed does not create a "new generation CT." Experts consider 3-D CT to be a worthwhile investment for hospitals with active services in the areas of orthopedics, craniofacial surgery, and neurosurgery, whereas cine-CT is recommended for orthopedics, pediatrics, and cardiology.

Doppler Echocardiography (Two-Dimensional)

Newly developed ultrasound instruments that combine two-dimensional imaging with Doppler display of blood flow now allow safe and definitive diagnosis of a number of cardiac problems, such as valvular stenosis and congenital defects. Some models have multicolor flow-mapping displays. A discrete cardiac color flow system costs $150,000 to $175,000 or more. Medicare covers the diagnostic use of this technology but not its use for monitoring. In addition to its uses in the heart, areas of application include study of major vessels such as the carotid and femoral arteries, evaluating organ profusion, and visualizing the vascularity of tumors. The enhanced ultrasound capacity is not a substitute for nuclear cardiology and angiography in cardiac diagnosis, but is rated a worthwhile investment for hospitals that have active cardiology services and are replacing an echocardiographic instrument or acquiring one for the first time.

Low-Osmolality Radiographic Contrast Agents

Here is an example of the cost-benefit tradeoffs that new technologies create for hospitals and physicians. New low-osmolality contrast agents are substantially safer than the standard media used in diagnostic imaging in procedures such as angiography and myelography. These new contrast agents are a notable advance over the current technology but about 15 times more expensive. If all hospitals adopted this as the standard of practice, the Commission on Professional and Hospital Activities in Ann Arbor, Michigan, estimates the cost could be as much as $1.4 billion annually (Shepherd 1988). For a typical 400-bed hospital, the commisssion estimates the annual cost at $657,066. As a result, hospitals are still using the new contrast agents sparingly and have not adopted low-osmolality as the preferred standard.

Magnetic Resonance Imaging

Few devices have had as much impact in diagnostic imaging as MRI. Its cross-sectional images provide diagnosticians with soft tissue contrast without the risk of ionizing radiation. Despite a capital investment cost of $2 million and more, about 600 hospitals and free-standing imaging centers had acquired MRI equipment by the end of 1986. Potentially, at least 50–100 percent as many MRI units could be marketed by 1990. HCFA approved MRI in late 1985 but does not cover "add-on" payments for special services under DRGs. However, most insurers provide coverage for outpatient MRI scans, which has greatly expanded the demand as well as improved financial feasibility. In imaging the central nervous system and in some musculoskeletal applications, MRI is the top-rated diagnostic modality. As for other applications, clinicians are still debating whether MRI is worth the additional cost. A primary benefit of MRI is earlier diagnosis, since MRI makes direct use of information in the body tissues. Three to four years ago it was thought desirable to buy MRI units with high field strengths (1.5–2.0 tesla) to permit MR spectroscopy (MRS) as well as imaging. High-strength units also had better images. However, MRS has been slow to develop, and even higher field strengths (4.0–8.0 tesla) may be needed.

Low-Strength Magnetic Resonance Imaging

Newer MRI units with field strengths as low as 0.02 tesla are now available, with costs ranging from $100,000 to $630,000. Better software provides high-quality images with much lower field strengths. Resonex, a company in Sunnyvale, California, has received FDA approval for an MRI device that does not require shielding. Cost is estimated at $1.2 million to $1.3 million, but installation costs should be significantly lower than the $1 million to $2 million in facilities investment needed for high-power MRI units that require extensive structural reinforcement and shielding. Low-strength MRI units can also be more easily installed in mobile labs.

Superconductivity could make MRI units even simpler and cheaper in the 1990s. There may even be 3-D MRI. It is predicted that in the next three to five years 3-D coronary MRI will achieve the resolution needed to allow noninvasive angiography. The clinical range of MRI applications continues to grow. Lower prices and reduced facility requirements are making MRI a more affordable diagnostic tool. Experts recommend that community hospitals of more than 300 beds should acquire MRI equipment, although financial feasibility is still an issue (Randall 1988).

Mammography

Thanks to active public information campaigns by the American Cancer Society and the American College of Radiology, the use of mammography scanning to prevent and diagnose breast cancer is growing nationally. Ob/gyn clinicians report pressure from insurers to do the tests more frequently and universally. Low-dose mammography is considered a "must" technology for any full-service diagnostic imaging department. In some markets, price-based competition has driven mammography prices below $50 per scan, whereas others charge $125 to $150. Some hospitals have developed profitable free-standing mammography screening centers, but more than one-third of the stand-alone centers have experienced low demand or poor financial results.

Outpatient Cardiac Catheterization

As early clinical studies emerge in support of the safety and efficacy of outpatient cardiac catheterization, use of this technology is predicted to be a future trend (New Technologies 1987). HCFA is reportedly considering making outpatient cardiac catheterization the preferred diagnostic test for Medicare patients. Already some hospitals and physicians are experimenting with mobile cardiac catheterization labs. Growing public attention to cholesterol and its role in heart disease may fuel demand for ambulatory cardiac catheterization services. Consistent with the diffusion of technology in other modalities (e.g., MRI), outpatient cardiac catheterization is likely to be applied to a wider range of cardiology patients, including asymptomatic patients, as a preventive health measure.

Single Photon Emission Computed Tomography (SPECT)

This diagnostic modality is a merging of nuclear medicine and CT technologies. It improves upon conventional planar radionuclide imaging, especially in cardiology and oncology applications. Improvements in radiopharmaceuticals will enhance SPECT further. For example, SPECTamine is a new brain imaging agent for stroke diagnosis. Medi-Physics, of Richmond, California, claims its product can accurately assess poststroke brain impairment within 48 hours of symptoms—before damage can be visualized by conventional CT scanning. Saint Agnes Medical Center in Fresno, California, was one of the first SPECT sites. At Saint Agnes, clinicians are experimentally using SPECT to differentiate Alzheimer's disease and to detect stress fractures in the spine that are too small to be discovered by CT or MRI. It is still too early to predict the impact of SPECT on competing imaging technologies. As an add-on, SPECT capability will cost $50,000 to $100,000. A complete system is estimated to cost from $165,000 to $285,000. Experts suggest that hospitals that are currently acquiring a gamma camera or nuclear medicine computer should consider only models that can be upgraded with SPECT in the future.

Tumor Markers

New tests for tumor markers based on advances in monoclonal antibody production offer the promise of improved effectiveness in cancer diagnosis. Current tumor markers include oncofetal proteins, hormones, enzymes, and metabolites, but most are not tumor-specific. OncoTrac is an example of the new generation of tumor markers based on monoclonal technology. The manufacturer, NeoRx Corporation, of Seattle, is seeking FDA approval for OncoTrac, which it claims will turn a metastatic melanoma anywhere in the body. Experts predict that by 1990 tumor markers will account for 7 percent of all markers used in vitro diagnostic testing (New Technologies 1987). Many community hospitals will be adding tests for tumor markers to the range of their laboratory diagnostic services.

Ultrasound

Although hardly a new technology, many other developments besides two-dimensional Doppler echocardiography are expanding the range and utility of ultrasound. Intraoperative and neonatal ultrasound have become more common. Endoscanning, which combines ultrasound with endoscopy, is rapidly developing. Ultrasound is being utilized in new methods for studying the heart, such as transesophageal echocardiography. Handheld "ultrasound stethoscopes" cost $9,000 but can provide diagnostic information on recent cardiac patients more quickly than portable ultrasound units. Computed ultrasonography, which uses microcomputer simulations of digitized data, has potential as well. For example,

Acuson Corporation, of Mountain View, California, provides, for about $130,000, a computed sonography unit that displays full-color images of blood flow.

Therapeutic Technologies

Advanced theraputic technologies and equipment assist community hospitals to provide the best quality of care. Among the most important of the new therapies and technologies for community hospitals are the following.

Balloon Angioplasty

Cardiac bypass surgery is rapidly being replaced by balloon angioplasty as the first-choice treatment for blockages of cardiac vessels. Bypass surgery thus becomes the backup treatment when angioplasty is unsuccessful.

Balloon angioplasty opens vascular strictures by inflating a tiny balloon within the vessel. Percutaneous transluminal angioplasty is the most frequently performed application of this technology. Percutaneous coronary transluminal angioplasty (PCTA) of renal and peripheral arteries is also gaining popularity, and all hospitals that perform conventional vascular surgery should also offer PCTA. PCTA is now an accepted therapy for multivessel heart disease in some patients.

Originally conceived as an alternative to coronary artery bypass graft (CABG) surgery, PCTA is now used in some patients who are not considered suitable candidates for surgery. Even with new developments in the use of laser angioplasty for cardiac surgery, experts believe that laser angioplasty will be added to PCTA and CABG, not replace either therapeutic approach ("Laser Angioplasty" 1987). Balloon angioplasty's minimal trauma and ease of application would allow some hospitals to offer PCTA that are not currently doing bypass surgery. It is even possible there may be ambulatory use of PCTA at some time in the future. Cardiac care experts insist that at present PCTA should be done only where an open-heart surgery team is immediately available in case emergency surgery is needed (New Technologies 1987).

Continuous Arteriovenous Hemofiltration (CAVH)

CAVH is used as an alternative or complement to conventional hemodialysis in treatment of acute renal failure and severe fluid overload. Unlike conventional dialysis, CAVH is continuous and does not require dedicated machinery or specially trained personnel. CAVH is not extremely efficient, but it is a short-term therapy that many hospitals with dialysis units may wish to offer.

Cochlear Implants

Because 60,000 to 200,000 patients in the United States could benefit from this therapy, hospitals with otolaryngology services may wish to make this technology available to their patients. Cochlear implants are multichannel and are a substantial improvement over single-channel devices for the profoundly deaf. The multichannel implant will not benefit all patients, nor is the single-channel implant as yet considered obsolete. The auditory nervous systems of some patients are in such a condition that multichannel devices would not work effectively. Hearing loss is a widespread phenomenon; by some estimates, 25–40 percent of older Americans have at least some hearing disability.

Gallstone Pump

One new technology for gallstone therapy is a nonsurgical procedure involving a gallstone pump. After a solvent, methyl tert-butyl ether, dissolves the stones, a computer-controlled pump flushes the gallbladder. The new pump represents a significant advance over previous techniques, which used hand pumps. The procedure requires only local anesthesia. The prevalence of gallstones increases with age (about 10 percent of the older population). Nearly 500,000 gallstone procedures are performed each year.

Lasers

A number of community hospitals are now considering developing a full-spectrum laser center that offers all laser modalities currently available, including the CO_2, argon, krypton, and neodymium:yttrium-aluminum-garnet (Nd:YAG) types. Medical lasers are proving beneficial in a wide range of therapeutic applications. It is estimated that 85 percent of all ophthalmologists are performing procedures with lasers. Every hospital should have at least one (if not two or three) of the laser modalities. New kinds of lasers include the free-electron laser, various dye lasers, and the excimer laser, which is being used experimentally to sculpt the cornea to correct myopia. One type of new laser has been approved for destruction of stones in the urinary tract, and another for eye procedures such as photocoagulation. Laser angioplasty is a significant extension of laser technology. "Closed lasers" that transmit argon laser energy through a metal cap on the end of a catheter are being experimentally used to unblock coronary arteries. "Laser stitches" are being used to close surgical wounds and may become commonplace in surgery.

Lithotripsy

Extracorporeal shock wave lithotripsy has demonstrated its effectiveness in the treatment of kidney and ureteral stones. Lithotripsy has substantially replaced conventional surgery for removal of stones in the kidney and ureter. It is essentially noninvasive, requires a short hospital stay or none at all, and is less costly than conventional surgery. With new developments in endoscopic ureterolithotripsy and laser lithotripsy for stones further down the urinary tract, percutaneous lithotripsy has become less important. The "second-generation" lithotripter made its way to the market in 1987 with the FDA's approval of Dornier's HM-4 model; this lowered the acquisition price of a lithotripter to about $1.5 million. As other manufacturers bring competing second-generation lithotripters to market, there is some concern that market saturation might occur until medicine discovers additional applications of lithotripsy. Dornier is engaged in clinically testing the effectiveness of its original water bath lithotripter (HM-3) on common bile duct stones.

Streptokinase Thrombolysis versus tPA

Controversy continues over whether streptokinase or the genetically engineered tissue-type plasminogen activator (tPA) is the therapy of choice for dissolving coronary arterial clots. Early studies showed streptokinase to be less effective than tPA, but cost has made this a controversial choice ("Quick tPA Approval" 1987). Streptokinase costs $180 per treatment versus $2,200 for Genentech's tPA. The problem is that tPA is not covered by private insurance or Medicare. Neither the federal government nor insurers have been willing to pay for tPA as a separate procedure, leaving patients the choice of paying out-of-pocket or providers the choice of supplying the procedure as a community service. To offset criticism, Genentech has recently offered to provide tPA at no cost to any patient who could not afford the treatment. The federal government is allowing Genentech to write off half the cost of the donated drugs.

Support Technologies

Information Systems

Integration is the current challenge for vendors of health care information. The goal is to allow data to flow freely from the lab to the finance department, for example—and with speed and flexibility. Information systems constitute a complex and rapidly developing sector of technology, and only brief mention will be made in this chapter of the relationships between information systems and other technologies.

Advances in local area networks promise to assist hospitals that have installed subsystems (e.g., a lab subsystem) incompatible with subsystems from other vendors. In 1987, 10 percent of U.S. hospitals significantly upgraded their information systems, most frequently the cost accounting system.

New ways of recording information about patients also bear watching. These include expanded applications of bar coding, the use of voice recognition technology for dictating reports, and the development of "smart cards" and "laser cards'' that allow patients to carry their personal medical records with them. Optical disks to store digitized information are likely to become important in medical records by the early 1990s, advancing the day of the "paperless" hospital. Information systems are becoming highly decentralized, and are being organized around system-specific nodes in the lab, x-ray unit, and other specialized areas. Personal microcomputers are predicted to achieve a tenfold increase in power and a fourfold decrease in computing cost within five years. Physician computer networks pioneered by Magliaro and McHaney, of San Diego, and Baxter Healthcare in Borgess Medical Center in Kalamazoo, Michigan, and St. Joseph's in Phoenix are linking hospitals to physician offices in more than a dozen communities. Computer networking helps channel patients to the hospital and enhances the practices of network physicians.

Home Care Technologies

A broad array of techniques and devices are migrating into home settings. Many hospitals with home health programs are offering high-tech services to their posthospitalization clients. AIDS has been a driving force in home care innovation. Cancers and pneumonias are now routinely treated with home chemotherapy and portable infusion therapy. Indwelling catheters allow home administration of hyperalimentation formulas and antibiotics. Improvements in technology enhances home care for ventilator-dependent patients, shortening hospital stays and speeding discharge to home care, assisted living facilities, or nursing homes. Home apnea monitoring will facilitate safer posthospital care for infants treated in newborn intensive care units.

Personal Emergency Response Systems

Medical alert systems such as Lifeline respond to the feelings of insecurity and dependency experienced by the chronically ill. A future generation of personal emergency response systems may be available in the 1990s, based on implantable biosensors now being tested in Europe and Japan.

NEW TECHNOLOGIES FOR TERTIARY CARE FACILITIES

America's academic medical centers, teaching hospitals, and regional medical centers are becoming citadels of advanced technology. Competition is driving tertiary care centers into increasingly specialized technology niches. With the diffusion of technology and trained medical specialists, community hospitals can enter fields like cardiac bypass surgery in states without certificate-of-need controls. Competition is spreading to ambulatory care with the development of very large "superclinics," such as Salick Corporations's 50,000-square-foot ambulatory cancer centers affiliated with major medical centers like Cedars-Sinai in Los Angeles.

Here are some emerging technologies that are now being tested in tertiary level facilities.

Diagnostic Technologies

Chorionic Villus Sampling (CVS)

CVS is a promising replacement for amniocentesis for prenatal diagnosis. Experts recommend that hospitals with large full-service obstetrics programs should add CVS. The only problem with the use of CVS is the undesired side effect of induced abortion experienced by a small number of patients. Hospitals may also wish to add flow cytometry to their programs, an existing technology recently applied to diagnosing fetal abnormalities.

Digital Subtraction Angiography

This technique failed to live up to its early promise, but it appears more successful with recently developed intra-arterial techniques. Hospitals with a substantial volume of noncardiac angiography and high volumes of diagnostic cardiology and heart surgery may wish to add this technology in order to broaden the diagnostic alternatives and relieve pressure on conventional angiography facilities.

High-Speed Cine-CT

Hospitals that want to provide state-of-the-technology cardiac diagnosis are closely watching the development of cine-computed tomography. The high-speed cine-CT system developed by Imatron of San Francisco costs $1.6 million and has been acquired by only a handful of medical centers to date. Some experts believe that applications of MRI in dynamic studies of the heart may supplant cine-CT in the future. In the short-term, ultrasound will provide sufficient diagnostic information for most cardiac centers, and experts do not recommend acquisition of cine-CT or MRI cardiac diagnosis at this time.

Therapeutic Technologies

Extracorporeal Membrane Oxygenation (EMCO)

EMCO treatment for respiratory failure is a high-risk procedure used in the case of newborns who might not otherwise survive. The risk of long-term neurological impairment for EMCO-treated patients suggests this technology is appropriate only in specialty children's hospitals and other hospitals with large neonatology programs.

Gallstone Lithotripsy

A new instrument, the biliary lithotripter, has recently become available from Dornier, the market leader in lithotripsy. Other alternatives to open surgery for gallstones are becoming widely used, including basket extraction after endoscopic sphincterotomy. Chemotherapy is being applied to gallstone therapy, and laser therapy for gallstones is under investigation.

Hyperthermia for Tumor Treatment

Hyperthermia, as an adjunct to radiation therapy, has become increasingly successful in destroying superficial tumors. Experts suggest that hospitals with comprehensive cancer programs should consider purchasing hyperthermia devices.

Implantable Cardioverter/Defibrillator

Automatic implantable cardioverter/defibrillators (AICDs) are demonstrating their effectiveness against arrhythmias. Since FDA approval in 1985, the devices have been implanted in several thousand patients. The device costs about $13,000 (this does not include the cost of implantation). About the size of a deck of playing cards, the implantable defibrillator autonomously responds to arrhythmias, pulsing electric charges to restore normal heart patterns.

Percutaneous Automated Diskectomy

Percutaneous automated diskectomy is a relatively simple method of removing herniated disks and can be done as a same-day surgery procedure under local anesthesia. The procedure is done using a small tube called a nucleotome. Percutaneous automated diskectomy is an alternative to chemonucleolysis (now falling into medical disfavor) and is less traumatic than laminectomy, an inpatient procedure. The cost of the equipment, which is available from Surgical Dynamics, of San Leandro, California, is $10,000.

Photoradiation Therapy (Photochemotherapy)

Photoradiation therapy, also known as photochemotherapy, combines laser light and a phototoxic drug to combat early-stage lung cancer and localized tumors in sites such as the urinary bladder, eye, esophagus, skin, and stomach.

Support Technologies

Electronic Imaging Transmission (Teleradiology)

Electronic transmission of images between facilities by standard telephone lines, microwave, or satellite radio communication is now a reality. The Mayo Clinic's satellite facilities in Florida and Arizona now utilize teleradiology routinely for clinical consultations from Rochester. Large imaging departments should now be planning image transmission between facilities by teleradiology.

Digital Image Management Systems and Optical Disk Storage

In a small but growing number of diagnostic imaging departments, "electronic images" are archived on optical disks instead of taking photos of images on cathode-ray tubes (CRTs) and archiving in traditional film storage. Some radiologists believe that the quality of CRT images is not yet sufficient for definitive diagnoses, but the availability of new 1,024-line CRTs should alleviate this concern. Large imaging departments should plan for availability, by 1995, of truly comprehensive picture archiving and communications systems (PACSs) or digital image management systems (DIMSs).

Bedside Computer Terminals

Tomorrow's nursing stations will be wherever nurses, with their pocket and bedside computers, are working. Decentralized hospital information systems that put electronic work stations at the bedside are now a market reality. Bedside computing reduces nurse charting time by as much as 30 minutes per nurse per shift. Health Data Systems, of San Bernadino, California, has developed the "Ulticare" system, which was pilot-tested at Michigan's William Beaumont Hospital and is now installed in a handful of other U.S. facilities.

CONTROVERSIAL TECHNOLOGIES

At the edge of technological innovation are a number of procedures and devices that are still being tested by medicine or have failed to meet expectations for efficacy or safety. Among these technologies are the following.

Positron Emission Tomography (PET)

Lack of insurance coverage for PET is only one of a number of limitations. PET shows real promise, especially for brain metabolism studies. The cyclotron technology is still underdeveloped, few clinical trials have been undertaken to assess PET's impact on patient care outcomes, and its chemical orientation may be difficult for physicians. PET is still an emerging technology.

Chemonucleolysis

Once considered a nonsurgical alternative to laminectomy for treatment of herniated lumbar disks, chemonucleolysis is now the subject of growing medical doubts regarding its clinical efficacy and safety. The therapy, which involves the injection of the enzyme chymopapain into the herniated disk, is now being abandoned by some physicians in favor of surgery. Indeed, percutaneous automated diskectomy may be a safer, more effective therapy than either chemonucleolysis or laminectomy. Some payers are reclassifying chemonucleolysis as an obsolete procedure (e.g., Blue Shield of California has withdrawn chemonucleolysis from its list of approved procedures).

Gastric Bubble

Hospitals are advised to use with caution the Garren-Edwards gastric bubble for treatment of the morbidly obese. Reports in the clinical literature indicate a higher rate of complications than originally anticipated.

In Vitro Fertilization

There are a growing number of techniques for treatment of infertility. At this early stage, safety has not been a significant problem, but the procedure is associated with low-weight births and a higher rate of complications for mother and children. A number of ethical issues have been raised about the concept of artificial fertilization and surrogate parenting (Taylor 1986). Many issues have yet to be clarified by new laws or by the courts, and controversy can be expected by hospitals initiating in vitro fertilization programs.

Percutaneous Nephrolithotripsy

With the development of extracorporeal shock wave lithotripsy, the use of percutaneous nephrolithotripsy as a stand-alone treatment for kidney stones is forecasted to decline rapidly. However, it will continue to have a place in the treatment portfolio of urologists as an adjunct therapy.

PLANNING CONSIDERATIONS FOR NEW TECHNOLOGY

For America's doctors, hospitals, and health systems, the challenge is to continue to provide medical care of the highest standard while maintaining a commitment to public service. Physicians and hospitals must protect resources for both technology investment and charitable care. Some high-tech services will be "cash cows" that generate profits—profits that can be used to subsidize other services. Hospitals must keep pace with technology in order not to be considered second-rate by physicians and the public. Finally, where state Medicaid programs are unable or unwilling to provide the poor with access to advanced technology, providers with a social conscience may be the only source of high-tech services.

Following are important planning considerations for new technology.

Technology Acquisition Process

Technology investments will be among the most important strategic decisions that doctors, hospitals, and health systems will make in the near and midrange future. Choices of technology focus ("niches") will shape health systems and their institutions for years ahead. The technology bazaar, with its competing products and systems, can seem overwhelming to the average physician or hospital executive. The technology acquisition process needs careful planning, medical participation, and tough-minded management. Take charge of the process and make sure the terms and conditions are set by the system or institution, not by the vendor.

Technology Forecasting

To maintain quality care and a competitive market position, hospitals and multihospital systems should maintain continuing awareness of new technologies. Technology forecasting is an extension of environmental monitoring. Multihospital systems should identify the clinical areas in which its member hospitals have a special interest. Technology forecasting can focus on member hospitals' centers of excellence, development plans, and diversification projects. The process of technology forecasting can be facilitated by hiring a full- or part-time chief technology officer (CTO) and by establishing technology planning committees. Technology forecasting should have a five- to ten-year time horizon.

Chief Technology Officer

Hospitals and multihospital systems may need a CTO. Hiring a CTO is recommended by Richard Foster, McKinsey and Company's managing director for technology and author of *Innovation: The Attacker's Advantage* (Foster 1986). The CTO's role is to coordinate and manage the organization's technology investment. Note, however, that few U.S. health care companies have a CTO,

at least not at high corporate levels. Only in industries driven by rapid technological change, such as computers and pharmaceuticals, is the position of CTO
or senior scientist given high management credibility.

In a multihospital corporation, the CTO would be responsible for activities
such as

- planning capital for technology acquisition (five to ten years) at system level
- budgeting capital for technology acquisition (three to five years) at system
  level
- acting as a control point for the system's capital pool for new technology
  and facilities
- maintaining technological awareness so as to identify emerging technologies
- tracking government and payers reimbursement policies for new technologies and acting as an advocate
- monitoring legislative and regulatory processes and acting as an advocate
  in legislation
- controlling regionalization of technology by local hospital units
- acting as a consultant to local hospitals on technology acquisition
- convening scientific and expert panels for technology assessment
- preparing and disseminating assessment reports on emerging technologies
  to system hospitals and physicians
- identifying obsolete technologies and medical procedures and planning their
  phaseout

Technology Assessment and Planning Committees

To identify and assess emerging technologies, multihospital systems and regional medical centers can establish expert panels to forecast tomorrow's state
of the art. The purpose of these committees is to identify opportunities for
technology acquisitions that would add new treatments or upgrade existing services and equipment. The planning focus is on the clinical centers of excellence
and the regional medical facilities. There are several alternatives for structuring
technology assessment and planning committees:

- a system-level technology planning committee to coordinate technology
  investment across the system
- specialty committees organized by centers of excellence
- clinical department committees for technology scanning and assessment

- ad hoc technology committees comprised of expert physicians drawn from across all medical specialties

The output of technology assessment committees consists of recommendations given to management and the board on technology planning and budgeting. Such recommendations can be enhanced by outside reviewers from biomedicine, bioengineering, and biotechnology (including experts from universities, academic medical centers, and biotechnology R & D organizations). Vendors are also an excellent source of information and consultation; despite their obvious biases, vendors know the technology.

Acquisition Process

Equipment consultants have a number of recommendations for managing the technology investment process to minimize risks to the buyer, including these:

- Make certain that maintenance costs are part of the vendor proposal.
- Include performance and documentation requirements in purchase negotiations.
- Define responsibilities for service.
- Ensure that contract policies give the purchaser the right to acquire equipment upgrades on favorable terms.
- Budget for anticipated enhancements.
- Ensure continued access to operational software or maintenance through an ownership agreement or escrow account.

ETHICAL, REIMBURSEMENT, AND LEGAL CONCERNS

Planning and acquiring new technology involves a complex set of ethical, financial, professional, legal, and tax issues.

Ethics

The field of bioethics is now well established. A number of nonprofit multi-hospital systems, such as the SSM (Sisters of the Sorrowful Mother) Health Care System in St. Louis, have professional ethicists employed in corporate offices or located in major institutions within the system. Ethical implications of emerging technologies should be assessed in tandem with clinical and market issues.

Technology raises two sets of ethical issues: (1) moral issues regarding technologies such as artificial fertility, genetic engineering, as well as life support; and (2) social equity issues regarding the accessibility of new technology to the poor. An underlying issue is the "technological imperative"—whether technology should be applied just because it is available. Some uses of technology are being justified as "expedient," such as transplantation of organs from anencephalic children or treatment of Parkinson's disease with fetal brain tissue. These uses raise concerns about technology's impact on the quality of life. Ethical issues also come to the fore when advanced technology is applied—or denied—to the terminally ill.

Reimbursement Policies

Reimbursement is a primary factor in the acceptance of health care technology. As long as payers consider a new technology "experimental," their refusal to pay for it means that only a few patients will have access to it—through clinical trials or by purchasing the treatment out of pocket. FDA approval is not enough. Major payers—insurance companies, government, and large employers—utilize expert scientific panels to judge when a technology is no longer experimental, has been shown to be safe and effective, and should be reimbursed when specified conditions are met. Industry newsletters such as the *Blue Sheet* and *Medical Technology Stock Letter* keep their subscribers continuously informed of the status of reimbursement for new technologies. Multihospital systems should maintain a continuing awareness of reimbursement policies regarding new technologies and pharmaceuticals and keep all their facilities informed.

Professional Standards

Professional standards are a powerful force in the diffusion of new technologies. Professional societies of physicians, nurses, and other health professionals define the "state of the practice" in their fields of practice. Their decisions to accept or reject a new technology are given great weight by payers and regulators—and by the courts. The Joint Commission on Accreditation of Healthcare Organizations (Joint Commission) is beginning to define hospital quality standards that may be technology-specific. The power of professional bodies to define "minimum technology levels" is increasing. For example, the American Society of Anesthesiologists (ASA) and the Harvard teaching hospitals recently set standards for operating room monitoring devices. The standards affirm the need for oxygen analyzers and ventilator "disconnect alarms," which are already in wide use. The new standards also recommend monitoring the CO_2 level of expired gas, as well as the use of pulse oximeters, computerized EEG, transcutaneous O_2 and CO_2 monitoring, and multiagent analyzers, including mass spectrometers and newer infrared monitors. Similiarly, high levels of monitoring are recommended for postsurgical recovery areas. Hospitals will not necessarily purchase all the recommended equipment, which ranges in price from $3,500 to $18,000, but they should expect that attorneys pressing liability actions will cite the ASA's recommendations as the "standard of care."

Legal Considerations

The primary area of concern from a legal perspective is hospital-physician joint ventures involving technology acquisition. Medicare reform in 1987 added new rules against physician inurement that more precisely define the boundaries and penalties for physician conflicts of interest. Federal tax reform legislation redefined treatment of losses from passive investments in limited partnerships, which has had the primary effect of making more hospital-physician ventures rely on financial feasibility, not tax advantages. Since these legislative changes, hospitals have found ways to reduce legal exposure on joint ventures while continuing to pursue them. If Congress believes that physicians are exploiting the current tax and regulatory policies in their own interest, substantial restrictions on physician participation in technology ventures may be enacted in the next three years.

Tax-Exempt Status

The ability of hospitals to acquire new technology may be curtailed if nonprofit facilities lose their tax-exempt status. The immediate threat is at the state and local level, where governments are hard pressed for new revenues. Utah has already enacted a statutory requirement that hospitals demonstrate their level of community (charitable) care before their local tax exemption is renewed. Two of InterMountain Health System's facilities in Utah were denied their exemption by local tax authorities. A number of other states are looking at the Utah statute. At the local level, a half dozen cities have enacted or are considering enacting local ordinances stripping hospitals of their property-tax exemption. In Pittsburgh, the university hospital donated $1 million to local officials as a trade-off for deferring such legislation. At the national level, Congress is considering legislation to reduce or eliminate hospital access to tax-exempt bonds. This would have a major chilling effect on technology acquisition by U.S. hospitals and could drive some community hospitals to shift to for-profit status.

CAPITAL FORMATION STRATEGIES

In today's reimbursement climate, it is increasingly difficult to fund capital equipment and facilities out of operational surpluses. For the future, physicians, hospitals, and health systems need to broaden their use of innovative capital formation strategies to fund technology investments.

Structuring Joint Ventures with Physicians

The most common, and most successful, hospital-physician joint ventures to date have been in diagnostic imaging. Ambulatory surgery centers are the second-most successful projects. Other popular joint ventures have included ambulatory care facilities, reference laboratories, medical office buildings, health promotion and wellness centers, medical hotels, and CCRCs. Not all have been "winners." Ambulatory care centers, health promotion centers, medical hotels, and CCRCs have proved to be high risk.

Ownership and control patterns in joint ventures are shifting away from percentage of investment to 50-50 shared control. Increasing physician control of ventures is intended to promote physician investment and commitment. The 50-50 trend signals a new era in hospital-physician relationships, a trend toward shared power outside the traditional hospital organization. In the past, the typical hospital has been unwilling to give up power to physicians at the board level. These new "parallel corporations," as Dr. Steve Shortell, of Northwestern University, calls them, provide an opportunity to redefine hospital-physician relationships outside of the relatively inflexible medical staff bylaws (Shortell 1986).

Innovative Financing

To acquire new technology, hospitals and multihospital systems are developing creative financing alternatives. For example, hospitals that purchase very new technology can negotiate reduced prices with vendors by acting as "beta sites" for evaluation and testing of new devices. A new wave of hospital-physician joint ventures are just being organized, and these may provide new models for capital formation. New organizations are being developed that will go beyond one project at a time, and hospitals and physicians are creating new out-of-hospital corporations that will own and manage a variety of joint ventures. In a variation of this theme, a southern California hospital in Torrance, California, has initiated a venture capital pool that is funded by the hospital and physician investors. The venture capital pool will be used to capitalize a variety of health-related ventures.

The "Torrance model" is being widely watched as a prototype for more advanced forms of hospital-physician collaboration in creative financing.

CONCLUSION: THE PROMISE OF TECHNOLOGY

New technology will reshape health care in the decade ahead. Improved diagnostics will pinpoint diagnoses earlier in the disease process. New therapeutics will deliver drugs directly to the cellular site. Pneumonias and other serious diseases will be treated with high-tech home care. Implanted biosensors will monitor the chronically ill, and implanted drug dispensing devices will provide precise dosages directed by an implanted computer chip. Computerized medicine will improve medical care with artificial intelligence, and computers at the bedside will automatically guide patient care. Patients and supplies will be transported by robots.

Yet the promise of technology is clouded by issues of ethics and economics. Will the poor have equal access to medical advances? Should the old have the benefit of heart transplants or high-cost superdrugs like tPA? Is competition among hospitals and physicians over specialized technology socially wasteful? How will humanistic concepts of the respect for human life be factored into genetic engineering and gene therapy? How will socially committed physicians and hospitals continue to make new technology available to the poor and the medically uninsured?

Physicians and their hospitals need to manage the technology acquisition process so as to gain optimal benefit from technological investment. New technologies will be expensive. Given limited capital resources, health care executives and multihospital systems need to know which technologies should be considered state of the art for the community hospital and which are as yet more appropriate for tertiary medical centers. Physician support is essential in technology planning. With so many new technologies emerging, hospitals and doctors need information on which controversial new techniques and tools are being proved worthy and which are not likely to gain medical (or payer) acceptance.

STRATEGIC IMPLICATIONS FOR PHYSICIANS

1. *Scan continuously for new technology.* Every medical staff should establish a technology scanning committee that meets at least four to six times per year to assess new technologies that might be acquired by the hospital (or by competitors). Providing technology assessments would be a highly valuable service. For major medical centers that are part of multihospital sys-

tems, information from the technology scanning process could be used systemwide and disseminated to other system facilities.

2. *Formalize regional referral relationships*. Transform informal medical referral patterns into hub-and-spoke regional networks with formal clinical protocols for patient transfer. To ease the fears of local hospitals and clinicians about losing patients, tertiary care centers should formalize commitments to return patients to local providers with appropriate aftercare protocols.

3. *Hospitals will compete for physician commitment with technology*. Hospitals will use technology as a strategy to market their services to physicians. Marketing the hospital's high-tech capabilities to the medical community (both to the medical staff and to community physicians who are referral sources) will be an increasingly popular strategy. As new technology is introduced, many community hospitals are moving aggressively to acquire new devices before competitors. Community hospitals are moving up the "technology pyramid" to acquire more sophisticated technologies that are magnets for physicians. These high-tech services capture the public's imagination as well, and they build up the hospital's market reputation as a state-of-the-art facility.

4. *Regionalize technology sharing*. Physicians should work to end the "medical arms race" between hospitals. This involves voluntarily regionalizing and rationalizing investments in advanced health technology among health facilities that share the same medical market area. Pooling capital equipment funds and centrally managing technology investment are fairly common among multihospital systems. Physicians and hospitals can collaboratively build capacity in selected specialties that will attract patients to their community, and they can also create regional networks by affiliating smaller facilities with specialized centers (e.g., cardiac surgery, oncology, and rehabilitation).

5. *Ethics committees will engage challenging issues*. Ethics committees of medical staff should be used to scan and provide early identification of ethical concerns arising from new technologies and to recommend hospital policies. Such committees can serve as forums for illuminating the ethical dimensions of technology-related issues. Medical leadership should play a key role in ethics committees at the hospital board level. Where possible, multihospital systems should employ medical ethicists or consultants to support the work of the ethics committees and to continuously monitor new technology for ethical concerns.

6. *Hospitals will build centers of excellence around key medical staff*. Physicians are central to plans regarding technological capacity. Equipment and expertise go hand in hand. Advanced medical institutions must have high-skill medical specialists in the clinical specialities that have been

targeted for major technological investment. Top-rated physicians will be the magnets used by hospitals to construct high-tech centers of excellence.
7. *Medical staff development plans need technology assessment.* A medical staff development plan, prepared with and for physicians, is a business plan for the medical staff. The plan identifies which clinical specialties need recruitment and outlines strategies such as the construction of medical office buildings or the acquisition of physician practices. Today, each hospital is identifying its "first team," that is, the 25–35 percent of the medical staff who will be the core physicians and have long-term relationships with the hospital. The medical staff development plan is intended to strengthen the hospital's medical staff capacity as an organization and to enhance the practices of committed doctors around which the hospital will build its future.

STRATEGIC IMPLICATIONS FOR HOSPITALS

1. *Reduce acquisition time with long-range planning.* Advance planning can reduce by months the lead time needed for technology acquisition, which routinely involves 18–36 months of planning, capital budgeting, equipment specification, vendor selection, installation, and testing. For hospitals in states with certificate-of-need regulations, the "franchise" on a controlled new technology can be gained by those institutions that have anticipated it and submitted the first application.
2. *Create high-technology centers.* Hospitals should develop an organizational capacity to identify, develop, and implement advanced technologies and create new, highly specialized niches. For example, Mount Carmel Health in Columbus, Ohio, established the Advanced Treatment and Bionics Institute (ATBI) in 1986 for the purpose of speeding technologies to patients. The hospital works in collaboration with the medical staff to provide physician sponsors with technical, administrative, financial, educational, marketing, and evaluation support. To date, 12 projects have been launched through ATBI, including photodynamic therapy, a new cancer treatment.
3. *Forecasting demand and break-even for new technology is critical.* The acquisition analysis is complicated by the many unknowns that must be factored into assumptions about technology utilization and reimbursement. Carefully estimate future technology utilization in consultation with physician experts. The demand forecast is the basis for preparing detailed revenue and expense statements to determine potential cash flow. Hospitals can purchase high-tech decision software to assess high-tech equipment. The Analytic Hierarchy Process is a decision system developed by Decision Support Software of McClean, Virginia, and recently used by Divine Prov-

idence Hospital in Williamsport, Pennsylvania, to assess an MRI acquisition. The software requires the user (buyer) to judge the relative importance of each decision criterion, and to specify a preference for each vendor relative to all criteria. The result is a prioritized overall ranking of the decision alternatives.

4. *Community hospitals are becoming new competitors in tertiary care.* Many community hospitals are invading the domain of teaching hospitals and academic health centers by developing clinical centers of excellence. Tertiary care centers should anticipate the future vulnerability of high-tech services, identify possible competitors, and assess the potential of competitors to take away market share. To forestall or coopt future competitors, a tertiary care center might attempt to bring them into a regional specialty care network (e.g., cancer, cardiac) in ways that enhance the local programs (e.g., continuing education, participation in clinical trials) but also continue to channel patients to the center.

5. *Medium to large hospitals should seek out technology niches.* Every hospital over 200 beds should have at least one high-tech center of excellence in which it provides state-of-the-art medicine. Larger facilities (300 beds and over) should maintain at least two specialized centers. Successful centers will affiliate with top medical specialists and provide the latest technology.

6. *Capital investment planning and budgeting is crucial.* Establish strategic and financial priorities for technology investment, and balance the use of resources with innovative financing. Hospitals should allocate 4–6 percent of the capital investment budget for new technology and related facilities. Remember to budget as much as 8–10 percent of the purchase cost of new equipment for technological upgrades. Long-range planning and capital budgeting should anticipate major capital outlays for technology and facilities over a five- to ten-year period—and for each institution as well as at the system level. To finance technology acquisitions, hospitals and multihospital systems should look for innovative capital formation strategies. Capital pools, in-house loan funds, taxable debt, philanthropy, venture capital funds, and joint ventures can all be used to capitalize technology investments. Congressional concerns about physician conflicts of interest may limit some hospital-physician joint ventures in the next two to three years.

7. *Managed care and PPSs will have a substantial impact on high-tech health care.* Over the next three to five years, loss of the Medicare capital pass through and the spread of managed care plans will reduce the amount of capital available for technological investment. Medicare will fold all capital payments into the standard case-based reimbursement formula. Medicare can be expected to limit and reduce fees for ambulatory procedures (it

already has for cataract surgery). The impact of managed care will be more gradual but no less significant. As managed care inpatients gradually come to constitute 30-40 percent of all inpatients in the 1990s, health care institutions will have less financial flexibility. Under fixed price (discount) contracts with managed care plans, hospitals will have less margin to invest in new technology. Reimbursement trends will make labor cost–substitution issues increasingly important in the next five years.

8. *Technology investment needs a higher level of strategic management*. Multihospital systems and tertiary medical centers should consider employing a chief technology officer, whose job would be to coordinate assessment, analysis, and regional development of technology across the system. The best medical specialists from across system facilities should be included in a technical advisory group that scans for technical advances, new equipment, and new medical procedures.

9. *Install Service Line Management*. The strategic emphasis on high-tech niches needs to be complemented by a strong service line management program. Create new "department heads" to manage key service lines such as cardiac care. These managers and their medical directors can then take the lead in developing hub-and-spoke referral networks of physicians and outlying hospitals for the purpose of channeling patients to the specialty services. Service line management will need financial, marketing, and planning support. Each service line should have its own five-year business plan, capital and technological investment plan, and marketing plan. Multihospital systems could create for their specialized services "generic" advertising and marketing campaigns to be shared by local hospitals operating in different markets.

BIBLIOGRAPHY

Activase: Biological Clot Dissolver. N.d. South San Francisco: Genentech.

"Cancer Care—At a Cost." 1986. *Health* (July): 11.

Cetus and Squibb Form Alliance. 1987. Emeryville, Calif.: Cetus Corporation, 18 June.

Cetus Awarded First U.S. Patent on "Mutein" Cancer Drug. 1985. Emeryville, Calif.: Cetus Corporation, 25 May.

Cetus Begins Human Testing of Breast Cancer Treatment. 1987. Emeryville, Calif.: Cetus Corporation, 18 May.

Cetus Corporation Combines Two Anticancer Products in Human Testing. 1987. Emeryville, Calif.: Cetus Corporation, 16 July.

Cetus Enters Third Genetically Engineered Protein into Human Testing for Cancer. 1986. Emeryville, Calif.: Cetus Corporation, 12 June.

Cetus Genetically Engineers Colony Stimulating Factor-1. 1985. Emeryville, Calif.: Cetus Corporation, 8 August.

Chesebro, J.H., et al. 1987. "Thrombolysis in Myocardial Infarction (TIMI) Trial, Phase I: A Comparison between Intravenous Tissue Plasminogen Activator and Intravenous Streptokinase." *Circulation* 76(1): 142–54.

Coile, Russell C., Jr. 1988. "The Promise of Technology: A Technoforecast for the 1990s." *Healthcare Executive* (November-December): 22–25.

"The Coming Battle over Gallstones." 1987. *Health Technology* 1 (November-December): 222–30.

Edwards, D.D. 1987. "After the Battle, tPA Declared a Winner." *Science News*, 21 November, 325.

"Extracorporeal Shock-Wave Lithotripsy (ESWL)." 1987. *Health Technology* 1 (March-April): 80–83.

FDA Approves Genentech's Drug to Treat Children's Growth Disorder. 1985. South San Francisco: Genentech, 18 October.

Foster, Richard. 1986. *Innovation: The Attacker's Advantage*. New York: Basic Books.

"Future Improvements in Magnetic Resonance Imaging." 1988. *Health Technology* 2 (January-February): 12–19.

Kolata, Gina. 1987. "Immune Boosters." *Discover*. (September): 68–74.

"Laser Angioplasty." 1987. *Health Technology* 1 (May-June): 128–30.

"Laser Lithotripsy of Ureteral Stones." 1987. *Health Technology* 1 (July-August): 174–80.

"Lasers in Medicine and Surgery." 1986. *JAMA* 256:900–907.

Licensing of Activase Marks New Era in Treating Heart Attacks. 1987. South San Francisco: Genentech, 13 November.

MacStravic, Robin S. 1988. "Pros and Cons of Marketing Technology." *Health Progress* (October): 36–39.

Merimee, Thomas J., et al. 1987. "Insulin-like Growth in Pygmies." *New England Journal of Medicine* 316: 906–11.

Miller, Julie Ann. 1986. "Interferon Helps Cells Help Themselves." *Science News* (February): 89.

"MRI: What Are Its Applications? What Will It Replace?" 1988. *Health Technology* 2 (January-February): 3–11.

"New Options Regenerate Interest in Diagnostic Ultrasound." *Health Technology* 2 (May-June 1988): 96–105.

"New Technologies for Your Hospital to Consider." 1987. *Health Technology* 1 (July-August): 138–48.

Noble, Holcombe B., ed. 1987. *Next: The Coming Era in Medicine* New York: Little, Brown.

"One Patient's Experience with Interferon." 1987. *FDA Consumer* (April): 11.

"Optical Disk Storage of Digital Images." 1988. *Health Technology* 2 (May-June): 119–21.

O'Rourke, Kevin D. 1988. "Two Ethical Approaches to Research on Human Beings." *Health Progress* (October): 48–51.

"Patients and Profits: When the 'Bottom Line' Dictates Care Levels." 1988. *Issues* 3 (January): 1–8.

A Progress Report on Biotechnology. 1986. 2d ed. Nutley, N.J.: Hoffmann-La Roche.

"Quick TPA Approval Boon for Genentech." 1987. *Health Business*, 13 November, p. 1.

Randall, Judith E. 1988. "NMR: The Best Thing Since X-Rays?" *Technology Review* (January): 59–65.

Rosenberg, Steven A., et al. 1987. "A Progress Report on the Treatment of 157 Patients with Advanced Cancer Using Lymphokine-Activated Killer Cells and Interleukin-2 or High-Dose Interleukin-2 Alone." *New England Journal of Medicine* 316: 889–97.

Safe and Effective Biosynthetic Growth Hormone: Clinical Trials, Research Opportunities Outlined. N.d.South San Francisco: Genentech.

Shepherd, Robert. 1988. " 'Cadillac Care': Advances in Technology Raise Cost-Control Questions." *Healthcare Financial Management* (November): 23–27.

Shortell, Stephen M. 1986. "New Models for Hospital-Physician Relations." In *The Corporatization of Health Care Delivery*, edited by Monica R. Dreuth. Chicago: American Hospital Publishing.

Sprague, Gary R. 1988. "Managing Technology Assessment and Acquisition." *Healthcare Executive* (November-December): 26–29.

Sun, Marjorie. 1987. "New Data Clinch Heart Drug Approval." *News and Comment*, 20 November, 1031.

Talpaz, Moshe, et al. 1986. "Hematologic Remission and Cytogenetic Improvement Induced by Recombinant Human Interferon Alpha (a) in Chronic Myelogenous Leukemia." *New England Journal of Medicine* 314:1065–69.

Taylor, P.J. 1986. Fertility God in the Gamete Laboratory. *Lancet*, 8 February, 332.

"Technology on Wheels: Evaluating the Options." 1987. *Health Technology* 1 (November-December): 231–38.

Weinstock, Cheryl Platzman. 1987. "Medicines from the Body." *FDA Consumer* (April): 7–10.

"Will tPA Force Changes in Cardiac Care?" 1987. *Science News*, 12 December, 376.

its own developmental dynamics. Below is a description of the outlook for the 1990s.

Health Maintenance Organizations

Look for HMOs to expand at an annual rate of 8–15 percent in the next three to five years. HMOs have slowed from their record growth of 1985–1987, both in enrollment and number of plans. At the end of the second quarter of 1988, there were 643 HMOs, with enrollment exceeding 31.3 million members. This record high enrollment represents only 1–2 percent growth in the first six months of 1988, which follows a five-year annual expansion pace of 15–25 percent. InterStudy's data show that HMO plans are now declining in numbers, mostly due to acquisitions and consolidations. Only a handful of new HMOs began operation in the first quarter of 1988 (*InterStudy Edge* 1988). In 1986 and 1985, there were 144 and 99 new plans respectively (McLaughlin 1987). Those years recorded annual enrollment gains of 23 and 26 percent as the trend towards managed care gathered momentum. If present trends hold, there should be 35 to 40 million Americans enrolled in 600–700 HMOs by the early 1990s. This projection assumes annual HMO growth returns to 8–15 percent, including the new and still experimental "open-ended HMOs." Open-ended HMOs and HMO hybrids (e.g., Prudential Plus) are fueling the HMO revival, with nearly 500,000 and 625,000 members respectively at mid-1988.

National HMOs

The growth of large national HMOs is a trend confirmed by the 1988 InterStudy HMO census. Two years ago, only Kaiser and HealthAmerica were active in 10 or more states. Now eight firms have HMOs headquartered in at least 10 states. National HMOs now enroll 60 percent of all HMO members in the United States. The number of HMOs affiliated with national firms doubled in 18 months, from 156 to 310. In 15 states, national HMOs now account for more than 75 percent of all HMO participants. Insurance companies are the driving force behind national HMOs. Of the eight national firms, five are at least partially sponsored by major national insurers and two others own insurance subsidiaries.

Preferred Provider Organizations

PPOs caught up with HMOs in terms of customer acceptance in 1987, spurred by 250 percent growth. In that year, enrollment reached 25 million, up from 16.5 million in 1986. The number of operational PPO plans has multiplied exponentially, from 369 in 1986 to 674 in May 1987 (directory according to the American Association of Preferred Provider Organizations). More than half of all PPOs are provider-sponsored, but insurance-sponsored PPOs will make major inroads in the 1990s and become the dominant type of PPO sponsor. Metropolitan, Prudential, Bankers Life, John Hancock, Mutual of Omaha, and Pacific Mutual Life are all actively developing PPOs. The managed care joint venture (Partners) of Voluntary Hospitals of America (VHA) and Aetna includes PPO development as a complement to their HMO projects.

Exclusive Provider Arrangements

EPAs are almost too new to count and have made little market impact as yet. A 1987 survey by the American Association of Preferred Provider Organizations, based in Washington, D.C., identified 37 such plans in the market. The EPA concept must still overcome buyer skepticism, and there are few track records. As self-insured employers experiment in new arrangements with providers, they want to be experience rated and to negotiate risk-sharing arrangements. In moving to EPAs, these aggressive companies are cutting out the traditional middlemen (insurers and third party administrators) or exercising much more control over the intermediaries regarding provider selection, rate negotiation, and utilization.

Open-Ended HMOs

These new hybrid health plans combine HMO features with indemnity insurance. Open-ended plans offer enrollees greater flexibility by providing payment for non-HMO providers if the enrollee chooses to opt out of the HMO network, but usually at a cost involving copayment or deductibles. As of March 1989, according to the InterStudy survey, eleven HMOs reported open-ended HMO enrollment of nearly 400,000. (The majority of enrollees were in Minnesota, which had five plans and 300,000 enrollees.) Other HMOs now offer the open-ended option; it is estimated that 40 to 45 plans may have 200,000 to 250,000 members who have selected this option (*InterStudy Edge* 1989).

MAJOR PLAYERS AND MARKET STRATEGY

The managed care marketplace has shifted dramatically in the last three years, driven by three trends: (1) the acceptance by employers of PPOs; (2) the shift of health insurers from fee-for-service to PPOs; and (3) the entry of Medicare HMOs and "competitive medical plans."

As managed care moves center stage in the health care marketplace, the market strategies of the major players—employers, government, insurers, and providers—will change in response. There are also some new players who will make an impact—third party administrators, union-sponsored and Taft-Hartley health plans, and government, e.g., Department of Defense's PPO contract with the Foundation Health Plan of Sacramento, California.

Entrepreneurs

Managed care market entry reflects a maturing of the HMO growth curve as well as saturation in some markets, such as Chicago, which has more than 30 HMOs competing for market share. In 1986, 99 new HMOs were started. The overwhelming majority were for-profit. More than 100 HMOs were launched in 1987, but the trend slowed dramatically in 1988. By year end, contraction and consolidation had begun to make an impact; there were five fewer HMOs than a year before, for a total of 643.

For-profit hospital chains are generally retreating from managed care ventures. New for-profit HMOs continue to enter the market, despite the well-publicized withdrawals from the HMO marketplace of American Medical International and National Medical Enterprises and the scaling back of its HMO efforts by Humana, which is only buying or building HMOs in regional markets where it has a strong hospital network. HMO investors have not been dismayed by depressed stock values for publicly held HMOs like Maxicare, whose stock plummeted to less than $1 per share, and U.S. Healthcare, which lost 50 percent of its market value in 1988. There continues to be a high level of entrepreneurial interest in HMO growth, but the trend is shifting away from new starts and toward expansion through acquisition and internal development.

Entrepreneurial PPO formation continues at a high level. Although the census of operational PPOs is still far from accurate, it appears that the number of PPOs has increased by 100 percent between 1986 and 1988. Early PPOs were typically sponsored by hospitals and physicians in a defensive response to HMO development. In the past three years, the PPO movement has increasingly been infused by the participation of major health insurers, such as Blue Cross.

Indemnity Insurance Companies

America's health care insurers are actively moving to coopt the managed care movement through HMOs, PPOs, and "managed indemnity" plans.

Virtually all major health insurers have managed care products of their own, such as Metropolitan's Met-Life or Prudential's Pru-Care. Metropolitan intends to be a 50-state player in the managed care competition, and it is buying or building HMO and PPO organizations in more than 30 major markets. To speed their entry in the HMO market, some insurers are buying established HMOs. For example, the Travelers bought 19 local HMOs from Whittaker in November 1986. Although enrollment in Travelers' HMOs jumped from 40,000 to 115,000 in 11 months, the company sold off a number of local HMOs outside its preferred markets. Travelers lost more than $20 million in its health care book of business in 1988. A sign of the times—12 other insurers and HMO competitors expressed interest in Travelers' sale offer.

Insurer-provider managed care ventures are just beginning to make a market impact, like the Partners plan created conjointly by Aetna and VHA. Early market acceptance has been slow, but Aetna and VHA intend to be in more than 100 major markets by 1990. The high cost of the HMO business is driving hospitals out of the game. With the Partners plan continuing to lose money, Aetna announced that it would provide all capital for acquisitions and growth beginning in 1989, thereby relieving VHA hospitals of additional levies for managed care investment.

Blue Cross will definitely be a major player in the managed care marketplace. How the "Blues" participate in managed care will have a critical impact on the nation's hospitals. In the past, most Blue Cross organizations contracted with all licensed hospitals and paid full charges (prevailing rates) or discounted charges. Some Blue Cross organizations utilize prospective payment and diagnostic-related groups to further reduce their hospital costs. Managed care offers the Blues a very different market strategy. Today most Blue Cross organizations have established a network of select providers for HMO and PPO options and offer employers discounts of 15–25 percent below price for standard indemnity plans. The HMOs affiliated with Blue Cross and Blue Shield account for 13.5 percent of all HMOs, according to the 1989 HMO census by InterStudy (*InterStudy Edge* 1989).

California Blue Cross is a trendsetter. It has eliminated the indemnity plan option for its own employees, who are now limited to the Blue Cross HMO or PPO alternatives. Now the California Blue Cross organization is trying the same strategy with major employers. To encourage employers to switch to the HMO or PPO option, California Blue Cross has imposed rate hikes on employers, in some cases ranging above 50 percent. The goal is to drive indemnity plan members into HMO and PPO alternatives where Blue Cross has more control over utilization and costs.

In New England, Blue Cross and Blue Shield of Rhode Island has adopted a new tactic in HMO market warfare. The Rhode Island Blues have imposed premium surcharges called "adverse selection factors" on employers who offer HMOs to employees. As a result, indemnity plan rates have increased substantially for some Rhode Island employers. An employer can lower the increase if it offers the Blue Cross and Blue Shield HealthMate plan, an experience-rated PPO that the Rhode Island organization recently introduced.

HMOs and PPOs

Once prime competitors, HMOs and PPOs are joining forces and converging in their operational and market strategies. The distinction between HMOs and

PPOs is breaking down. Some HMOs are broadening their product line to compete with PPOs. Beginning in 1987, a number of independent HMOs, like Maxicare and Pacificare, began to offer employers the "triple option"—an HMO package, a PPO alternative, and a standard indemnity health plan—in response to a trend initiated by some Blue Cross organizations and major health insurers. This trend will grow in popularity with major employers in the 1990s for its ease of administration (single-vendor).

HMOs are still growing at 8–15 percent annually. Consolidation is now widespread in the HMO industry. Maxicare of Los Angeles purchased two HMOs in the past 18 months and as a result became one of the top five managed care systems in the nation (*InterStudy Edge* 1989). However, "digesting" the acquisitions has depressed earnings, and Maxicare's stock is trading at a fraction of its maximum price two years ago. As previously noted, open-ended HMOs are a new phenomenon on the managed care scene. Their rapid acceptance in the Twin Cities suggests these managed care hybrids will take market share away from both HMOs and PPOs in the decade ahead.

A "second generation" of PPOs is entering the marketplace, according to Peter Boland (1985b). These new PPOs are more like HMOs: They select providers carefully, control utilization, and have stronger disincentives in order to reduce out-of-plan use by enrollees. Some larger PPOs are beginning to buy smaller plans. Admar, of Orange, California, with 1.2 million members, purchased SelectCare Management, of Torrance, California, a PPO with 200,000 members. Admar gained not only the new members but also a strong utilization review system and more control over its provider network. SelectCare had contracted only with major medical groups.

Major Purchasers

Major employers will have a major influence on the future development of managed care alternatives, just as they have had from the beginning of the HMO movement. Early HMOs were started by industrial employers like Kaiser Permanente. In the Twin Cities region, local employers enthusiastically sponsored HMO development in the early 1970s. Today, an estimated 49 percent of Twin Cities residents are members of HMOs.

Managed care is a major strategy in employer health cost control. A survey of 1,208 major employers by EQUICOR (Equitable Life/Hospital Corporation of America) reports that use of HMOs and PPOs is the main method by which business hopes to control health costs in the future (Gardner, Kyzr-Sheeley, and Sabatino 1985). Chrysler Corporation is a case in point. Joseph Califano, a former secretary of Health, Education and Welfare and now a board member of Chrysler, stated that the major auto maker hopes to have 80 percent of its work force enrolled in PPOs and HMOs by the early 1990s (*Health Care Competition*

Week 1987a). In the 1987 open season alone, Califano reported, membership in these plans increased from 33 to 50 percent among Chrysler employees, with PPO enrollment growing faster than HMO enrollment.

Today, employers are demanding more control over HMO costs (Kittrell 1986). In the Chicago area, half of large local businesses negotiate HMO premiums and rewrite HMO plans to meet employer specifications, according to James Mortimer, president of the Midwest Business Group on Health. With more than 50 HMOs and PPOs fighting for a piece of the action, Chicago is a "buyers market" for major employers negotiating with managed care plans.

Government

The federal government is attempting to encourage Medicare enrollees to convert from fee-for-service medicine to HMOs.

At-risk contracting for Medicare is gaining ground. Under the Tax Equity and Fiscal Responsibility Act of 1982, Congress gave the Department of Health and Human Services new authority to contract with HMOs on an at-risk basis, paying the HMOs 95 percent of what Medicare typically spends on the average Medicare enrollee in the community served. Although still far below the 20 percent of eligibles that the government hopes will convert by 1990, Medicare HMO enrollment is moving upwards. From September 1985 to December 1986, enrollment jumped from 552,096 to 1,025,466 (McMillan and Lubitz 1987).

The 41 Medicare HMOs are not universally happy with the program. In a survey by InterStudy in early 1987, more than half of the participating HMOs reported their Medicare contracts have been unsuccessful financially, primarily due to inadequate Medicare payments (Baldwin 1987b). The federal government may contract with PPOs if capitation requirements can be eased to allow PPOs to qualify for Medicare risk-sharing contracts. These PPOs could be insurance company sponsored or hospital-physician joint ventures with an insurer partner, who would take the role of principal risk taker.

Medicare-insured groups are an experiment in turning over control to the purchasers. As an alternative to Medicare HMOs, HCFA is negotiating with Chrysler and other major corporations, as well as unions, to place their Medicare-eligible retirees under a company-managed Medicare plan. The first experiments will test this concept. HCFA announced a preliminary agreement with the Amalgamated Life Insurance Company to take over Medicare for 5,000 union retirees in the Philadelphia area (Hanna 1987). The Amalgamated Clothing and Textile Workers includes 130,000 retirees and their spouses. These risk-sharing contracts would give the company or union the opportunity to gain greater control over the Medicare supplemental costs they fund for retirees.

Consumers

Who joins a managed care plan? The mythology of the managed care industry is that HMOs are favored by young, healthy wage earners who are building families and careers; older persons with more chronic health problems and long-term relationships with their physicians tend to favor indemnity health plans. There is some validity to these generalizations, but only some. More recently, marketers have asked, Who joins PPOs? A preliminary RAND analysis of six large employers offering a PPO option suggests that PPO enrollees fall some-where between these two stereotypes: They are older and have higher incomes than HMO enrollees but not as old or wealthy as those who still prefer indemnity health plans, with their greater flexibility of provider choice (Ginsburg 1987).

Hospitals

One third of the nation's hospitals had contracts with HMOs and PPOs, according to a fall 1986 survey by the AMA (Rahn 1987a). Few hospitals gained more than 5–10 percent of their inpatients from HMO and PPO sources in 1985–1988. For example, St. Mary's Hospital in San Francisco has 100 managed care contracts in place, mostly PPOs, producing 18 percent of total revenue. But 60 percent of its managed care business comes from only 5 or 6 contracts (Hanna 1987). The percent of managed care inpatients is growing rapidly. A national survey in 1989 predicted that all hospitals will have HMO and PPO contracts and that HMO/PPO plans will cover 50 percent of inpatients by 1992 (Coile 1989).

Physicians

Physicians may be "mad as hell" about managed care, but few are joining anti-HMO organizations like San Antonio-based Physicians Who Care. More than half of the nation's doctors have signed agreements to treat HMO and PPO patients (Rundle 1987). Physicians who saw the managed care handwriting on the wall have formed their own managed care organizations. Lifecare, an HMO in Santa Clara, California, was started by physicians; today it has more than 100,000 members, second only to Kaiser in California's Silicon Valley.

MANAGED CARE IN THE 1990s: TRENDS TO WATCH

If this is the outlook for managed care, what does it all mean? Here are key trends that will shape the future of managed care in the decade ahead.

1. *Enrollment Growth*: Managed care plans (HMOs and PPOs) will enroll 35–40 percent of the civilian population of the United States by 1992 (up from 25 percent in 1987) and more than 50 percent by the mid-1990s. Medicare enrollment will be a driving force in managed care growth, rising from 5 percent in 1987 to 15–20 percent in 1992 and to 35–40 percent by 1995.
2. *Contract Care*: If government-pay patients and "managed indemnity" are included, 75–85 percent of all inpatients may be "managed care" patients in the future—patients whose reimbursement is prospectively limited by negotiated contract or government regulation. Thus, only about 25 percent of patients will pay "charges," and some of these patients will be self-pay or no pay. The growth of managed care will increasingly limit hospital financial flexibility, as control shifts to the managed care buyers.
3. *Ownership*: Controlling interests in managed care plans will be held predominantly by insurance companies. Large national HMOs will control 60 percent of the future managed care market by 1990 (up from 49 percent in 1987), and national PPOs will gain share against local PPOs.
4. *Private Regulation*: Although the public sector continues to deregulate some aspects of the health care marketplace, the real trend to watch is private regulation of health providers by payers through benefit limits and utilization controls. Managed care plans will be most intrusive, limiting provider control over patient care decisions.
5. *Quality and Cost*: Providers must be price competitive, but quality will also be a primary concern of managed care plans. Managed care plans will deeply probe quality records and carefully select high-quality providers.
6. *Preferred Providers*: There will be two types of providers in tomorrow's marketplace: (1) major hospital and medical group HMO and PPO contractors, who will be the preferred providers, and (2) all others. Providers in the second group will have to compete for a shrinking number of fee-for-service patients and discretionary health care dollars.

LOOKING FORWARD: A WATERSHED TIME FOR MANAGED CARE

The 1990s will be a watershed era for managed care. It is the broadest organizational and business concept yet suggested for the emerging hybrid organizations that combine features of HMOs, PPOs, and EPAs. New combinations of prospective payment, case management, capitation, risk sharing, service and benefits mix, incentives, and prices are constantly being created. Don't count on today's patterns as final. The entire managed care concept is still experimental.

More to the point, in the managed care marketplace, it is the *buyers* who will manage the care as well as the costs. All major payers—employers, unions, insurance companies, and government—want more direct involvement in all aspects of financing and delivery of services. Managed care plans will contract with cooperating providers in new ways that will realign the health care buyer-supplier relationship. The history of alternative delivery systems has been that innovative buyers reshaped the market with like-thinking providers.

The challenge of managed care does not lie on the far horizon. For physicians and hospitals who believe that managed care will be the dominant form of reimbursement in the 1990s, opportunities to be part of the managed care movement are presenting themselves now.

STRATEGIC IMPLICATIONS FOR PHYSICIANS

1. *Managed care plans will channel patients.* The lifeblood of tomorrow's medicine is managed care. Physicians will receive 40–50 percent of their revenues from managed care plans by 1995. In some regions, such as the West, the trend will begin sooner. Managed care plans will channel patients to selected providers in their network. Affiliation with a managed care plan will be a critical factor in physician success. Designation by a popular HMO or PPO could make a 25–50 percent difference in clientele.
2. *Preauthorization for all medical treatments will be required.* In a managed care environment, physicians will have to obtain health plan approval in advance for many treatments. The increasing "private regulation" of medicine will mean more time justifying treatments and fighting retroactive denials by managed care plans and utilization review intermediaries.
3. *Doctors will select patients on the basis of their managed care plans.* In the future, doctors will become highly selective in accepting new patients. One of the criteria will be the patient's health plan. Some doctors may not like the discounted prices of particular plans and be unwilling to accept new patients with that coverage. Conversely, physicians may lose patients if they have no affiliation with or designation by their patients' HMOs or PPOs.

STRATEGIC IMPLICATIONS FOR HOSPITALS

1. *Every hospital should have a hospital-affiliated IPA for managed care contracting.* Larger hospitals and health systems should create their own IPAs and PPOs. Small and mid-sized hospitals should participate and invest in managed care networks with other local and regional hospitals.
2. *Hub-and-spoke HMOs and PPOs will become prevalent.* Perhaps the most promising opportunity today is the creation of regional PPOs by collabo-

rating hospitals in order to manage local medical markets. Such PPOs will be the secret to market dominance in the 1990s. They will contract with managed care buyers and major employers to channel patients to the network of doctors and participating hospitals. Ideally, a regional PPO would have an HMO option for employers or third party administrators who want one vendor for all their health service coverage.

3. *Hospitals and health systems must control and gain ownership of managed care plans through purchase or joint ventures.* Otherwise, they will find themselves relegated to the role of vendors competing for patients principally on price. Wall Street investors were rediscovering HMOs at the end of 1989 at the same time many HMOs were losing money; this may provide an opportunity for investment at below-market prices in the 1990s. The window of opportunity for local hospitals and physicians to invest in HMOs and PPOs is closing and may be shut by 1992.

4. *Now is the time to invest in managed care through acquisition and consolidation.* The managed care market will expand dramatically at an annual rate of 25–35 percent in the next five years. Between 1990 and 1995 the market should begin to reach saturation, resulting in more consolidation and some market shakeout of managed care plans. Smaller plans, those with fewer than 40,000–50,000 enrollees, will be prime targets for acquisition.

BIBLIOGRAPHY

Bachman, Sara S., David Pomeranz, and Eileen J. Tell. 1987. "Making Employers Smart Buyers of Health Care." *Business and Health* (September): 28–34.

Baldwin, Mark F. 1985a. "New Rule Lets Other Healthcare Plans be Reimbursed Like HMOs." *Modern Healthcare*, 1 February, 64–65.

_____. 1985b. "Boston HMOs Ready for Stepped-up Battle." *Modern Healthcare*, 10 May, 42–46.

_____. 1985c. "HMO Firms Deal Directly with HCFA." *Modern Healthcare*, 7 June, 66.

_____. 1985d. "Poll: HMO Quality Satisfies Members." *Modern Healthcre*, 7 June, 66.

_____. 1986a. "Enrollment in Typical HMO Up 30% in '84—Survey." *Modern Healthcare*, 17 January, 24.

_____. 1986b. "Hospital, Physician Groups Oppose Budget Office's Shared Payment Plan." *Modern Healthcare*, 19 December, 10.

_____. 1987a. "IPA-Model Growth Leads Expansion." *Modern Healthcare*, 30 January, 46.

_____. 1987b. "Most Medicare HMOs Unhappy with Program." *Modern Healthcare*, 24 August, 26.

Barkholz, David. 1985. "Hospitals in Metropolitan Life's PPO Report Dramatic Business Increases." *Modern Healthcare*, 6 December, 46.

_____. 1986a. "AHS to Market Managed Insurance." *Modern Healthcare*, 28 February, 16.

_____. 1986b. "SunHealth Alliance Plans Entry into Healthcare Insurance Arena." *Modern Healthcare*, 28 February, 48–50.

_____. 1986c. "Company Grows by Focusing Efforts." *Modern Healthcare*, 28 March, 70.

_____. 1986d. "HealthAmerica Plans Utilization Cuts." *Modern Healthcare*, 28 March, 70.

Berenson, Robert A. 1987. "Hidden Compromises in Paying Physicians." *Business and Health* (July): 18–22.

Boland, Peter. 1985a. "Purchase Concerns to Prevail in Future PPAs." *Hospitals*, 16 May, 101–4.

_____. 1985b. *The New Healthcare Market: A Guide to PPOs for Purchasers, Payors and Providers.* Homewood Ill.: Dow-Jones Irwin.

Cherskov, Myk. 1987. "Insurers Set to Fight Managed Care Plan Fraud." *Hospitals*, 5 February, 42.

Coile, Russell C., Jr. 1989. "Financial Megatrends 1990," Healthcare Forum (November-December).

Donlon, Thomas M. 1986. "Unbundling of Claims Services with Self-Insurance." *Business and Health* (January-February): 11–13.

Duis, Terry. 1985. "Hospital Heads Should Analyze HMO, PPO Affiliation Proposals." *Modern Healthcare*, 5 July, 142–44.

Ellis, Randall P. 1986. "Biased Selection in Flexible Benefit Plans." *Business and Health* (May): 26–30.

"Employers Seek HMO Accountability." 1985. *Modern Healthcare* 26 April, 32.

Etheredge, Lynn. 1986. "The World of Insurance: What Will the Future Bring?" *Business and Health* (January-February): 5–9.

Feezor, Allen. 1987. "No Future Guarantees for Self-Insured Plans." *Business and Health* (April): 16–19.

Firshein, Janet. 1986a. "What's the Secret of HMO Success?" *Hospitals*, 5 April, 69–70.

_____. 1986b. "HMO Suit Sparks Concern over Medicare Reimbursement." *Hospitals*, 20 September, 74–75.

_____. 1987. "HCFA Outlines 1987 Legislative Medicare Agenda." *Hospitals*, 20 February, 50–52.

Fox, Peter D., and Maren D. Anderson. 1986. "Hybrid HMOs, PPOs: The New Focus." *Business and Health* (March): 20–27.

Fritz, Dan, and David V. Repko. 1986. "A Blueprint for Forging New HMO Relationships." *Business and Health* (July-August): 38–39.

Gardner, Steve F., B.J. Kyzr-Sheeley, and Frank Sabatino. 1985. "Big Business Embraces Alternate Delivery." *Hospitals*, 16 March, 81–84.

Ginsburg, Paul B., Susan D. Hosek, and M. Susan Marquis. 1987. "Who Joins a PPO?" *Business and Health* (February): 36–38.

Goldsmith, Jeff C. 1985. "Insurer's Change in Approach May Threaten Hospitals' Margins." *Modern Healthcare*, 1 February, 49–56.

Graham, Judith. 1986a. "Mutual of Omaha Introducing PPOs." *Modern Healthcare*, 28 February, 16.

_____. 1986b. "Insurers to Launch PPOs as a Way to Contain Costs, Protect Markets." *Modern Healthcare*, 11 April, 40.

————. 1986c. "N.J. Hospitals Plan Delivery Systems." *Modern Healthcare*, 6 June, 26.

————. 1986d. "Initial Public Offerings Slow as HMOs Fail to Extract Substantial Profits." *Modern Healthcare*, 20 June, 62.

Greene, Jay. 1987. "HMOs Posted Large Gains in Enrollment, but Most Saw Profits Decline during 1986." *Modern Healthcare*, 5 June, 118–26.

Hanna, Sam. 1987. "Employees Report Large Differences in HMOs." *Health Care Competition Week*, 5 October.

————. 1987. "Travelers Puts up Eight HMOs for Sale." *Health Care Competition Week*, 19 October.

"HMOs Post Income Gains." *Modern Healthcare*, 28 February, 38.

"The 'I' in IPA Fuels HMO Growth." 1986. *Hospitals*, 5 January, 73.

Inguanzo, Joe M., and Mark Harju. 1985. "What's the Market for HMOs and PPAs?" *Hospitals*, 1 September, 74–75.

The InterStudy Edge. 1989. InterStudy Edge, January.

The InterStudy Edge. 1989. Vol. 1. Excelsior, Minn.: InterStudy. (Reported in *Medical Benefits*, March 30, 1989, 1.)

Kenkel, Paul J. 1987. "Concern over Financial Strength of HMOs Leads Some States to Stiffen Solvency Requirements." *Modern Healthcare*, 28 August, 80.

Kenney, James B. 1985. "Using Competition to Develop a Buyer Driven Market." *Business and Health* (November): 39–42.

Kittrell, Alison. 1986. "Employers Turn to Managed Care, Utilization Review to Control Costs." *Modern Healthcare*, 9 May, 96–98.

Luft, Harold S. 1985. "HMOs: Friend or Foe?" *Business and Health* (December): 5–9.

Luhr, Richard A., and Peter D. Fox. 1987. "Considering PPOs for Small Business." *Business and Health* (June): 48–49.

McLaughlin, Neil. 1987. "HMOs' Dramatic Rate of Growth to Shift to Frost Belt, Rural Areas." *Modern Healthcare*, 16, January, 38–41.

McLaughlin, Neil. 1987a. "Experts Say HMOs' Capital Needs to Be Limited to Takeover Attempts." *Modern Healthcare*, 12 March, 154–56.

————. 1987b. "Chains Likely to Give a Repeat Performance and Struggle through 1987, Analysts Predict." *Modern Healthcare*, 10 April, 86.

McMillan, Alma, and James Lubitz. 1987. "Medicare Enrollment in Health Maintenance Organizations." *Health Care Financing Review* 8 (Spring): 87–93.

"Managed Care Pricing Strategies Shifting." 1985. *Hospitals*, 16 May, 85–86.

Polakoff, Phillip L., and Paul F. O'Rourke. 1987. "Managed Care Applications for Workers' Compensation." *Business and Health* (March): 26–27.

Powills, Suzanne. 1986. "HMOs' Quality Comes under GM's Watchful Eye." *Hospitals*, 20 July, 40.

Powills, Suzanne, and William Weinberg, 1985. "PPAs: A New Payment System Evolves." *Hospitals*, 1 May, 43–46.

"PPOs Make HMOs 'Fight for Their Lives.' " *Modern Healthcare*, 22 November, 54.

Rahn, Gary. 1986. "Hospitals Increase HMO Development: Report." *Hospitals*, 20 September, 73–74.

Rahn, Gary. 1987a. American Hospital Association, and Mary Traska. "Formal Hospital/HMO Contracts Increase: Survey." *Hospitals*, 20 July, 47–51.

_____. 1987b. "Managed Care." *Hospitals*, 20 August, 42–44.

Richman, Dan. 1985a. "Hospitals Should Mull Implications of HMO, PPO Contracts—Experts." *Modern Healthcare*, 5 July, 138–140.

_____. 1985b. "Chicago HMOs Promise Lower Rates but Employers Skeptical about Savings." *Modern Healthcare*, 22 November, 54.

_____. 1986a. "HMO Enrollment Heading Higher, but Experts Disagree on How Fast." *Modern Healthcare*, 3 January, 78–80.

_____. 1986b. "Investor-Owned HMOs' Enrollments Up: First-Quarter Net Income Results Mixed." *Modern Healthcare*, 20 June, 30.

_____. 1987. "PPOs Outstripped HMOs Last Year in Number of Locations and Enrollment." *Modern Healthcare*, 5 June, 130–136.

Rundle, Rhonda. 1987. "Doctors Who Oppose the Spread of HMOs and PPOs Are Losing Their Fight." *Wall Street Journal*, 6 October, 1–22.

Sharkey, William H., Jr. 1986. "Insurers Finding New Niche in Cost Management Programs." *Business and Health* (January-February): 16–18.

Steiberm, Steven R. 1987. "What's an HMO? 51% of Respondents Don't Know." *Hospitals*, 5 February, 78.

Stowe, James B., and Richard H. Egdahl. 1987. "Measuring Purchaser Value from Managed Care." *Business and Health* (August): 20–22.

Sutton, Harrly L., Jr. 1986. "Community Rating: An Historical Perspective." *Business and Health* (July-August): 41–44.

Tatge, Mark. 1985. "HMO Enrollment up 26.7% to 1.68 Million." *Modern Healthcare*, 7 June, 138–41.

Traska, M.R. 1985. "Baby Boomers Help HMOs Grow to 42 States." *Hospitals*, 16 May, 84–97.

_____. 1986a. "HMO Chains Grow Faster than Independent Plans." *Hospitals*, 5 April, 69.

_____. 1986b. "Alternate Care." *Hospitals*, 20 July, 55–57.

_____. 1987a. "More Changes Predicted for Managed Care." *Hospitals*, 20 January, 32.

_____. 1987b. "Hospitals to Feel Heat as Plans Handle Change." *Hospitals*, 20 January, 44.

_____. 1987c. "HMOs: A Shake-up (and Shakeout) on the Horizon?" *Hospitals*, 5 February, 40–48.

_____. 1987d. "Hancock's HMO Sale a Move Away from Delivery." *Hospitals*, 5 July, 43–46.

Valentine, Steven, and Robert Joffe. 1985. "PPOs Growing Rapidly in CA Market: Study." *Modern Healthcare*, 1 February, 58–60.

Wallace, Cynthia. 1985. "IPA Growth Potential Gains Followers." *Modern Healthcare*, 5 July, 92.

_____. 1986a. "HMO Is Targeting Small Employers to Fuel Expansion Throughout State." *Modern Healthcare*, 14 March, 38.

_____. 1986b. "HMOs Converting to For-Profit Status Could Face More Rigorous Reviews." *Modern Healthcare*, 11 April, 42.

_____. 1986c. "PPOs Luring Enrollees from HMOs." *Modern Healthcare*, 6 June, 26.

_____. 1986d. "Hospitals May be Required to Make Concessions to Attract HMO Business." *Modern Healthcare*, 6 June, 44.

_____. 1987e. "HMOs Battle for Market Share throughout Southern California." *Modern Healthcare*, 20 June, 44–46.

_____. 1986f. "Bids for HealthCare USA and Peak Signal Consolidation among HMOs." *Modern Healthcare*, 18 July, 36.

_____. 1987. "Maxicare Plans to Increase Premiums an Average of 6%." *Modern Healthcare*, 5 June, 14.

Winsberg, Gwynne R. 1985. "The Hidden Costs of HMOs." *Business and Health* (December): 18–21.

Yanish, Donna Leigh. 1986. "Kaiser Shifts Strategy to Retain Position in Prepaid Plan Market." *Modern Healthcare*, 9 May, 68–72.

Chapter 8

Promoting Health

For all its reputed conservatism, Western medicine is undergoing an amazing revitalization. Patients and professionals alike are beginning to see beyond symptoms to the context of illness: stress, society, family, diet, season, emotions. Just as the readiness of a new constituency makes a new politics, the needs of patients can change the practice of medicine. Hospitals, long the bastions of barren efficiency, are scurrying to provide more humane environments for birth and death, more flexible policies. Medical schools, long geared to skim the cool academic cream, are trying to attract more creative, people-oriented students. Bolstered by a blizzard of research on the psychology of illness, practitioners who once split mind and body are trying to put them back together.

—Marilyn Ferguson, *The Aquarian Conspiracy: Personal and Social Transformation in the 1980s*

Ever since Hippocrates lectured on health under the Plane tree, health care providers have sought to promote health. Health is now widely recognized to be as much a result of life style as high-tech medical care. Health promotion has moved into the center of modern health care. From counterculture to mainstream, the "wellness" movement emerged during the 1970s, an outcome of consumerism and a rising consciousness about the links between health habits and well-being.

It's working! Heart disease is down substantially, and so is the rate of cardiac mortality. Once people recognized the dangers of Type A high-stress behavior and the hazards of cholesterol, they changed their lives and life styles. Public awareness of these health risks has led to a decline in beef consumption and a rise in seafood consumption. Salads and "designer vegetables" grace American tables (and hospital cafeterias) from Maine to California. More than 20 percent of average Americans report they exercise hard at least three to four hours per week, and a majority attest they walk or exercise regularly for their health. The running boom has peaked, but ''striding'' (walking vigorously) is selling millions of pairs of fitness shoes to the sedentary.

A NEW PARADIGM FOR MEDICINE

Thirty years ago, Rene Dubos, a research microbiologist, suggested in *Mirage of Health* that the advances he and others had made in the development of antibiotics and therapeutics had less to do with the real health of populations than a variety of economic, social, nutritional, and behavioral factors (Dubos 1967). Five years later the U.S. Surgeon General's landmark report clearly revealed the link between smoking and diseases such as emphysema, chronic bronchitis, hypertension, and lung cancer. A new awareness of the contribution of life style, environment, and genetics infused medicine in the decades following.

Sometimes called the *wellness movement*, this new orientation broadened the paradigm of traditional biomedicine. Since the Dubos essay on health, a body of research findings has accumulated that demonstrates the validity of a more comprehensive approach to health, one which recognizes the many antecedents and cofactors in the disease and healing processes. Although not fully accepted by all physicians, the holistic concept of health is gaining stature. Dozens of studies by employers have begun to quantify the beneficial impact of health promotion programs in terms of reduced health care utilization and lower health care costs (Bly 1986).

THE WELLNESS CONTINUUM

Health promotion is more than an adjunct of acute care. It involves an array of programs and services designed to enhance satisfaction and well-being. Many of the services of the wellness continuum listed in Exhibit 8-1 are only health related, and the physician or hospital may simply be a referral source rather than a direct provider.

WELLNESS MOVEMENT WELL ENTRENCHED

By 1987, health promotion programs were offered by more than one-third of U.S. hospitals. If the definition is broadened to include community health ed-

Exhibit 8-1 The Wellness Continuum

Family life education
Parenting
Childbirth education
Child development
"Tough love" adolescent counseling
Coping with older parents
Retirement planning

Healthy life style
Safe driving
Diet and nutrition
Stress reduction
Accident prevention

Health habits
Smoking
Cardiovascular risk reduction
Alcohol and drug abuse
Arthritis

Health screening
Comprehensive physical exam
Computerized health risk assessment
Cholesterol
Chest x-ray
Diabetes
Cardiac fitness
Alcohol and drugs
AIDS

Occupational health
Worksite accident prevention
Back hardening
Drug testing
Worksite health and safety risk appraisal
Employee health risk management
Worksite health education classes

Fitness
Health clubs
Swim centers
Aerobics
Stretching
Yoga
Race or marathon medical support

Rehabilitation
Sports medicine
Physical therapy
Pain management
Back clinic
Cardiac rehabilitation

Health support groups
Recovered alcoholics
Adult children of alcoholics
Diabetics
"Mended hearts" cardiac patients

ucation, nearly all hospitals are involved in some aspects of health enhancement. The curve is still rising. A 1985 survey showed more than 26 percent of American hospitals offered wellness programs, up 6 percent from 1983 (Longe 1986). Health promotion programs continue to be most popular in the upper Midwest (30 percent) and the Southwest (29 percent), although the West trails only slightly

(24 percent). In the South, the percentage has nearly doubled from the 8 percent reported in 1985.

The wellness movement is clearly becoming institutionalized, and wellness programs are now an integral part of the spectrum of hospital-based services. In many hospitals and health systems, health promotion programs are strongly linked to occupational health activities. More than 40 percent of U.S. hospitals now provide occupational health programs, up from the 33 percent reported in a 1985 survey by the National Research Corporation of Lincoln, Nebraska. Again, the Northeast led in occupational health initiatives, with 44 percent of the hospitals reporting programs. Fewest offerings were found in the Southwest (14 percent) (Jenson 1989).

Larger hospitals in metropolitan areas are more likely to provide health promotion and occupational health programs. More than half of large hospitals (over 300 beds) offer such programs. Urban hospitals are more than twice as likely to offer health enhancement services, but smaller hospitals (100–199 beds) and nonmetropolitan hospitals are moving to expand their wellness efforts.

WHY ISN'T HEALTH PROMOTION PROFITABLE?

With all this wellness and fitness, why aren't health providers more successful in profitably conducting health promotion services? From the beginning of the health promotion era, hospitals and physicians have sought to tie wellness to mainstream health care. It has been a struggle! Despite many efforts, few hospitals have managed to do better than break even on health promotion programs. To many health-minded consumers, hospitals symbolize disease, despite attempts to change the public's perception.

Why haven't hospitals and physicians been more successful in health promotion? At least a dozen good reasons are presented in Exhibit 8-2.

DRIVEN BY DIVERSIFICATION

The development of health promotion programs was an early experiment in diversification. Stephen M. Shortell, of the Kellogg School of Management at Northwestern University and author of a recent study on hospital diversification, suggests that the phasing down of hospital-sponsored health promotion is part of a wider "back to basics" trend for U.S. hospitals. Health care executives saw health promotion as a "feeder system" for hospital-based facilities, such as rehab and the laboratory. In fact, experience has shown that health promotion

Exhibit 8-2 12 Reasons for the Failure of Hospital-Sponsored Health Promotion

1. Limited insurance coverage for any health-related service besides acute illness services.
2. Employer skepticism about the benefits to be gotten by paying employees to be "healthy."
3. Inability of providers to profit from "prevention" efforts that kept consumers away from doctors and hospitals.
4. Consumer skepticism about whether health-promoting services can best be obtained from the disease-oriented medical care system.
5. Poorly located and marketed hospital-based programs that cannot compete with private-sector health clubs and fitness centers.
6. Paying "hospital" overhead for nonacute programs which has hampered profitability.
7. Lack of special advantages for health promotion as a result of hospital sponsorship.
8. Lack of linkage or perceived benefits to medical staff.
9. Direct competition with medical staff in some areas (e.g., executive physical examinations).
10. Lack of hospital expertise in conducting, managing, or marketing health promotion and fitness.
11. Undercapitalization and inadequate support, leading to cash flow problems and continuous financial struggles.
12. Existence of excellent competing programs in the community that outcompete hospitals on price (YMCA), location, or amenities (health clubs and fitness centers).

and health care are very different, and there have been relatively few inpatient referrals.

INTEGRATING HEALTH PROMOTION INTO HOSPITAL CONTINUUM

Hospital executives are beginning to learn how to effectively integrate health promotion programs into the hospital's continuum of care:

- *Screening programs* have the lowest costs and highest returns among health promotion and wellness activities. One-day community health screening efforts cost as little as $500 to $5,000. Many hospital-sponsored screening programs utilize volunteers. Lab costs are minimal with volume testing. Cholesterol screening, one of the hottest kinds of screening today, is reportedly yielding, for every 100 tests, 1–5 referrals for physician follow-up and additional testing.
- *Community health education programs* are widespread and low cost. Many programs utilize in-house speakers from the medical and nursing staffs.

Outside speakers are used successfully for one-day "theme" events. Stor-
mont-Vail Medical Center in Topeka, Kansas, headlined a one-day conference on women's health with national columnist Ellen Goodman. The
session drew more than 250 women. Fees for such educational programs
range from $5 to $25.

- *Disease-oriented education programs* tie into hospital-sponsored ambulatory
  services or are linked by physician referral to the medical staff. Alameda
  Hospital, of Alameda, California, a 145-bed community hospital, has proac-
  tively utilized community health education to stimulate demand for hospital
  and physician services. Its Health Directions lecture recently drew 250 local
  residents for a program on cardiac care. Six hundred turned out for the
  hospital's Fit or Fat series. Another program, No Butts about It, is for
  people who want to stop smoking; it consistently fills up, and the hospital
  reports an 83 percent success rate. Why Weight, a weight control program
  just launched, is already full. A CPR class marketed jointly with the local
  Red Cross trained 110 community residents. Coming up—cardiac technology and stress reduction. The hospital's market research has found "word
  of mouth" to be among the strongest market strategies in its local service
  area. The public education efforts reinforce the hospital's value to the community and inform local residents of hospital programs.

- *Occupational health programs* are a natural complement of health promotion. Employers spent more than $12.4 billion on care for disabled
  employees and $400 million on industrial medicine, according to a recent
  report. Some free-standing industrial medicine centers have been successful, but others, such as the one sponsored by HealthWest of Chatsworth, California, have been $500,000 losers, despite extensive planning
  and market research. Hospitals today are eschewing expensive capital
  investments in free-standing centers. Instead, hospitals are taking screening and health education programs directly to the worksite and collab-
  orating with employers in the development of corporate health risk
  management programs.

ELDERCARE: THE NEXT MARKET FOR HEALTH PROMOTION

Older Americans are health care's main customers for hospital, physician,
and health-related services. The elderly consume more than 40 percent of national
health expenditures, from high-tech transplants to home and ambulatory care.
A hospital that is designing health promotion services for the elderly may provide
some or all of the following (Dychtwald and Zitter 1986):

- health education classes (e.g., coping with chronic illness)
- self-care instruction (e.g., use of medication)
- accident prevention counseling (e.g., home safety modification)
- healthy living classes and workshops (e.g., weight loss)
- behavior change programs (e.g., smoking cessation)
- peer support groups (e.g., Alzheimer's support groups)
- emergency medical training (e.g., CPR)
- physical fitness (e.g., senior aerobics)
- life enhancement programs (e.g., retirement planning)

Many senior health promotion programs are packaged with senior membership plans. Geriatrics consultant Peter Yedidia of San Francisco–based Geriatric Health Systems estimates that more than 40 percent of U.S. hospitals now offer senior membership plans. Fees range from $5 to $25 per month. Some plans emphasize health promotion, whereas others add Medicare benefits coordination. This market is heating up, with multiple hospitals in the same markets competing for senior loyalties. Expect hospitals to step up health promotion benefits and services under senior membership plans in the next 18–24 months in order to stay competitive.

THE HEALTHWISE HEALTH AND WISDOM WORKSHOP

The concept of senior membership programs is a hot button in health care marketing. New programs are springing up everywhere. How can a hospital differentiate its senior plan from those of competitors? What will help create a lasting impression in the minds of senior consumers? How can the hospital generate a sense of consumer loyalty by means of its senior plan? Perhaps through a Health and Wisdom Workshop, suggests Don Kemper, founder of Healthwise, based in Boise, Idaho. Hospitals using this franchised program typically offer the 90-minute seminar as an orientation to its senior membership program. Participants are given copies of *Growing Wiser*, a 400-page guide to senior health promotion that covers a wide array of senior health concerns. The guide is an introduction to a series of Growing Wiser health education and self-care classes oriented to senior health promotion that the hospital may offer as follow-up.

STAYWELL—A MODEL EMPLOYER HEALTH PROGRAM

Staywell demonstrates the contribution that a health promotion program can make to an employer's bottom line. In a long-range study, Minneapolis-based

Control Data Corporation reported savings of 20 percent in employee health expenses by employees participating in a long-range health promotion program. Control Data recently completed a five-year evaluation of the cost and impact of its corporate health promotion program, trademarked as Staywell. To assess impact, 1,500 employees enrolled in Staywell were matched with 1,500 "control" workers who had similar health benefits but who were not enrollees.

No doubt about it, Staywell lived up to its name! The results constituted powerful evidence for the benefits of promoting employee health: health costs were 20 percent lower for Staywell participants. Staywell reduced smoking, encouraged fitness among the sedentary, slimmed the overweight, and promoted higher seat belt use. The result: healthier life styles, lower health expenditures. For example, smokers had 18 percent higher health costs; "couch potatoes" had health expenses that were 14 percent greater than formerly sedentary workers who had raised their exercise levels under Staywell.

According to David R. Anderson, manager of R & D for Staywell, the program is part of a long-range business strategy. The Staywell program grew out of Control Data's decade-long development of Plato—a constellation of computer-assisted instruction (CAI) programs. Starting with six modules of wellness-oriented CAI, Staywell has developed a continuum of health instruction, both instructor led and self-study. From a core of offerings in smoke cessation and weight reduction, the scope of Staywell has broadened to include life style, safe driving, and consumerism.

Initially home grown for Control Data employees, Staywell blossomed into a national network of more than 50 hospital distributorships. Sponsors include Memorial (Long Beach, California), Intercommunity (Covina, California), and other community hospitals from coast to coast. Staywell's hospital distributors profit by selling "turnkey" health promotion programs to local employers and by contracting to provide the Staywell instruction programs directly to employees.

Health risk management is Staywell's newest market initiative. It's computerized health assessment program uses new software to develop employee health profiles. Health risk management finds high-risk employees through screening, then targets them for intensive education and risk reduction to avoid high-cost hospitalizations. The formula is to find employees at high risk and work with them, a proactive strategy that plays well to employers who are frustrated with rising health costs.

Staywell appeals to corporate health benefits managers who have already achieved short-term gains in cutting health costs and now want to invest in healthier workers and retirees for the long term. Staywell has competition from the Travelers Insurance Company's Taking Care and from Johnson and Johnson's health promotion program. All three major employers are targeting other Fortune

500 companies as well as midsized firms with a sophisticated perspective on health promotion investments.

SAINT AGNES' CORPORATE HEALTH RISK MANAGEMENT PROGRAM

America's major corporations are beginning to recognize the value of promoting health. The cost of employee medical benefits is rising at an alarming rate which now threatens to erode the profitability of some of the largest U.S. corporations. The problems employers face are:

- Employers' health-related expenses constitute the fastest rising cost of doing business in the United States.
- U.S. businesses pay approximately one-half of the nation's health care bills.
- Corporate expenses for health care are rising at a rate that, if unchecked, could eliminate all the profits of the average Fortune 500 company in eight years.

As a consequence, health care cost containment measures are becoming an increasingly important priority in our nation's board rooms. Employers are taking a more proactive approach to reducing these costs. The practices that businesses are adopting include preadmission authorization, direct contracting with providers, utilization review, increasing the employees' share of costs through higher deductibles and copayments, and establishing self-insured health benefit plans.

One of the latest and most promising techniques to reduce health care spending is corporate health risk management, an innovative approach that applies the well-established principles of traditional risk management to the health of the employee group.

Ron Kelsey, writing in the *Hospital Entrepreneurs' Newsletter*, provides an account of a program (Health Risk Management) developed and marketed by Saint Agnes Regional Medical Center, a regional tertiary facility in Fresno, California, where Kelsey was the vice president of corporate marketing. Saint Agnes contracted with a major California manufacturing company in 1986 (Kelsey 1988).

In its initial contact with the employer, Saint Agnes solicited issues and concerns from each level of management. Senior managers feared that employees might suspect the program was a guise for drug testing or that employees might be terminated if tests showed them to be at high risk. To alleviate this fear, each employee was given a copy of Saint Agnes' policy on confidentiality, which guaranteed that laboratory and personal risk data would be reported only to them at their home addresses.

Personal Health Risk Assessment

A total of 262 employees took part in the Health Risk Management program. Their personal health risks were evaluated through a medical-statistical data base analysis using a life style risk factor model developed by Swedish Health Management Systems in Denver. The health risks of the entire work force were also compared with a sample from the national population (cases per 100,000), adjusted to match the age, race, and sex composition of the study group.

The analysis focused on a number of modifiable life style–related risk factors. These factors are typically responsible for a significant portion of an employer's total health care costs and are most amenable to change through personal or organizational interventions: uncontrolled hypertension, chronic heavy drinking, high-risk cholesterol levels, current cigarette smoking, excess body weight, inadequate exercise, and failure to use seat belts.

Saint Agnes used the information to generate a summary report for management that identified the percentages of employees at risk for the seven evaluated factors. Typically, 25 percent of employees fell into a high-risk category and then received special counseling, a physician referral, or both.

Corporate Cultural Assessment

Saint Agnes' corporate health risk assessment of the California manufacturer showed that its employees viewed smoking as the norm and that exercise did not have a high value. More than 50 percent of those surveyed indicated that lack of communication was a stress-inducing factor within the corporate culture. Nutritional norms also were far less than optimum, as 42 percent of the employees considered doughnuts and coffee a typical breakfast. Alcohol and drug use was another potential problem: 6 percent of the employees categorized themselves as heavy consumers (15 or more drinks per week) and nearly 25 percent expressed interest in confidential services relating to alcohol or drug use.

The questionnaire also showed that 60 percent of the employees believed they could improve their health by changing life styles. Programs that attracted the greatest employee interest were personal wellness, nutrition, weight control, stress management, and personal exercise. Not surprisingly, employees were more reluctant to change their smoking and drinking habits. Approximately 75 percent did not want to make changes in alcohol consumption and 65 percent were not interested in smoke cessation programs.

Financial Impact of Risk Identification

The report by Saint Agnes showed that the health risk estimates for stroke, heart attack, and death secondary to motor vehicle accidents were significantly higher than those for the matched group from the national data base. To establish a base line for measuring the economic impact of the risk factors, Saint Agnes conducted a claim and loss experience analysis detailing how the manufacturer had historically spent its health care dollars by service type, diagnosis, and benefit group. Turnover and absentee rates were evaluated to serve as benchmarks for any subsequent intervention efforts.

This analysis indicated that 48 percent of the manufacturer's total health care costs resulted from treatment of employees with health concerns, diseases, or disabilities resulting from the seven modifiable risk factors. The percentages of high-risk employees for these factors were as follows:

- chronic heavy drinking: 6.6 percent
- uncontrolled hypertension: 25.8 percent
- high cholesterol levels: 12.9 percent
- excess body weight: 27.0 percent
- cigarette smoking: 30.0 percent
- inadequate exercise levels: 21.3 percent
- failure to wear seat belts: 39.3 percent

Without intervention programs to reduce risk levels, the projected three-year health care cost resulting from these risk factors would be more than $600,000 for the employer. The information, broken out for each risk factor for one- and three-year periods, can then be compared with intervention program costs to yield valuable "bottom-line" savings for each proposed activity.

Corporate Risk Management Plan

Saint Agnes developed a health risk management plan for the corporation that outlined the potential economic impact for each of the seven identifiable health risks and presented more than 20 intervention alternatives. For each factor, the hospital recommended a program that offered the greatest potential net savings. For example, the hypertension risk factor would cost the company nearly $100,000 over three years; the risk management plan recommended an onsite treatment clinic that would generate net savings of $50,000 per year.

After reviewing Saint Agnes' detailed management report, the company began intervention techniques that addressed several different life style issues. Even though employees indicated they did not want management intervention in their smoking habits, they became motivated to change after receiving their personal risk profiles. Other intervention techniques included providing weight management classes that emphasized nutrition, restocking company vending machines with healthier snacks, monitoring seat belt use at the parking lot gate, and encouraging workers to participate in employee assistance plans for alcohol and drug problems.

Early results from the corporate health risk management program are promising, with savings approaching or exceeding targeted goals. The program demonstrates that many health risks are reducible or preventable through life style modification. This is a new and effective way to combat rising health care costs in a new partnership between physicians or hospitals and employers. Corporate health risk management is a management tool for quantifying the advantages of health intervention and directing employers to specific actions that will generate the greatest savings. More important than short-term savings are the long-term returns that result from a healthier, more productive, and profitable work force—and a healthier group of retirees tomorrow.

"HEALTH FAIR" STORES: THE RETAILING OF AMERICAN HEALTH CARE

U.S. hospitals have searched long and hard for a way to "retail" health care products and services to the mass market of American consumers. They need wait no longer. A new concept in marketing health-related products has been developed in Texas that may provide enterprising hospitals and multihospital systems with a way to "manage their markets" through retail health stores.

The concept is simple: Mall + Medicine + Cross-Sell = Health Fair. Health Edco, of Waco, Texas, is the originator of the Health Fair store. Their intent is to franchise the stores nationally, placing them in the country's top 100–200 shopping malls, with each store owned and operated by a local hospital or multihospital system. Once the top mall locations are taken, competitors will be locked out by exclusive, protected-territory arrangements and thus be forced to imitate the Health Fair concept in second-tier retail locations.

Picture a brightly lit retail store in a suburban shopping mall around the corner from Bloomingdales or another major anchor tenant. Shoppers are attracted by well-designed displays of books on parenting and personal health. Studies show that the average mall shopper spends three to five seconds deciding whether or not to go into a store. The upbeat, colorful decor of the stores invites customers to browse and buy. This is more than a health-oriented bookstore, much more. Parenting and family health are top-selling items, followed by health promotion and self-health. The average Waldenbooks or Brentanos bookstore will carry 400–600 health books; Health Fair stocks 5,000. There are home health and self-testing items, gift items, videotapes, and children's educational products.

Health Fair has other marketing secrets besides finding ideal mall locations. To begin with, the stores cross-sell hospital programs and services in a dozen different ways. In fact, they are essentially retail extensions of the affiliated hospitals. Store clerks are trained health professionals. In-store cholesterol testing gives results within moments, followed by a referral to a hospital program and clinician. Physician referral is on-line from the store countertop computer through computerized physician referral services. Specific hospital services, such as weight control, sports medicine, mammography, or diabetes clinics, can be promoted through in-store displays, signs, bag stuffers, and video displays. Enrollments and appointments can be made in the store through direct-line dialing or the countertop computer. Hospital-sponsored health insurance can be sold, similar to the way Sears sells Allstate.

Imagine the many possible tie-ins between store and hospital. For each newborn, the hospital gives the parents a coupon for a free infant car seat. Where is the coupon to be exchanged? At the Health Fair store, of course. Concerned about your troubled adolescent or aging parent? Readers browsing Health Fair bookshelves see not only pertinent literature but the telephone numbers and promotional materials of related programs of the hospital, such as adolescent psychiatry or hospital-sponsored case management for seniors. Coupons are provided in the store for discounts on hospital-based services. Hospital inpatients upon discharge are given discount coupons for durable medical equipment or self-testing devices—good only at the hospital's Health Fair store, naturally. A Health Fair store would be a natural asset for any hospital with a senior membership plan, community education classes, or marketing outreach programs.

Health Fair is more than a concept. Two Health Fair stores have been piloted by the Baylor Health System of Dallas and will wear the Baylor "brand-name." More Health Fair stores were opened in Houston and a half-dozen major metropolitan areas in 1988, with a dozen more planned for 1990.

Each Health Fair store is a joint venture between Health Edco and the sponsoring hospital or system. The store is sited in a top-quality mall location to reinforce the hospital's market presence in desired neighborhoods. A top-quality mall provides selective, high-traffic visibility for promotion of the health care provider's name and services. In turn, the hospital encourages its thousands of inpatients and outpatients, employees, and preferred customers to use the Health Fair store for health promotion and education. A mall location marks one of the hospital's preferred market zones and keeps its brand name visible 365 days a year.

Think of Health Fair as providing a seven-day-a-week promotion for the hospital and its portfolio of diagnostic and therapeutic services. Health Edco estimates there are only 800 top-quality mall locations across the country. The window of opportunity for retailing health care just opened.

TOMORROW'S WELLNESS MARKET

Each year about one in ten Americans is hospitalized. Are the other nine individuals candidates for health promotion? It isn't that simple, as American physicians and hospitals are learning. Like most "markets," the potential audience for health promotion is actually a constellation of niches.

Health promotion has a high potential for success. Much has been learned about development, distribution, and marketing the ultimate intangible: personal health. The most promising target market segments for health promotion services in the future are the following:

- *Employers*: As employers face 10–40 percent hikes in health insurance premiums and a potential $1–2 trillion of unfunded liability for retiree health benefits, they are coming to recognize the long-range investment value of health promotion.
- *Government*: Like employers, the federal government is coming to recognize the investment potential of health promotion; in the short term, elected officials must respond to the growing political clout of the senior lobby, whose number one issue is health.
- *Seniors*: The elderly constitute the fastest growing segment of the population and are the most concerned about their health. Senior membership plans bundled with health promotion will be one of the most competitive venues in the health care marketplace in the next one to three years.
- *Discretionary Purchasers*: Caught in a tightening revenue squeeze, America's hospitals need programs that will be used discretionally by more well-heeled consumers. Products and services that promote self-health and better living will sell very well, especially in the highly affluent 55–64 age group.
- *Hospital and Medical Office Employees*: Health promotion should start at home. This will reduce hospital-paid health benefits expenditures and demonstrate the value of health promotion. Hospitals should make a special effort to successfully engage employees in health promotion activities.

LOOKING FORWARD: THE MARKET FOR HEALTH PROMOTION HAS ARRIVED

Health promotion has come a long way from public health pamphlets in physician offices and hospital waiting rooms. Today it is an established product line in the portfolio of the average community hospital and a service of many physicians. To be successful, health promotion does not need million-dollar fitness or education facilities. Most importantly, it begins with an attitude that promoting the community's health is part of the value core of medicine and the civic mission of the hospital. Managing successful health promotion activities requires a skillful blend of marketing and management.

Health promotion programs are an investment in the future—a managed care future. As managed care grows, it is changing the fundamental assumptions of the health industry. No longer will health care providers only be rewarded when patients become ill. Through risk sharing and the "gatekeeper" concept, hospitals and physicians will become more deeply committed to protecting and promoting the health of their long-term customers. This is good economics and good public policy—and a smart investment. Not all health promotion efforts will show profits, but some things should be done from the heart. Health promotion is one!

STRATEGIC IMPLICATIONS FOR PHYSICIANS

1. *The definition of the practice of medicine is becoming broader.* Mainstream medicine is coming to accept a more holistic view of health and disease. Young physicians are trained to take a broader social and financial history of their patients. Therapies routinely include life style modification as well as prescription drugs. Medical practice is being reshaped by an accumulating body of knowledge of the antecedents and cofactors of disease.

2. *Physician risk sharing will encourage health promotion.* Health maintenance organizations will increase their use of physician risk-sharing as a way of controlling health plan expenditures. As physicians are placed in situations where they share a financial risk for the health costs of their patients, they have a direct economic incentive to promote a healthier life style which relies less on health services to maintain good health.

3. *Patients need to become partners in the therapeutic process.* If life style is a significant factor in health, then the patients must become the therapeutic partners of their doctors. Educating patients may be one of the most important roles for physicians.

4. *Doctors must learn communications skills to be more effective in persuading patients to remain under treatment and modify their life styles to reduce health risks.* With respect to many health risk factors, such as hypertension, more than half of the patients with diagnosed chronic diseases are not following a therapeutic regimen. Noncompliant patients are "time bombs" of acute disease. They are dangerous—and costly—in a managed care environment in which physicians are at financial risk. Physicians of the future may use robot telephone calls to their noncompliant patients encouraging follow-up visits to maintain medical supervision.

STRATEGIC IMPLICATIONS FOR HOSPITALS

1. *Hospitals will become health centers.* Every hospital of the future will offer a broad array of programs and services to enhance health as well as to treat disease.

2. *Risk sharing will provide incentives for promoting health.* Hospitals and physicians will increasingly be asked to take a share of financial risk in contracting with HMOs or directly with major employers. Hospitals will now have a long-range incentive to keep potential patients healthy and out of the hospital as much as possible. Only as a result of these direct incentives will hospitals begin to think of themselves as "health maintenance organizations."

3. *Walk the talk.* According to management consultant Nancy Austin, coauthor of *A Passion for Excellence*, the successful manager must "walk the talk." Take this advice: Health care organizations should be healthwise and healthy! Hospital employees work in a high-stress, high-risk environment. A hospital with a health maintenance self-concept should demonstrate its commitment by providing a healthy worksite and health-enhancing programs for its own work force.

BIBLIOGRAPHY

Bly, J.L. 1986. "Impact of Health Promotion on Health Care Costs and Utilization." *JAMA*, 19 December, 35–40.

Dubos, Rene. 1967. *Mirage of Health*. New Brunswick, N.J.: Rutgers University Press.

Dychtwald, Ken, and Mark Zitter. 1986. *The Role of the Hospital in an Aging Society*. San Francisco: Age Wave.

Ferguson, Marilyn. 1981. *The Aquarian Conspiracy: Personal and Social Transformation in the 1980s*. Los Angeles: Jeremy Tarcher.

Jenson, Joyce. 1989. "Hospital Diversification Proliferates in Past 5 Years." *Modern Healthcare*, 19: 48.

Kelsey, Ronald R. 1988. "Corporate Health Risk Management: Employers' Newest Tool To Reduce Health Care Costs." *Hospital Entrepreneurs Newsletter* 4.

Longe, Mary E. 1986. "Hospital-Based Community Health Promotion: A Status Report." *Family Community Health* (May): 72–78.

Peters, Tom, and Nancy Austin. 1985. *A Passion for Excellence*. New York: Random House.

Chapter 9

Behavioral Medicine

It is understandable that we know very little about health, since there is always a strong need to respond to and care for those who are sick. It is far simpler, much easier, more exciting and more personally satisfying to look for the dramatic medical 'magic bullets,' for dramatic surgical rescues, than it is to weigh, judge, and confirm the more complex determinants of health like behavior. . . .

—Robert Ornstein and David Sobel, *The Healing Brain*

Behavioral medicine will be the next growth opportunity for U.S. health care for the next three to five years. Already, the stakes are high. The annual cost of behavioral health services may exceed $100 billion each year for inpatient and ambulatory care of psychiatric and chemical dependency services. It is widely recognized that alcohol is a contributing factor in 30–50 percent of all hospital admissions. In the report *The Fifty Billion Dollar Drain*, researchers estimated that alcohol and drug abuse adds $27 billion to the annual cost of health insurance. This amount may be just the tip of the iceberg.

Mental health care is a ballooning market. Major employers and health insurers are experiencing double-digit increases in mental health costs despite employee costsharing, precertification, and diagnostic-related groups. Large companies are now paying 7–15 percent of their health costs for psychiatric treatment, according to the federal Bureau of Labor Statistics. A recent report in *Benefits News Analysis* states that 15–20 percent of health plan costs are now allocated to mental health services (Freudenheim 1986).

Behavioral health is a growth market but one which is coming under increasing buyer scrutiny. The growth potential is still strong, at least for providers who anticipate the trends and strive to satisfy major employers and insurers.

Increased buyer control of behavioral health care is a threat but also an opportunity. As a result of increasing control, behavioral medicine providers will have to cut inpatient stays, shift to ambulatory care, unbundle services, increase prices, seek niches such as adolescent psychiatry, develop and sell case management programs, and enter into risk-sharing, prepaid contracts.

RECESSION-RESISTANT MARKET

Behavioral health—psychiatric and chemical dependency services—has been among the most recession-resistant segments of health care, even with its high margins. Except for Medicare, most payers still pay charges. Employer-paid private insurance reimburses 80-90 percent of all psychiatric and drug dependency care.

Increasing competition in health care markets has not driven down behavioral medicine prices. Although Medicare has included psychiatric and chemical dependency care within its prospective payment system (PPS), the federal payment level is highly profitable. Experts believe Medicare erred when it set a single rate for psychiatric care provided in both nonpsychiatric and specialized psychiatric units (Taube et al. 1985). Hospitals with defined psychiatric units were allowed to apply for an exemption from DRG-limited payment and bill for charges in the cost reimbursement system. The result has been sizeable gains for hospitals.

DIMENSIONS OF THE BEHAVIORAL HEALTH MARKET

For the producers—community and psychiatric hospitals, psychiatrists, psychologists and related therapists—psychiatric and chemical dependency care is a growth market with high profitability. Profit margins can range as high as 28–30 percent for the hospital, according to industry analyst Kenneth Abramowitz of the New York investment firm Sanford C. Bernstein and Company (Kittrell 1986). Ambulatory behavioral medicine services can be lucrative. Psychiatry is one of the highest-earning medical specialties.

In an era of slipping admissions and declining lengths of stay in med-surg units, which are the hospitals' bread and butter, psychiatric and chemical dependency care have become among the strongest contributing profit sources. Providers need to expand their behavioral medicine business as a hedge against rising (and uncompensated) Medicare lengths of stay for many med-surg services.

HIGH-LEVEL COMPETITION—AND SPENDING—IN
BEHAVIORAL MEDICINE

Investor-owned health care companies have targeted this niche and are pursuing behavioral medicine intensely. Growth in psychiatric facilities is slowing from the high point in 1985, when the psychiatric bed supply expanded 41 percent. The chains made capital investments totaling more than $500 million in 1985 for expanded facilities and services. In 1985, the for-profit chains increased the number of their psychiatric beds by 30 percent while their nonprofit competitors boosted the number of their beds by 51.2 percent, according to *Modern Healthcare's* annual "multis survey" (Barkholz 1986). Expansion continued at a bullish pace in 1986, with a 22 percent increase. Now the chains are slowing their expansion and seeking higher profitability. In 1987, supply grew by 13 percent among investor-owned chains, while nonprofit systems increased the number of new beds by 12 percent. The slowing pace of expansion suggests that inpatient psychiatric care is entering a period of controlled growth.

The chains continued increasing the bed supply in 1987–1988, but not at the 1985–1986 pace. Community Psychiatric Centers of Santa Ana invested $60 million to add eight new facilities in 1987 and six more in 1988. Charter Medical Corp added 10 facilities in 1987, at a cost of $160 million. Hospital Corporation of America (HCA) added 10 facilities, boosting the number of its hospitals to 53. Psychiatric construction was 15 percent of HCA's $500 million capital budget for 1987. Psychiatric Institutes of America added 10 facilities in the past year, bringing its inpatient facilities to 57. The nonprofit health systems matched the pace of the proprietaries, increasing the number of behavioral health facilities by 27.9 percent in 1986, for a national total of 266 facilities with 24,192 beds.

Who are the biggest providers in behavioral medicine? In 1987 Charter Medical operated more facilities than any national psychiatric chain, with 63 facilities, followed by National Medical Enterprise's (NME's) Psychiatric Institutes of America (57), HCA's Psychiatric Company (53), and Community Psychiatric (40). HCA was the largest provider of inpatient psychiatric care in 1988, in terms of the number of beds (6,217).

Despite the slowdown in construction, demand continues at a high level. Patient revenues at HCA rose 20.8 percent to $412 million in 1987. However, HCA's revenues were topped by Charter's, which totaled $559 million, an increase of 34 percent. NME experienced an 83 percent occupancy rate at its psychiatric facilities in 1987. As a result, NME is still expanding capacity and will operate 4,150 beds at the end of 1988. By 1989, all major chains were beginning to slow their investment in new facilities, and the inpatient market was becoming saturated by 1990. For the 1990s, growth will shift to ambulatory programs and residential treatment facilities.

REPOSITIONING INTO BEHAVIORAL MEDICINE MARKET

Some investor-owned companies are withdrawing from the general acute hospital market while expanding their behavioral health business. American Medical

International (AMI) and NME have divested a number of their general acute hospitals and increased the number of their psychiatric beds and facilities. Having abandoned their "supermed" ambitions and written off their HMO and insurance ventures, both companies are now repositioning themselves in the health care marketplace and concentrating on a limited number of high-potential niches like behavioral medicine.

Behavioral health services are a prime focus of the diversification efforts being made by health systems in anticipation of slow growth in inpatient demand and a greater emphasis by employers and insurance companies on outpatient care. As the major behavioral medicine buyers increase their scrutiny of inpatient care, both nonprofit and for-profit chains are rapidly diversifying into ambulatory, day-hospitalization, and long-term residential care facilities for behavioral medicine. New programs providing specialized services target adolescents and geriatric patients.

Psychiatric providers are developing complementary service lines, such as residential treatment facilities and day treatment centers. Behavioral medicine plays a role in the multilevel campus concepts of some hospitals. For example, HCA is placing new psychiatric facilities on the campuses of its acute care community hospitals. HCA is also forming joint ventures with other providers to build institutions in new markets. For the University of California at Davis, HCA is building a new 78-bed psychiatric facility adjacent to the university's medical center and medical school.

THE THREAT OF OVERBUILDING

Is there a danger of overbuilding and market saturation in behavioral medicine? In some regions, signs of overbuilding and impending market saturation are becoming apparent. In Houston, for example, the HCA operates three psychiatric facilities, and added a fourth in 1987. Even so, Gulf Pines, HCA's newest facility, achieved a 50 percent utilization rate within the first year. In addition to Gulf Pines, four other psychiatric hospitals opened in 1986, and another 130-bed facility opened in 1987. In 1988 Humana Hospital of Baywood doubled its psychiatric beds to 60 and opened a chemical dependency unit.

Houston has gained 1,095 new psychiatric beds since September 1985. Marketing is intense and so is competition. Advertising seems to help. HCA's facilities are averaging 77–85 percent occupancy. Humana's Baywood facility is full. The Houston area Healthcare Business Coalition reported to *Modern Healthcare* that psychiatric care was three times the national use rate. If the Houston use rates return to the national level, the Harris County Mental Health Association forecasts a surplus of 500 psychiatric beds by 1990.

MANAGEMENT CONTRACTS

The rapid proliferation of new behavioral medicine facilities has created a "management gap" and fostered a growth market for contract management firms. Of the nation's 6,000 general acute care hospitals, 1,418 operated inpatient psychiatric units in 1986, up 4 percent. Community hospitals operated 897 alcohol and chemical dependency units, an increase of 41 percent, according to the American Hospital Association (AHA 1987).

Contract management of hospital psychiatric services is expanding rapidly. In 1987, the number of managed psychiatric units grew 17 percent; a total of 185 units are under management agreement, up from 157 in 1986. Business is booming for companies like Psychiatric Institutes of America, which operates 43 psychiatric facilities and has management agreements with 30 psychiatric units in general acute hospitals, up from 15 last year. Mental Health Management, of McClean, Virginia, manages 77 units, mostly in general acute hospitals. CompCare, of Irvine, California, runs 30 psychiatric units and owns three facilities, and Republic Health Corporation of Dallas owns 16 facilities and manages 32 psychiatric and substance abuse units in community hospitals.

Nonprofit health systems are acquiring psychiatric units to complement their regional "cluster" marketing strategy of providing comprehensive services. Samaritan Health Services of Phoenix acquired Camelback Hospitals, a nonprofit, two-unit psychiatric chain. HealthOne Corporation of Minneapolis and Comprehensive Care Corporation jointly own a 247-bed psychiatric facility. Expect more nonprofit multi-hospital systems to buy or build behavioral medicine facilities in the 1990s and to develop comprehensive service systems.

The growing capacity of these health systems in behavioral health programs and facility management will allow them to participate in future managed care risk contracting for alcohol, drug, and mental health services.

SHIFTING EMPLOYER ATTITUDES CREATE A MARKET

Rising demand for behavioral health services reflects changing employer attitudes toward alcohol and mental health problems in the workplace. Employers now have more holistic views about health care and health benefits. Sophisticated employers recognize the importance of a long-term investment in the work force. High productivity is due as much to behavioral health as to physical health.

As employer attitudes broadened in the 1980s, major companies liberalized behavioral health benefits. After years of ignoring the problem, businesses began to deal in a more enlightened way with employees who suffered from psychological problems or chemical dependency. Health benefit policies were revised, so as to authorize treatment on both an inpatient and outpatient basis. Although there were limits on days of care and physician visits per year, demand soared.

Today, behavioral health coverage is widespread. According to a survey of 39 major companies with 14 million employees by the Health Insurance Association of America (1986), over 99 percent of the employees had coverage for inpatient mental health care and 97 percent had complementary coverage for outpatient services. Most employee mental health benefits were capped by total dollar limits, but employers had raised the limits in the five-year study period.

Attitudes have shifted in the American workplace. Employers now conceptualize emotional problems and alcohol and drug dependency as diseases, not as deviant behaviors or life styles. One response is the widespread adoption of employee assistance programs. These confidential employer-paid programs aid workers with alcohol, mental health, or drug abuse problems, and they have been well received by both management and the rank and file. Instead of firing workers with high absenteeism or poor safety records, employers now send them to rehabilitation programs—often in hospital-based psychiatric and drug units. According to a three-year study of employee assistance programs by the Alcohol, Drug Abuse, and Mental Health Administration, such programs successfully send 70 percent of workers back to the worksite.

MEDICARE REIMBURSEMENT FOR BEHAVIORAL MEDICINE

The federal government's implementation of DRG-based payment for psychiatric services has opened the door for the provision of needed behavioral health services to the elderly. Medicare's experience with case management for psychiatric diagnoses has not been entirely successful. Due to the continuing policy dispute over the efficacy of psychiatric DRGs, Medicare expenditures for behavioral medicine services are paid to many hospitals through cost reimbursement, not DRG-based case management.

To compensate for the inequity between costs of psychiatric care in defined psychiatric units and costs in med-surg units, the federal government has allowed an exemption from the prospective pay system for psychiatric hospitals and general hospitals with psychiatric units. They may charge Medicare on a cost reimbursement basis rather than accept the preset price under Medicare's DRG system. A large number of hospital psychiatric units and specialized psychiatric hospitals have sought the exemption.

THE PSYCHIATRIC DRGs: ARE THEY DIFFERENT?

Real discrepancies exist in the daily cost, per-case cost, and length of stay for psychiatric treatment between psychiatric units and general med-surg units.

It has been argued that DRGs are too simplistic to be applied to psychiatry. Research confirms that psychiatric DRGs explain only 3 percent of the variance in hospital lengths of stay. Health service researchers have applied themselves to the question: Are psychiatric DRGs inferior to general medical DRGs (Frank and Lane 1985)?

Analysts from the Johns Hopkins University found that both medical and psychiatric DRGs had a wider range of variation when compared with surgical DRGs, which involved much more predictable treatment patterns (Davis and Breslau 1984). The problem, the analysts believe, is that both medical and psychiatric are widely variable. The psychiatric DRGs are no worse than the medical DRGs in predicting appropriate cost or length of stay.

Attempts to construct a "better psychiatric DRG" have been frustrating, according to a HCFA research team. The alternative DRGs could only predict 22 percent of the variation in psychiatric lengths of stay (Frank and Lane 1985). The researchers suggested HCFA should search for an alternative basis for prospective payment, such as the mixed model the Veterans Administration is piloting, which uses a DRG-based system for acute care and per diem for long-term care. This finding may encourage HCFA to stay with Medicare's cost-based reimbursement for inpatient psychiatric care while it gains experience and research continues.

CASE MANAGEMENT OF BEHAVIORAL HEALTH

Buyers are posing a challenge for behavioral health care management. With mental health expenditures rising rapidly, buyers want insurers and providers to manage cost-effectively psychiatric and chemical dependency care. The solution is a case management approach. Think managed care, throw in prospective payment and provider risk sharing, and the stage is set for a dramatic shift in the already turbulent health care marketplace.

The changes could either throw into tumult one of the major profit centers of America's health care providers (alcohol, drug abuse, and mental health services) or create a new business opportunity—the managing of these services on a prospective basis.

Payers are now searching for a way to cut soaring expenditures for behavioral health services. Employer claims for behavioral health soared 15 percent in 1985–1986 and cost employers $156 per employee in 1986. Costs rose to $169 per employee in 1987, another 8 percent hike and have continued to climb.

The solution may be a special form of managed care—prospective contracting for case management of behavioral medicine services—which is both a threat and an opportunity for health care providers.

Payers Believe Costs Are Out of Control

From the perspective of payers, the cost of psychiatric and chemical dependency care is a runaway train. Already, government and private health insurance plans report their spending on psychiatric benefits is shooting up 10–20 percent a year, faster than for any other medical benefits. Large companies are spending 7–15 percent of their health care dollars on psychiatric care, with drug and alcohol cases absorbing more than a third of these costs (Blue Cross 1986).

Take Tenneco, a multinational company whose experience is typical. At Tenneco, behavioral health costs in 1986 were 8.1 percent of company health expenditures. Dependents filed only 17 percent of the claims for behavioral health, but their costs equaled 52 percent of the budget due to high use of inpatient care. Behavioral medicine may be a growth market for providers, but because of the expenditures payers are looking for someone to blame.

Expanding Costs Alarm Employers

Employer understanding of the problem has increased as major corporations become more sophisticated in analyzing their health benefits experience. Health care coalitions of employers now number more than 150. Many of the voluntary organizations of buyers are pooling their health care claims data to analyze the causes of their rising health costs.

The Florida Health Coalition, representing 29 of the largest employers in the state, believes these costs are way out of line, and launched a search for a company to develop a managed care system for behavioral health services as a way of coping with what it considers to be a "tremendous increase" in behavioral costs in 1985–1986. Coalition executive Stephen White reported that between 20–30 percent of employee health benefit dollars are spent on behavioral health services, based on data collected from the Florida employers ("Florida Coalition" 1986). The coalition selected Preferred Health Care, a Wilton, Connecticut, psychiatric case management firm. Preferred was established by 130-bed Four Winds Hospital of Katonah, New York. The Florida employers expect similiar results to the experience of CIBA-GEIGY (see "Case Study in Case Management" below).

EMPLOYER COST SHIFTING

Can behavioral health costs be curtailed? One potential solution for employers is to increase the employee's cost share for behavioral health services. For the past several years, cost shifting has been a leading strategy to reduce the expense to America's major businesses. According to an annual employer survey done by the Health Research Institute of Walnut Creek, California, employers continue to cope with health care cost rises by increasing employee deductibles and coinsurance levels (Hembree 1985). Most employee health policies cover 80 percent of inpatient costs, plus a specified number of ambulatory care visits. Some employers are now shifting behavioral health costs to employees by picking up only 50 percent of inpatient costs.

Employers are now realizing that cost shifting is only partially effective. William Hembree, director of the Health Research Institute, suggests there exists a pattern of health care use that cost shifting alone cannot fix. Employees fall in three groups. The first group consists of employees who do not use the employer's plan, negating the value of any deductible or coinsurance program. The second group—and probably the largest—includes employees who infrequently use the plan. Cost shifting will influence their health care utilization, but this group is responsible for relatively minor expenditures. The third group is made up of a small number of employees with serious health care problems. Such employees quickly run up health expenses beyond the thresholds of coinsurance and deductibles. But the crux of the problem, believes Hembree, is that these employees are too emotionally involved in their problem to worry about comparative shopping (Kittrell 1986).

CASE STUDY IN CASE MANAGEMENT

A potentially promising solution may be a combination of case management, prospective payment, and risk sharing.

Few employers, barely 1 percent in a recent survey of 1,500 major companies, have utilized case management (O'Sullivan and Brody 1986). It is complex and needs to be grounded in a solid and well-analyzed data base of claims experience. If the payer sets rates too high, providers take advantage. If rates are pegged below average costs, few providers will want to participate.

The administrative complexity of rate setting is multiplied when alcohol, drug abuse, and mental health are involved. As one discharge planning expert recently wrote, "Although much has been learned about the underlying biological, genetic and biochemical aspects of mental illness over the last decade, psychiatry still less precisely predicts outcome as a function of its ministrations than many other medical specialities. The human mind has proven far more difficult to treat than the heart, lungs, and kidneys" (O'Sullivan and Brody 1986).

That's not all. Many of the mentally ill also have physical problems. Their inability to take on responsibility may impede the self-care necessary to manage physical health problems (e.g., diabetics not controlling their diets). Difficulty in following the doctor's orders or in maintaining physical health may be compounded by schizophrenia, psychotropic medication, or drug abuse.

Case Management Works

Setting rates and standards for behavioral health patients won't be easy for either buyers or sellers. But it has been done successfully in one of America's most competitive health care markets: the Twin Cities. Group Health, a major Twin Cities HMO, developed a prototype case management system for chemical dependency patients in conjunction with the Metropolitan Clinic of Counseling (MCC).

At the time of the design and implementation of case management (in 1977), adult psychiatric inpatient lengths of stay averaged 28 days and adolescent stays ranged from 60 to 73 days. MCC developed a triage system for assessing mental health needs and planning treatment strategies, established a structured outpatient program, and contracted with a local hospital for short-stay inpatient care. It worked! Average length of inpatient stay has fallen to 10 days. MCC handles 65 percent of its capitated population of 325,000 exclusively as outpatients, and the remaining 35 percent receive some degree of inpatient care.

Two new programs have been developed to handle tougher problems. An ambulatory detoxification program handles withdrawals of one-third of its alcoholics on an outpatient basis, as well as 50 percent of opiate addicts and 80 percent of benzodiazepine addicts. MCC's "dual disorders" program manages patients with coexisting mental health and chemical dependency problems, primarily with outpatient therapy and support from Alcoholics Anonymous, buttressed by the use of antipsychotic, antidepressant, or antimania drugs. Individuals with dual disorders are at high risk for relapse.

Capitating an outside provider worked for this Twin Cities IPA- model HMO. The total cost of providing mental health and chemical dependency care has declined since 1977, when the HMO plan spent 22 percent of all benefits for alcohol, drug, and mental health care. The plan spent only 4–5 percent of benefits for ADM care in 1985. The number of inpatient days per 1,000 enrollees dropped from 125 in 1977 to 37 in 1982. The average length of stay for inpatient chemical dependency dropped from 23 days in 1976 to 10 days in 1983, and the average inpatient mental health stay was cut from 19.2 days to 10.3 days in the same period.

Similar results for a case management approach are reported by an Atlanta-based HMO (Merrill 1985). Under a managed care system for mental health, hospital use averaged 17 days per 1,000 enrollees, compared with another HMO that employed a traditional concurrent review system and used 77 inpatient days for every 1,000 employees.

Case Study in Case Management

Business is impressed with early results from the application of case management to psychiatric care. A case study in point is the CIBA-GEIGY Corporation, of Ardsley, New York. CIBA-GEIGY is a member of the Fairfield-Westchester employers health care coalition and is a sophisticated health care purchaser. Like other employers, CIBA-GEIGY watched its mental health costs soar in the early 1980s, rising from 9.5 percent of the company's overall health costs (in 1982) to 12.3 percent (in 1983). The average length of psychiatric stay was 29.5 days. Given its broad health benefits coverage—365 days annually with 80 percent coverage after 30 days for mental health services and a $250,000 lifetime limit—CIBA-GEIGY was vulnerable to high utilization (Rodriguez and Maher 1986).

By 1984, the company took steps to curtail its rising mental health expenses. Worksite health promotion and employee assistance programs were stepped up, and more efficient health claims processing was put into place. CIGA-GEIGY contracted with Preferred Health Care (PHC), a for-profit psychiatric review firm in Katonah, New York, to provide case management for its "outliers" (cases with long lengths of stay or indeterminate prognoses).

PHC's case management approach includes telephone-based preadmission and continuing care review. Its case managers are certified mental health professionals. In the pilot project, which involved 24 inpatient and three outpatient cases, PHC cut the average length of stay from 29.5 days in 1983 to 26 days by the end of 1984. PHC was then given the job of managing all inpatient mental health care, and it was able to further lower the average inpatient stay to 22.7 days by mid-1985. This was accomplished with an average of four phone calls or direct meetings between the PHC case manager and the treating psychiatrist or psychologist. Actual costs for evaluated care were 26 percent below expected costs. CIBA-GEIGY, naturally, is a satisfied customer.

PHC is not alone. Its prime competitor, American Psychiatric Management (APM), now provides capitated coverage for over 2 million insureds. Both companies started in the East, but the trend is spreading. PHC has recently negotiated a contract with GTE in California.

Case Management of Behavioral Medicine: The Opportunity

There are multiple business opportunities in the management of alcohol, drug abuse, and mental health services:

• establishing a PPO for alcohol, drug abuse, or mental health services

- entering into provider contracts with a behavioral health PPO as a member of a PPO network
- entering into an EPA for behavioral medicine services with an employer, insurer, or third party administrator
- establishing or expanding a claims review service for concurrent and retrospective claims review for behavioral health services
- establishing, acquiring or expanding employee assistance programs, with a prospective payment option for employers and other major purchasers

No doubt about it, case management of behavioral health care can be risky, but experienced case managers in firms like PHC and APM have been remarkably successful in bringing behavioral health utilization under control. They have demonstrated that case management is feasible and can be profitable in this area of health care. Now the future of this business opportunity is in the hands of management-minded physicians, hospitals, and health plans.

MENTAL HEALTH HMOs: MANAGED CARE AND BEHAVIORAL MEDICINE

As employers take a more active role in the provision and payment of mental health care for their employees, new kinds of managed care plans are emerging in response: mental health HMOs and PPOs. These "single-business" managed care plans are organizing networks of mental health providers that include lower-cost service and setting alternatives. The successful plans will be those that are sensitive and responsive to the specific mental health care needs of employers.

Mental health HMOs and PPOs are specialized organizations. They have developed computerized case management systems and protocols for the management of a wide range of mental health, alcohol, and drug abuse diagnoses. These new managed care plans hope to succeed by sharply reducing the use of inpatient psychiatric care and by emphasizing ambulatory and nonhospital treatment. Mental health HMOs and PPOs make wide use of nonphysician mental health professionals, outpatient treatment (especially for substance abuse), residential care, and partial hospitalization. Outpatient services are the gateway to inpatient services in the mental health managed care model.

The following principles will contribute to the success of managed care plans specializing in behavioral medicine, according to Jim Bakhtiar, medical director of Heights Psychiatric Hospital and Chairman of the Department of Mental Health at Lovelace Medical Center, Albuquerque, New Mexico (Masters 1988):

- Understand demographics, populations, and the incidence and prevalence of mental illness.

- Understand the types, roles, costs, knowledge base, and most appropriate use of mental health professionals.
- Develop comprehensive services, including inpatient, outpatient, partial hospitalization, emergency, and residential care services.
- Monitor patient care and costs within the system through the use of information systems.
- Develop quality assurance and utilization review programs for every aspect of the comprehensive care system.
- Interface and coordinate outpatient and inpatient services to allow for continuity of care.

Managed mental health care is a high-potential market. Already, LifeLink, a mental health HMO based in Orange County, California, covers more than 1.5 million customers in southern California. Nearly 500,000 of these insureds were subcontracted by HealthNet of California, which transferred its responsibility for mental health benefits to LifeLink. This is not a business for the timid. LifeLink is at financial risk for the enrollees. Utilizing expertise gained in managing Treatment Centers of America, LifeLink has developed a select network of behavioral medicine providers to which it channels patients. Case management is continuous. It begins with the development of a formal treatment plan for every patient and includes ongoing monitoring of the progress of care.

Managed mental health plans use hospital services much more sparingly than traditional insurance companies. The National Association of Private Psychiatric Hospitals (NAPPH) found that only 2 percent of the patient days of its members were paid by managed care plans in 1987. The average inpatient length of stay for psychiatric diagnoses is already falling. NAPPH data show the average length of stay in 1987 was 30.6 days, down from 33 days in 1986. Managed care plans will push the average inpatient length of stay for psychiatric admissions into the low 20s by the early 1990s.

TREATMENT GUARANTEES

Treatment guarantees! That's the last thing anyone expected in behavioral health. In a full-page ad in the *Wall Street Journal*, CompCare, of Irvine, California, introduced its "care promise" of free retreatment for patients who successfully complete its chemical dependency program but have a relapse within five years. The marketing campaign is targeted at payers, especially employers, insurance companies, managed care systems, and volume purchasers. About 15 percent of patients treated at CompCare facilities need more treatment, the company reported to *Modern Healthcare* (Wallace 1986).

The guarantee concept is catching on. In Salt Lake City, the Wasatch Canyons Hospital, a 104-bed psychiatric hospital of the Intermountain Health Care system, has launched a media campaign featuring its treatment guarantee. The Salt Lake City region became intensely competitive after deregulation in 1985, when eight new psychiatric facilities were built in an 18-month period. Patients may participate for as few as two days to qualify for the retreatment promise. This is a bold marketing initiative to counter low occupancy among the nine local facilities. The guarantee program may give Intermountain a competitive edge.

EMERGING MARKETS: ADOLESCENT PSYCHIATRY

Adolescent psychiatry is a market niche with real growth opportunities, but an appropriate marketing approach is critical to success. Bridgeway Hospital, in North Little Rock, Arkansas, developed the "YouthCare" concept when it saw the potential need for adolescent behavioral health services in its region. The only local program focused on adolescent depression. There were no services for teenage alcohol, drug, or behavioral problems.

Bridgeway's radio and print ads convey two themes: "Kid problems are our business" and "Is your kid loaded?" An R.N. was placed in charge of inquiries, and a tracking form was used for every phone call. The hospital also initiated direct sales calls to mental health professionals, physicians, and psychiatrists. A statewide referral network of social service agencies was developed.

Behavioral medicine ad campaigns were a successful investment. YouthCare's average length is 35 days, with revenues of $30,000 to $35,000 per admission. The ads resulted in ten admissions per month (the costs were covered with one or two admissions). Census rose in nine months from 17 to 95 percent and has averaged 80 percent in succeeding months even though other local hospitals have now entered the market.

CONCLUSION: BEHAVIORAL MEDICINE PRESENTS NEW OPPORTUNITIES

The last frontier of science is the human brain, and the next frontier for health care, in the 1990s, is behavioral medicine. Psychiatrists, behavioral psychologists, and physiologists are working to understand the mind-body connection. As this connection is better understood, better treatments will follow. Behavioral medicine—including psychiatric, alcohol, and drug abuse services—is a high-potential market for health care organizations. Now it's up to the innovators and market leaders to develop the new programs (specialized behavioral health HMOs and PPOs), assume the risk for service delivery, put in place the case management and review systems, and set the standards for tomorrow's alcohol, drug abuse, and mental health care.

STRATEGIC IMPLICATIONS FOR PHYSICIANS

1. *Behavioral medicine will be a growth field.* As medical and scientific understanding of the mind-body connection increases, behavioral medicine will continue to expand. New knowledge and more case finding will cause a rise in the numbers and types of mental health–related disorders and patients.
2. *Behavioral medicine is rapidly growing in importance for occupational health.* The rising incidence of stress-related claims under workers' compensation is one sign of the market shift. Broadening employer attitudes make employees more willing to refer themselves for treatment for behavioral problems. Mental health, alcohol, and drug abuse problems may be responsible for 40 percent or more of all occupational medicine patients in the future.
3. *A direct threat to psychiatrists and other physicians working in behavioral medicine is the increase in status of nonphysician therapists.* New managed care HMOs and PPOs prefer to use the lower-priced therapists as an alternative to physicians who often charge $100 or more per therapy hour.
4. *The growth of managed mental health care will change the rules and reimbursement for behavioral medicine.* Managed care plans will prefer ambulatory care, outpatient treatment centers, and nonhospital alternatives. These plans will be very active in monitoring and controlling physician treatment. Expect an expansion of this form of private regulation through reimbursement policies and treatment procedures that will limit the independence of judgment of physicians treating mental health, alcohol, and drug abuse patients.

STRATEGIC IMPLICATIONS FOR HOSPITALS

1. *Hospitals, physicians, and other behavioral health providers should consider participating in risk-sharing arrangements.* Given the trends, providers should experiment with capitated behavioral medicine on a fee-for-service basis where reimbursement is calculated according to a pre-negotiated schedule of fees and discounts. The variation in behavioral health services and lengths of stay is very broad. This could provide a

good opportunity—or be a deep pool of lost costs. For those who can manage risks, the rewards could be substantial.

2. *Behavioral medicine is an emerging market. Now is the time to explore and move rapidly.* Today's marketplace is not for the timid. The market for capitation and case management in behavioral health could solidify within two to three years—or sooner. Don't miss this window of opportunity.

3. *An employee assistance program can provide a good base from which to expand.* Recent data from the federal Bureau of Alcohol, Mental Health and Drug Abuse showed substantial benefits for employers resulted from investment in employee assistance programs (Medical Benefits 1986). There was no significant difference in performance between in-house employer programs and outside contractors. Take advantage of this opportunity by building or buying a franchised employer assistance program or by joining an established network of such programs.

4. *Lower inpatient use should be expected with case management.* The buyers are already shifting away from reliance on inpatient services and toward ambulatory care. Expect more intense payer scrutiny and heavier concurrent review of behavioral medicine inpatients which could cut inpatient lengths of stay by 50 percent by 1995.

5. *Diversification of behavioral health services is a reasonable strategy.* The CIBA-GEIGY experience showed that 65 percent of behavioral medicine patients could be managed entirely with ambulatory care, and inpatient admissions and lengths of stay fell dramatically. Expect a similiar impact on inpatient facilities, and diversify now into ambulatory, day hospitalization, and long-term residential care.

6. *Innovation could make the difference.* One of the "medical hotels" operated by GuestHouse of America, of San Antonio, Texas, is now being used for residential treatment of behavioral medicine patients in conjunction with a nearby hospital's comprehensive behavioral health program.

BIBLIOGRAPHY

AHA. 1987. *Hospital Statistics*. Chicago: AHA.

Barkholz, David. 1986. "System Shows Strong Growth in Number of Psychiatric Beds." *Modern Healthcare*, 6 June, 108–12.

Blue Cross Association. 1988. "High Cost of Mental Health." *Blue Cross Short Shots*, 9 January.

Care Institute. Comprehensive Care Corporation. 1986. *The Fifty Billion Dollar Drain*. Irvine, Calif.: Care Institute, Comprehensive Care Corporation.

Cox, John R. et al. 1985. "Chemical Dependency: Medical Issue or Political Problem." In *HMOs Confronting New Challenges: Proceedings of the 1985 Group Health Institute*. Washington, D.C.: Group Health Association of America.

Davis, Glenn C., and Naomi Breslau. 1984. "DRGs and the Practice of Psychiatry." *Medical Care* 22:595–96.

Drucker, Jack, et al. 1985. "Who's Afraid of Mental Health?" In *HMOs Confronting New Challenges: Proceedings of the 1985 Group Health Institute*. Washington, D.C.: Group Health Association of America.

"EAPs Are Effective—Three Year Study Finds." 1986. *Medical Benefits*, 30 September, 5.

"Florida Coalition Seeking Mental PPO to Slash Treatment Costs." 1986. *Health Care Competition Week*, 22 December, 6.

Frank, Richard G., and Judith R. Lave. 1985. "The Psychiatric DRGs: Are They Different?" *Medical Care*. 23:1148–55.

Freudenheim, Milt. 1986. "Business and Health: Mental Health Costs Soaring." *New York Times*, 7 October, 30.

Health Insurance Association of America. 1986. *A Profile of Group Major Medical Expense Insurance in the United States*. Washington, D.C.: Health Insurance Association of America.

Hembree, William E. 1985. "Getting Involved: Employers as Case Managers." *Business and Health* (July-August): 11–14.

Hospital Statistics: 1985 Edition. 1985. Chicago: American Hospital Publishing.

Kittrell, Alison. 1986. "Employers Turn to Managed Care, Utilization Review to Control Costs." *Modern Healthcare*, 9 May, 96–97.

Masters, Guy. 1988. "Managed Mental Health Care." *PPO Postscript* (Arthur Young/Brighton Consulting, Los Angeles) 6 (July): 1–2.

Merrill, Jeffrey C. 1985. "Defining Case Management." *Business and Health* (July-August): 5–9.

"Mushrooming Psych Costs." 1986. In *Short Shots*. San Francisco: Blue Cross of California.

Ornstein, Robert, and David Sobel. 1987. *The Healing Brain*. New York: Simon and Shuster, 27.

O'Sullivan, Anne, and Michael Brody. 1986. "Discharge Planning for the Mentally Disabled." *Quality Review Bulletin* (February): 55–67.

Owens, Arthur. 1986. "Earnings: Have They Flattened Out for Good?" *Medical Economics*, 8 September, 162–81.

Rodriguez, Alex R., and John J. Maher. 1986. "Psychiatric Case Management Offers Cost, Quality Control." *Business and Health* (March): 14–17.

Taube, Carl A., et al. 1985. "Prospective Payment and Psychiatric Discharges from General Hospitals with and without Psychiatric Units." *Hospital and Community Psychiatry* 36:754–60.

Taube, Carl, Eun Sul Lee, and Ronald N. Forthofer. "DRGs in Psychiatry." *Medical Care* 22:597–610.

Wallace, Cynthia. 1986. "Psychiatric Management Firms Capitalize on Growing Market." *Modern Healthcare*, 10 October, 68–69.

Chapter 10

AIDS, Ethics, and Economics

AIDS is a very new disease and most doctors are very confused about its treatment. Most have not been trained generally to accept the patient as full partner in the healing process. . . . The doctor's challenge with an AIDS patient seems to be to keep you alive until a cure is discovered. Regrettably, hospitals also go along with this, in their competitive attitude towards who has the largest market share of AIDS patients. The AIDS patient with insurance is clearly a cash cow. The AIDS patient is also today's leper, the focal point of attitudes similar to those of 100 years ago.
—Hank Koehn, *"My Passage through AIDS: A Prominent Los Angeles Businessman Reflects on His Life and His Fate"*

AIDS is a "wild card" disease that is causing a crisis of global proportions. It is the greatest challenge U.S. physicians, hospitals, and health providers have ever faced. By 1990, an estimated 100,000 AIDS cases will have been diagnosed across the nation. By 1991, some 270,000 Americans may have AIDS. The RAND Corporation estimates the five-year health costs of AIDS care (1986–1991) may range from $15 billion to $113 billion (Pascal 1987). Is the AIDS crisis a doomsday scenario or a "growth market" that will fill empty hospital beds and physician waiting rooms?

It is both. AIDS is a growing problem with no cure in sight. Yet it will create a surge of demand for hospital, long-term care, home health, and physician services. AIDS is creating an emerging market that needs innovative management and financing strategies.

AIDS: A CATASTROPHE WAITING TO HAPPEN

AIDS is a catastrophe waiting to happen to the health industry. America's hospitals and medical profession are woefully unprepared for the "AIDS wave."

In a national survey of 300 health executives, physicans, and industry observers done for the *Healthcare Forum* (Coile and Grossman 1987), the experts predicted that in the 1990s the following will occur:

- AIDS will reach global epidemic levels.
- Every community hospital will have AIDS cases.
- There will be too many AIDS patients to "mainstream" into standard med-surg units.
- Hospices and home health agencies will be the preferred settings for AIDS patients.
- Some health workers will demand—and get—"combat pay" for handling AIDS cases.
- As the AIDS crisis worsens, a number of caregivers will refuse to treat AIDS patients.
- Insurers and employers will mandate AIDS testing.
- The cost of AIDS care will overwhelm local resources.
- Congress will enact a Medicare-type program for AIDS victims.
- Community hospitals will support a "federalization" of AIDS, segregating patients into public facilities.
- Having numerous AIDS patients will hurt a hospital's image and census.
- Some hospitals will refuse to admit AIDS patients who have no health insurance.
- Hospitals and concerned health agencies will develop community plans for dealing with AIDS.

AIDS IS NOT A "MANAGEABLE PUBLIC HEALTH PROBLEM"

As of May 31, 1989 the number of AIDS cases reported worldwide reached 157,191 according to the World Health Organization (Hilton 1989). Given widespread underreporting, the organization believes the actual number exceeds 400,000. In the United States, the total number of people who have gotten AIDS exceeds 100,000, and of these nearly half are already deceased. An estimated 1.5 million Americans are "healthy seropositives," that is, people whose blood carries the AIDS infection but who have not developed the disease (Boffey 1988).

Despite the mounting AIDS toll, some experts have suggested that AIDS is a "manageable public health problem" no worse than polio or tuberculosis— and one for which a cure will soon be found. There is an "AIDS hysteria," according to one California hospital executive, and "there are other communicable diseases that are not as fearsome to the public though just as contagious'' (Coile and Grossman 1987).

As the AIDS problem worsens, expect that public paranoia about AIDS will rise. A majority of the *Healthcare Forum* panel predicted that in some localities public health officials will quarantine and even lock up dangerous AIDS patients. The continued promiscuity of a Canadian flight attendant diagnosed with AIDS and known to U.S. Public Health Service officials as "Patient Zero" pushed authorities to consider mandatory confinement before his death. Patient Zero was considered to be responsible for acquiring and spreading AIDS in New York in 1976 and may have started the U.S. invasion.

AIDS Will Test the Limits of Provider Compassion

As the AIDS problem continues to spread, some hospitals will refuse to admit AIDS patients without adequate health insurance, referring them to public facilities. This practice of "patient dumping" is illegal if the patient's condition is life threatening. One rural California hospital was sued for allegedly testing a man for AIDS against his will, refusing him an operation, and advising him to seek treatment in San Francisco. Preop blood testing for a hernia operation showed him to be HIV positive, although the patient had not given permission for an AIDS test. According to the lawsuit, the patient was told by a hospital physician that he would die if he had the operation there or at any other local hospital. After threat of legal action, the hospital did consent to perform the surgery (Weber 1988).

As the number of AIDS patients grows, every hospital can expect to see some. However, AIDS patients are still clustered in a handful of major metropolitan areas, predominantly on the East Coast, the West Coast, and Texas. Although all states now report AIDS cases, the numbers are small and many AIDS patients with sexually transmitted AIDS probably acquired the disease out of their home state.

The number of patients with blood-acquired AIDS is small. That there are any is a tragic result of the use of unscreened blood in the early 1980s before HIV testing of blood became universal in 1985. More than half of all hemophiliacs may be carrying the AIDS virus now. Blood-acquired AIDS is a significant problem for hospitals, physicians, and blood banks. A San Francisco AIDS patient won a $500,000 judgment against the Irwin Memorial Blood Bank for negligence, the first of an estimated 200 liability lawsuits pending against blood banks. Blood bank officials fear that AIDS personal injury lawsuits could threaten the financial viability of a number of the nation's major metropolitan blood banks.

AIDS Units: Modern Leper Colonies?

Fear of AIDS and lack of insurance among AIDS patients has led to a pattern of channeling AIDS patients to a small number of hospitals, mostly public facilities. Under pressure of demand, these facilities are specializing in AIDS treatment. Health executives believe that numerous AIDS patients may hurt a hospital's image. "But it's not right," protests an Arizona hospital administrator (Coile and Grossman 1987).

Right or not, an AIDS image problem could lead to a self-defeating cycle in which patients shun hospitals willing to treat AIDS cases and force AIDS patients into a dwindling number of hospitals still willing to accept them. Many hospital executives are haunted by the specter of the plague house. This scenario is dreaded in all regions, especially the South, according to the *Healthcare Forum* survey.

PROVIDERS FEAR RISING AIDS COSTS

A major problem for physicians, hospitals, and other providers of AIDS care is reimbursement. Few hospital managers believe that specialized AIDS units in community hospitals can be profitable or even break even. Fear of losses is high, especially after the closure of American Medical International's all-AIDS facility in Texas. The cost of AIDS care will exceed the resources of local hospitals and philanthropy as the AIDS problem spreads and losses mount. Three of four health care executives believe that losses on AIDS patients will inevitably rise unless there is a major infusion of public funds, most likely from the federal government.

Compounding the burden of AIDS costs will be the rising burden of liability insurance protection against AIDS for health workers. Such protection may become enormously expensive for the industry, as indicated by the judgment against the San Francisco blood bank. This could be an especially difficult problem for self-insured health care organizations.

AIDS Discrimination

With the widespread use of AIDS testing by insurers and employers, AIDS discrimination problems are mounting. The high cost of AIDS is an actuarial problem for insurers, who routinely reject any insurance applicant who tests HIV positive. Employers are beginning to use AIDS tests to screen out potential employees (Ricklefs 1987; Pear 1988). A number of wrongful dismissal cases are now pending, such as that filed by James Dorsey, an unemployed teenager who enrolled in classes at a U.S. Job Corps training program, then was dropped when the program learned he had tested positive for AIDS antibodies.

Some states, including California, Florida, Massachusetts, and Wisconsin have laws that restrict the use of AIDS tests for employee screening and require that lab results be kept confidential. A California ballot initiative defeated in November 1988 would have required that public health officials be informed of all positive AIDS tests and that all sexual partners of those who test HIV positive be traced and informed.

The courts are siding with AIDS patients against discrimination by health care providers. In New York City, an administrative judge awarded $26,647 to a man refused treatment by his longtime dental clinic. A California judge ruled against Centinela Hospital in Inglewood after the hospital excluded a gay man from an alcohol rehabilitation program. Delaware's attorney general forced the Nemours Foundation to drop its policy of transferring out seropositive patients from its Wilmington hospital.

AIDS Bailout: Scenario for a Federal AIDS Takeover

If no cure emerges within five years, AIDS will be a national—not a local—problem. Hardpressed state and local governments will lobby for a federalization of AIDS care. In the face of mounting AIDS caseloads and mounting losses, U.S. hospitals will lobby Congress to create a "Medic-AIDS" program to underwrite care for all people with AIDS.

Several potential solutions could be enacted. One option would be creation of a Medicare-type program for AIDS patients. Another would be to automatically qualify AIDS patients without insurance for state Medicaid programs. Still another would be to fund a national network of public AIDS facilities, perhaps reopening the former U.S. Public Health Service hospitals as specialized AIDS treatment centers. This solution would segregate AIDS patients, thereby bringing back an old trend—specialized facilities like the tuberculosis sanatoria of 50 years ago.

AIDS COSTS: CAN PROVIDERS SURVIVE THE AIDS WAVE?

AIDS costs give health care providers much cause for concern. Hospital stays are lengthy, between 15 and 25 days, and AIDS patients may be hospitalized three to six times over the course of their disease. AIDS patients need specialized home care and hospice services, and many nonhospital costs are poorly reimbursed. Treatment costs are boosted by the complexity of dealing with multiple opportunistic infections at the same time.

A major concern for all providers of AIDS care is reimbursement. Breaking even on AIDS care and achieving a reasonable net return is possible depending on case mix, as community hospitals and specialized AIDS units are demonstrating. Profitability is linked to insurance coverage. AIDS patients with private or group insurance are able to meet their costs. Patients dependent on Medicaid are often losers for the hospital, because Medicaid rates are low and AIDS lengths of stay are long.

The reimbursement situation is more difficult for public hospitals (Aleshire 1987). AIDS patients in public hospitals mostly depend on Medicaid or are uninsured. County hospitals in Los Angeles lost an average of $4,626 in uncollectable charges for each AIDS patient, according to a 1986 study (Scitovsky and Rice 1987). Most of these write-offs were due to the low Medicaid rate in California. A private hospital in Los Angeles responding to the same survey reportedly lost $2,345 in uncollectable costs for each AIDS patient treated.

CASE STUDY OF A SUCCESSFUL AIDS UNIT

In August 1985, Sherman Oaks Community Hospital opened a special treatment center for AIDS patients. The ten-bed unit was the first AIDS center in a community hospital. The rationale for a separate AIDS unit, according to N. Marc Goldberg, the hospital's chief executive officer, was to focus research and treatment of the disease while assuaging the fears of other patients at the hospital by isolating AIDS cases (Leach 1985; "Special Unit" 1985).

Goldberg started planning for the unit as the number of AIDS cases in the Los Angeles area topped 1,000 in 1985. The hospital estimated that 135,000 persons may have been exposed to the AIDS virus in Los Angeles and that up to 20,000 new cases may be generated by 1991. Staffing at the Sherman Oaks AIDS unit is one nurse per three patients, compared with an average of one per six on other med-surg units. The nurses are specially trained to deal with the medical and psychological needs of AIDS patients.

The hospital developed special personnel policies for staff working on the AIDS unit or involved in AIDS care. High-risk groups, including pregnant employees or others deemed to be at risk for infection, are not assigned to the AIDS unit. Sherman Oaks does not pay a wage differential to employees for working on the AIDS unit. No hospital employee may refuse to treat AIDS patients; refusal can lead to disciplinary action. Sherman Oaks has an active volunteer program that provides assistance to the AIDS unit.

Medical staff acceptance and support has been excellent. The AIDS unit is headed by nationally known AIDS specialists and provides access to the latest in treatment advances. The hospital is engaged in several FDA studies of various drugs for future AIDS treatment. All physicians are requested to identify AIDS patients upon admission. Any concerns by the medical staff about the AIDS unit have been alleviated by the quality of the program. The fact that AIDS patients are isolated on a special unit is seen as an advantage by doctors and patients.

Has there been a public relations backlash from the AIDS unit? Goldberg reports that the public's response has been "extremely supportive." Other patients feel more comfortable in a hospital where the AIDS victims are in their own unit rather than placed on all floors. AIDS patients have been very laudatory because their special needs are being recognized and cared for. Non-AIDS patients have been very supportive, Goldberg believes, "because they admire the hospital's willingness to step out front and do the scientific things that are necessary to meet the needs of the patients and at the same time take all precautionary measures to allay any fears and anxieties of the non-AIDS patients" (Leach 1985).

The AIDS unit at Sherman Oaks was designed after study of the pioneering AIDS unit at San Francisco General Hospital. The Sherman Oaks unit is under the co-direction of Eugene Rogolsky, M.D., and Joel Weisman, D.O., who are among the most experienced American physicians in providing AIDS treatment. The specialty unit has affiliated itself with UCLA and other academic medical centers for the purpose of collaborative AIDS research and education.

Sherman Oaks has an unusually high number of specialized programs for a 165-bed community hospital. In addition to the AIDS unit, the hospital has a nationally recognized burn center, an acute care oncology unit, a sports medicine orthopedic surgery unit, a 16-bed ICU, and a telemetry unit. The hospital is part of the NuMed system, and has a history of innovation and entrepreneurship.

Sherman Oaks treats 300–400 AIDS patients per year at a cost averaging $20,000 per hospitalization and two admissions per patient. The hospital does not have a Medicaid contract, and most of its patients have private insurance. Reducing the cost of AIDS care is a continuing concern, and Sherman Oaks is working with several community groups and other health organizations to create a hospice for AIDS patients.

PROFILE OF THE AIDS "MARKET"

The health industry's fearful view of AIDS is too limited. America's hospitals, health systems, and insurance plans face the AIDS crisis with foreboding. Hospitals are afraid that treating AIDS cases may drive non-AIDS patients away, infect hospital workers, and result in major financial losses. Physicians are afraid of infection and wary of AIDS patients despite warnings from the AMA that failure to treat is unethical (Pear 1987). Health workers are afraid of accidental exposure to the AIDS virus. There is a national shortage of latex gloves. The

CDC has warned hospitals that every patient must be treated with AIDS precautions.

Not since the polio epidemic of the 1950s has the U.S. health industry ever faced such a challenge. Americans are fortunate they have a well-developed health industry, top-quality facilities, and concerned health care professionals. Managing the AIDS crisis will test the intelligence, compassion, and business savvy of many health care executives in the near future. Like the Chinese epigram, within the AIDS crisis lies opportunity. Every hospital must manage the AIDS challenge if it is to be successful in the next five years.

Has AIDS Created a "Market"?

Despite its surging growth, AIDS is not considered by many to provide an entrepreneurial market opportunity. Early experiments with specialized AIDS facilities have been mixed. Few providers are breaking even on AIDS care, and a number of hospitals have experienced losses on per-stay AIDS reimbursement. American Medical International's AIDS hospital in Houston was a financial failure that was closed in late 1987.

Will AIDS hurt or help hospitals? The national survey on managing the AIDS crisis published in *Healthcare Forum* in December 1987 found that many health care administrators feared that numerous AIDS patients could hurt the market image of a hospital and jeopardize its finances (Coile and Grossman 1987). The national survey panel was concerned that AIDS could overwhelm local resources, and roughly three out of four (73 percent) believed losses on AIDS patients will inevitably rise unless hospitals receive a major infusion of public funds, most likely from the federal government.

This perspective is too narrow. AIDS has created a "market" in the literal sense of the term. Like many trends, on closer inspection the spread of AIDS is neither all blight nor a blessing in disguise. AIDS has given rise to a group of customers with substantial health needs. Many have an ability to pay. Although the percentage varies throughout the country, between 60 and 70 percent of AIDS patients have health insurance. Even those who lose their insurance when they stop working or are without private insurance usually qualify for Medicaid.

Scope of the Growing AIDS Problem

By January 4, 1988, the Centers for Disease Control reported that more than 50,000 cases of AIDS had been identified. Six weeks later, that number had swelled to nearly 52,000. By January 1989, U.S. AIDS cases numbered nearly 75,000. AIDS is broadening into what many fear will be a full-fledged national epidemic. At this point, every state has AIDS patients. Many AIDS cases are clustered in a handful of major metropolitan areas on the two coasts: New York, northern New Jersey, San Francisco, and Los Angeles. More metropolitan areas are feeling the impact of AIDS, including Dallas, Houston, Chicago, Minneapolis, and Atlanta. The disease is slowly spreading into suburban and rural areas. Even Missoula, Montana, had three cases of AIDS identified by December 1987; there were 13 cases statewide.

How many Americans are at risk for AIDS or are already carrying the virus? No one really knows yet, because there has been no widespread testing for the disease. Pilot studies are only now being carried out to develop preliminary data. A recent estimate by AIDS researcher Fred Hellinger predicts a total of 71,000 AIDS cases in the U.S. by 1990 and 114,000 cases by 1992. In 1989, the CDC have tested the blood of one-third of all newborns for AIDS, but no names are attached to the blood samples.

Public health officials estimate that between 1 million and 1.5 million U.S. residents may be already infected with HIV-I (Human Immunodeficiency Virus). Some researchers believe a second virus from central Africa (HIV-II) is an additional deadly agent (Pascal 1987). The first reported American case of AIDS due to HIV-II was recently reported in New Jersey.

Defining "AIDS"

The definition of AIDS is both clinical and bureaucratic. The disease, as officially defined by the CDC, involves suppression of the immune system conjoined with the presence of one or more opportunistic infections. The CDC, in September 1987, broadened the definition to include people with some AIDS symptoms, a condition labeled *AIDS-related complex* (*ARC*), and these patients are now officially considered to have AIDS.

People with AIDS are considered "disabled" under the policy of HCFA (Pascal 1987). This disability condition is deemed by the federal Social Security Administration to be equivalent to the Title II Listing of Impairments. Thus an unemployed individual who has a CDC-defined AIDS diagnosis and applies for disability under Title II (Disability Income) or Title XV (Supplemental Security Income) will be given disability status immediately, thus qualifying him or her for Social Security payments.

GROWTH POTENTIAL: AIDS FORECAST FOR 1991

Like any health care market, people with AIDS are actually a diverse cluster of market segments, each with a unique set of demographics, insurance protec-

tion, clinical needs, and service expectations. People with AIDS include: homosexual and bisexual men, intravenous drug users, heterosexual men and women,
and children and adults infected through the use of blood products.

If the experts are right, the growth of the AIDS market will be explosive (see
Table 10-1). A growing concern is the potential for a teenage AIDS epidemic
(Smilgis 1987). America's teenagers know the facts about AIDS but they are
not changing their sexual behavior to avoid the disease, according to a study by
the Children's Defense Fund.

Although AIDS has been diagnosed in fewer than 1,000 of those aged 13–
21, the 15,000 cases identified in the 20–29 age group indicate that many
contracted the disease while in their teen years. According to the Children's
Defense Fund study, 80 percent of males and 70 percent of females are sexually
experienced by age 20. Yet only 30 percent of the young men use condoms, an
important AIDS preventive measure. Of those teens with AIDS, 9 percent got
it through heterosexual intercourse (twice the adult rate). Almost 50 percent of
the youths became HIV positive through homosexual activities, and 12 percent
were IV drug abusers. A rapid spread of teen AIDS in the 1990s could hit inner
cities hardest. The growing number of IV drug abusers acquiring AIDS could
eventually lead to the spread of the disease through heterosexual activities among
ghetto youth.

AIDS: THE PRIMARY CONCERN OF THE INSURANCE INDUSTRY

Before 1985 few insurers thought about AIDS. According to a recent industry
report, *AIDS and Life Insurance,* by the American Council of Life Insurance
(ACLI), few companies kept records of AIDS-related deaths, disabilities, or
health care claims. By 1987 insurers had moved quickly to limit their AIDS-
related liability. They have instituted AIDS testing for prospective policyholders

Table 10-1 AIDS Forecast for 1991

	1988	1991
Homosexual and bisexual men	40,000	190,000
Intravenous drug users	10,000	55,000
Heterosexual men and women	1,500	24,000
Blood-infected children and adults	700	2,000

Source: U.S. Centers for Disease Control, 1988.

in all states except California (Washington, D.C., also does not permit AIDS testing). A bill to repeal the California prohibition on testing is in the California legislature, and insurers have threatened to stop writing new policies for Washington residents until testing is permitted.

How big is the AIDS liability for U.S. insurers? At the end of 1986, an estimated $20 billion in individual life insurance and more than $30 billion in group insurance could be claimed as a result of the deaths of individuals currently infected with HIV. A report predicts that claims for AIDS-related deaths on the basis of policies already in force could exceed 10 percent of the life insurance industry's total claims by the mid-1990s.

The life insurance industry's fears are heightened by a forecast of the mortality potential of AIDS. Early estimates by the CDC and others were that between 10 and 20 percent of HIV-positive individuals would progress to AIDS. That estimate was later revised upwards to 50 percent. By 1989, AIDS experts were beginning to believe that, over a 7–15 year period, the progression rate may be closer to 100 percent.

PROVIDERS WANT TO KNOW IF AIDS IS AN EPIDEMIC

The estimates of the spread of AIDS will continue to be highly uncertain until scientists have more experience with the disease. Many unknowns are involved. These are the questions that hospitals and health care providers need to have answered if they are to plan for the AIDS wave:

1. *How many people in the general population are already carrying the disease?* Scientists do not really know how many in the general population are HIV positive. Until more broad-based samplings of the population are carried out, officials can only speculate. The current estimate is that 1 million to 1.5 million Americans are virus positive (Pascal 1987; Boffey 1988). Six pilot studies are being undertaken to determine the relative exposure of high-risk groups.
2. *Of those who test HIV positive, how many will develop full-blown AIDS?* Initially, AIDS researchers believed that 5–19 percent of seropositives would develop AIDS. More recent data suggest that 75 percent of HIV positives will develop AIDS within seven years; 50 percent will do so within five years (Pascal 1987).
3. *How will the disease spread differentially among the high-risk groups and how many of the general population will become infected?* The spread of AIDS varies markedly by high-risk group. Very generally, transmission of the disease appears to be slowing among homosexual and bisexual men, but it is exploding in the ghettos, spreading among intravenous drug users

and heterosexual men and women and their children. Also, hospitals are more aggressively notifying patients who may have received AIDS-con-taminated blood products. As more blood recipients are tested, more AIDS cases will be identified in the short term. Hospitals in northern California began notifying thousands of patients in 1988 to see their physician if they were transfused or received blood products between 1977 and 1985. An estimated 1,500 units may have been contaminated.

4. *Are current estimates of AIDS accurate?* A study by Anthony Pascal (1987), a senior health care researcher at the RAND Corporation, questioned the CDC consensus forecast of 270,000 AIDS cases by 1991, which was established at the Coolfont conference sponsored by the U.S. Public Health Service in 1986. According to RAND research, the midrange estimate for AIDS in 1991 is 440,000 cases with an upper-range potential of 775,000. The researchers fear substantial underreporting of AIDS cases and the potential for AIDS to jump risk-group boundaries and be as infectious as other sexually transmitted diseases.

THE COST OF AIDS TREATMENT

The annual cost of AIDS health care was more than $1 billion in 1989 and may exceed $2 billion by 1990. The financial aspects of the AIDS wave are still being charted by health economists. One of the most widely quoted estimates was reported by Ann Hardy of the CDC in 1985 (Scitovsky and Rice 1987). She calculated the national cost of hospitalizing all AIDS patients could reach $1.473 billion in lifetime care. That estimate was based on an assumption of lifetime hospital use of 168 days per AIDS patient, an average survival time of 392 days from diagnosis, an average charge of $878 per hospital day, and a total treatment cost of $147,000 per AIDS case. Hardy's estimates were based on a small sample of AIDS patients in a single hospital in Atlanta. Since 1985, the use of hospitalization has been declining, as has the average length of stay. Using a case management approach, San Francisco is managing AIDS care for $35,000 to $40,000 per case.

More recently, Anne Scitovsky and Dorothy Rice prepared updated cost es-timates for the CDC based on an analysis of costs and utilization at the AIDS unit of San Francisco General Hospital (Scitovsky and Rice 1987). The re-searchers differentiated between AIDS conditions, finding that patients with Pneumocystis carinii (a form of pneumonia) had an average length of stay of 11.89 days, whereas those with Kaposi's sarcoma, a rare cancer, or other AIDS-related conditions averaged only 3.70 days. Based on their analysis of the San Francisco data, they predict 3.2 admissions per AIDS patient. The average charge per hospital day was predicted to fall in the range between $740 and $950 per day, with hospital stays averaging between 13 and 25 days. Outpatient and home care expenditures added between $2,000 and $4,000 per patient to the cost of AIDS treatment. Out-of-hospital AIDS treatment costs may average 10 percent of total AIDS costs, according to a study at Boston's New England Deaconess Hospital (Scitovsky and Rice 1987).

Compiling studies from other regions, Scitovsky and Rice demonstrated that the San Francisco data generated valid estimates. Cost data from an analysis of Medicaid cases in California suggest that AIDS patients may experience between 5.6 and 6.7 hospital stays over the course of the disease (Scitovsky and Rice 1987). Other studies done in Florida and Michigan show 3.2 to 4.2 admissions per AIDS case, with hospital stays averaging 20.1 to 21 days.

New York has the most AIDS cases of any city. Data from New York on 1,573 AIDS patients showed that AIDS cases treated in 1985 without intensive care averaged from 17.2 to 18.2 days of stay at a cost per hospital day of $518 to $575. However, the 8.4 percent of New York patients who did require intensive care stayed on average 29.1 days at a cost of $1,000 per day. Drug cases averaged 17.4 days of stay at a cost of $587 per day; nondrug patients averaged 18.0 days at a cost of $573 per day. Stays were longer and costs higher in city-operated hospitals in New York, with average stays of 25.4 days and per-day costs of $800.

Los Angeles AIDS costs were similar. In an analysis of 976 AIDS cases by the Hospital Council of Southern California, hospital stays averaged 17.3 days at a cost of $963 per day. These studies were based on 1985 data, and more recent information suggests that hospital stays are shortening but costs per hospital day are rising. So are outpatient and home care costs, as the treatment emphasis swings away from hospitalization.

CASE MANAGEMENT REDUCES COST OF AIDS CARE

The cost of treatment for AIDS patients can be substantially reduced through more extensive employment of managed care benefit programs that maximize use of less costly out-of-hospital services. Case managers at San Francisco General Hospital's AIDS unit have reduced per-case costs to between $35,000 and $40,000. Case management is quickly catching on with AIDS providers and health insurers.

Blue Shield of California reports it has achieved a savings of $8,000 per case for a number of persons with AIDS who are enrolled in Blue Shield's individual case management program (Blue Shield of California 1987). The program is designed for Blue Shield members suffering from a catastrophic or long-term illness, including AIDS. It facilitates movement of patients to alternative treatment sites such as the home and reduces hospital inpatient care. In an 18-month period during 1986 and 1987, Blue Shield paid an average of $52,455 for each of 20 AIDS patients served through case management. Without the program, Blue Shield estimates per-case costs at $60,000 or more.

The key to case management success in AIDS is flexibility. The case manager has the power to arrange payment for medically necessary services, whether the services or settings are specifically covered in the AIDS patient's health insurance contract. Case management is more than efficient resource allocation. It is concerned with quality and customer relations. Even more important than dollar savings, says a Blue Shield spokeperson, "we are playing a key role as the patients' advocate and assisting them when they are least able to help themselves."

TREATMENT TRENDS

As the health industry's experience with AIDS grows, treatment patterns are shifting. Inpatient stay is falling. In the future AIDS stays may range from 10 to 15 days. More use of out-of-hospital care is encouraged by case management.

Treating AIDS with new drugs is done on an outpatient basis or at home. AZT (azidothymidine) is extending the lives of AIDS patients, although AZT has not reduced the mortality level. Although expensive (its $10,000 annual cost was recently reduced to $7,500), the drug increases ambulatory visits and lab work for frequent monitoring. AZT may be shortening hospital stays as well. Pentamadine isethionate is being used at home for care of AIDS patients suffering from Pneumocystis carinii pneumonia. The drug costs $120 per month and the home equipment can be purchased for $200.

More drugs to fight AIDS and opportunistic infections are on the way. The FDA has approved more than 100 studies to test 40 potential agents that attack retroviruses like HIV. More than 80 trials are also underway to test nearly 30 compounds for efficacy against cancers and other infections. Two drugs to treat Kaposi's sarcoma should gain approval by 1990. Both use slightly different forms of alpha-interferon. All new drugs must undergo three levels of trials before FDA approval, but the agency is speeding up review of drugs for AIDS treatment and giving them priority over other applications.

AIDS ALTERNATIVE TREATMENT SETTINGS

Home care will be one of the primary settings for AIDS care in the future. Continental Health Affiliates, a home health agency in Englewood Cliffs, New Jersey, has already treated more than 500 AIDS patients at an average cost of $5,000 per case. Continental applies traditional principles of home care to AIDS patients, including infusion therapy and pain management. In San Francisco, the Pacific Presbyterian Medical Center recently purchased the San Francisco Home Health and Hospice agency which is one of the leading providers of AIDS home health services in the area.

Hospices will be an important AIDS resource. The Shanti Project in San Francisco is a grass-roots hospice designed for AIDS patients which has received considerable support. In New York City, hospices are playing a key role in AIDS care. A recent national survey of hospices found that so far only 23 percent had treated AIDS patients, but 97 percent indicated a willingness to do so on request. In the future hospices may bifurcate, suggests bioethics consultant John Golenski of the Berkeley-based Bioethics Consultation Group. Some hospices will specialize in AIDS, and traditional hospices will refer AIDS patients to the specialized programs (Golenski 1987).

TRENDS FOR THE FUTURE

The nature of the AIDS epidemic is rapidly shifting. These will be among the AIDS-related trends to track in the next three to five years:

- *New Risk Groups*. The disease is migrating into new risk groups. These include the elderly, some of whom may have been infected by contaminated blood between 1977 and 1985 and only now be developing the disease. Another growing risk group consists of children born to AIDS-infected parents. A recent survey by the New York City Health Department showed that 1 out of every 61 babies born in the Bronx tests HIV positive.

- *Inner-City Scourge*. Most at risk for AIDS in the future may be the low-income residents of inner cities. AIDS is being transmitted from intravenous drug abusers to non–drug abusers through heterosexual transmission. This trend gives health authorities much cause for alarm. Public health officials fear the disease could become prevalent among teenagers, who often neglect safe sex practices.

- *Bed Shortage*. Already New York City is experiencing a hospital bed shortage driven in part by the AIDS caseload (the nation's largest). As AIDS care becomes more specialized, the limited number of "AIDS beds" in a community may fill rapidly.

- *AIDS Patient Channeling*. Although a growing number of hospitals will treat some AIDS patients, a pattern is emerging of channeling AIDS patients to a limited number of hospitals with AIDS programs. Those patients with private insurance will be referred to community hospitals with specialized AIDS units and medical staff. AIDS patients on Medicaid are being channeled into public hospitals.

- *Alternative Delivery Systems for AIDS*. Bioethics consultant John Golenski suggests that alternative delivery systems for AIDS will be developed (Golenski 1987). These programs will utilize managed care and case management and emphasize outpatient services, home care, and hospices. Specialized AIDS alternative delivery systems may even contract with insurers, HMOs, and the government.

CONCLUSION

Managing the AIDS situation is one of the biggest challenges that each doctor and health care executive will face in the 1990s. Even with a cure, the numbers of AIDS patients will double in the decade ahead. Without a cure, the problem may reach grave proportions in cities such as New York and San Francisco by the early 1990s. To manage this mounting public health threat will require a combination of innovation and compassion from America's physicians and health care institutions.

STRATEGIC IMPLICATIONS FOR PHYSICIANS

1. *Every doctor should acquire an AIDS knowledge base*. AIDS is not a specialized condition that only physicians with gay practices or inner-city locations will see in the 1990s. Blood-acquired AIDS is a condition that could affect large numbers of Americans (including the elderly) who otherwise would have minimal exposure to the AIDS virus. Every physician should become knowledgeable about AIDS treatment. Doctors attending pregnant women should provide counsel and test for AIDS. All doctors should add AIDS cues to their routine history examinations.
2. *Physicians should assist their hospitals and staff in developing and maintaining a system of responsible precautions in providing AIDS care*. Such assistance will include continuing education, policies and procedures, and quality assurance. Since universal precautions were ordered by the Occupational Safety and Health Administration in 1987, hospitals may become complacent with respect to AIDS precautions. Overcoming paranoia or complacence in the workplace will require active medical staff participation.
3. *AIDS case management will blend the clinical and economic aspects of medicine*. Probably never again will U.S. health providers have the luxury of providing all care at any cost. Disciplined case management is essential to keep costs within reason and make efficient use of scarce AIDS resources.

STRATEGIC IMPLICATIONS FOR HOSPITALS

1. *Hospitals must plan ahead.* AIDS will become more visible in the 1990s. Every hospital, board, and medical staff will need to address AIDS-related issues. The number of AIDS cases is growing rapidly, especially in the inner cities. Planning at the community level will begin to address regional needs and rationalize current treatment patterns. Some state hospital associations and regional hospital councils may begin to voluntarily designate regional AIDS treatment centers. Every hospital needs an AIDS plan.
2. *Experimentation will be essential in dealing with the disease.* To solve the AIDS crisis, America needs new drugs, treatment methods, financing, levels of care, safeguards for health care workers, use of health personnel, fund raising and philanthropy methods. These and other innovations are being developed now in those hospitals that are taking on the challenge. AIDS may change the manner in which health care is rendered. It provides an opportunity to experiment with self-care, holistic health, and using friends and relations as trained caregivers.
3. *AIDS care networks will be created.* AIDS will change the health system in important ways, especially for doctors and hospitals. The AIDS crisis will cause doctors and health facilities to become involved in a broad network of community providers and multiple levels of care outside the walls of the traditional hospital. Home care will grow in response to the increasing number of AIDS patients.
4. *AIDS is creating a market the U.S. health industry must manage.* Management of this market is more than good social policy. It may mean hospital survival, especially for those public and community hospitals with high AIDS caseloads. Inability to cope with the burdens of AIDS could financially break such hospitals. The Catholic Hospital Association's report *No Room in the Marketplace* demonstrates the burdens that socially minded hospitals are already carrying. The growing AIDS problem could cause many inner-city and public medical centers to founder.

BIBLIOGRAPHY

Aleshire, Peter. 1987. "AMA Warns AIDS-Patient Dumping Will Overwhelm Public Hospitals." *The Tribune* (Oakland, Calif.) 13 September, A11.

Blue Shield of California. 1987. *Case Management Reduces Cost of AIDS Care*. San Francisco: Blue Shield of California.

Boffey, Phillip M. 1988. "Spread of AIDS Abating, but Deaths Will Still Soar." *New York Times*, 14 February, 1–22.

Coile, Russell C., Jr., and Randolph M. Grossman. 1987. "FutureTrack: The AIDS Wave." *Healthcare Forum* (November-December): 41–43.

Golenski, John. 1987. Personal communication with the author.

Hilton, Bruce. 1989. "AIDSWEEK: 50% Cut for AIDS." *San Francisco Chronicle*, 16 July, A–5.

Koehn, Hank. 1987. "My Passage through AIDS: A Prominent Los Angeles Businessman Reflects on His Life and His Fate." *Los Angeles Times*, 14 August, V1, 5.

Leach, Eric. 1985. "Hospital in Sherman Oaks to Open AIDS Isolation Unit." *The Daily News*, (Van Nuys, Calif.) 11 August, 1–9.

Pascal, Anthony. 1987. *The Costs of Treating AIDS under Medicaid: 1986–1991*. Santa Monica, Calif.: The Rand Corporation.

Pear, Robert. 1987. "AMA Rules That Doctors Are Obligated to Treat AIDS." *New York Times*, 13 November, 10.

_____. 1988. "Study Finds Most Insurers Screen Applicants for AIDS Virus." *New York Times*, 18 February, 1, 15.

Ricklefs, Roger. 1987. "AIDS Cases Prompt a Host of Lawsuits." *Wall Street Journal*, 7 October, 31.

Scitovsky, Anne A., and D. P. Rice. 1987. "Estimates of the Direct and Indirect Costs of Acquired Immunodeficiency Syndrome in the United States, 1985, 1986, 1991." *Public Health Reports* 102 (January-February): 5–17.

Smilgis, Martha. 1987. "The Big Chill: Fear of AIDS." *Time*, 16 February, 50–53.

"Special Unit Established for AIDS Patients." 1985. *FAH Review* (November-December): 28.

Weber, David. 1988. "AIDS: Providers Struggle with AIDS Care." *HealthWeek*, 6 June, 18–22.

Reshaping Medical Practice and Health Care Management

Chapter 11

Physician Bonding

The key lies in the willingness and ability of hospitals and physicians to give up old ways of thinking and behaving and to build a new kind of social contract—a social contract based on paradox, ambiguity and change, risk, and the pursuit of "responsible excellence."

—Stephen M. Shortell, "The Medical Staff of the Future: Replanting the Garden"

THE EVOLVING HOSPITAL-PHYSICIAN RELATIONSHIP

For many reasons, ranging between altruism and survival, hospitals and physicians are developing new relationships (Table 11-1). Everyone is wary, yet the future is clear. Hospitals and physicians will be locked together in an increasingly complex web of clinical and financial ties. In a word, they will be *bonded* together in mutual dependency, converging interests, and joint economic arrangements.

Hospitals Will Select a "First Team" and Doctors Will "Marry" a Hospital

It's choosing time in hospital-physician relationships. In a recent Delphi survey done for *Healthcare Forum*, a national panel of health experts predicted that in the next three years each hospital would quietly identify its "first team" of preferred physicians and seek to lock them into long-term relationships (Coile 1987). Doctors are examining their hospital affiliations, picking from among the choices, and settling into "marriages" that will last years or an entire lifetime.

Physicians in the 1990s will have closer ties with fewer hospitals. Experts predict each physician will be driven into a "monogamous relationship" with a single hospital for reasons such as these:

Table 11-1 Ranking Hospital-Physician Bonding Alternatives

Type of Bonding Strategy	Hospital Cost	Hospital Impact
Computer networking with physician offices	Moderate	High
Diagnostic imaging center	High	Moderate
Group purchasing for physicians	Low	Moderate
Equipment purchase or lease-back	Moderate	Low
Group practice development	Moderate	High
Hospital-sponsored group practice	High	High
HMO contracting or IPA	Moderate	High
HMO development	High	Moderate
Medical director (full-time)	Low	Low
Medical institute or center of excellence	High	High
Medical office buildings	Moderate/high	Moderate
New physician practice subsidy or guarantee	Moderate	Moderate
PPO contracting organization	Low/moderate	High
Physician billing service or collection	Low	Low
Physician practice acquisition	Moderate/high	Low/moderate
Physician practice building or marketing	Moderate/high	High
Physician practice management	Moderate	Low
Physician recruitment	Low/moderate	Moderate/high
Physician referral service	Low/moderate	Moderate/high
Physician retirement or financial planning	Low	Low
Physician service bureau	Low/moderate	Low
Real estate limited partnership	Moderate/high	Low
Research or teaching subsidy	Moderate/high	Moderate
Superstar physician recruitment	High	High
Venture capital pool	High	Unknown

- A single-payment Medicare system would eliminate the split between physician and hospital payments for a stay of care.
- Using a self-insurance pool, a hospital could cover the malpractice costs of its medical staff.
- Physicians could influence quality-of-care decisions regarding technology acquisition and staffing levels.
- Joint ventures, cooperative advertising, and other shared projects would benefit both physicians and hospitals.

Gerald McManis, president of McManis Associates, based in Washington, D.C., forecasts a new era in which physicians and hospitals will share the risks and rewards of health care delivery on a much larger scale than a single joint venture (Coile 1988). Rather than sharing rewards on a piecemeal basis, McManis encourages formation of socioeconomic guilds in which hospitals and a large number of doctors would be stockholders. The guilds would own several projects and would likely develop financial arrangements with insurance companies, community hospitals, and tertiary care centers.

As medical groups grow and develop market clout, hospitals can expect the most influential physician groups to seek preferred hospital treatment—perhaps even a seat on the board—in exchange for affiliation and referrals. One California group practice consisting of 35 doctors recently "shopped" the 20,000 patient days they control. The group went looking for a new hospital affiliation when the old hospital included a rival medical group in a managed care deal. The physician move was a signal of the changing times. Loyalty and commitment have a price.

Physicians want more say in quality-of-care decisions. Shrinking hospital reimbursement and tight hospital budgets make the budgetary decisions all the more critical to them. As hospitals give more consideration to cost-containment procedures, hospital CEOs can expect that doctors will seek a high-level role in key committees or at the board level. Doctors want a voice in policy decisions regarding technology acquisition, staffing levels, and hospital diversification.

Most physicians have time to play an active role in only one or two medical institutions, Bruce Spivey, M.D., president of Pacific Presbyterian Medical Center, stated in a recent interview with *Modern Healthcare* (Perry 1988). Dr. Spivey observed, "If you're on the active staff of too many places, you've got too many meetings to go to" (p. 43).

WHAT DOCTORS WANT WHEN THEY AFFILIATE
WITH HOSPITALS

Doctors are shopping for hospitals, and they are as discriminating as "Morris the cat"—finicky, in a word. They have become more conscious of the strategic importance of the right hospital relationship. How do doctors select hospitals? Richard Nordstrom and his colleagues at a California university analyzed 30 factors affecting physician attitudes towards hospitals (Nordstrom, Horton, and Hatcher 1987). Seven kinds of attributes emerged as especially influential. The results are highlighted in Table 11-2.

MARKETING HOSPITALS TO PHYSICIANS

Physicians still control 70 percent of admission decisions. That is down from 88 percent in the early 1980s, according to Atlanta-based market research consultant Paul Keckley (Perry 1988). Channeling patients into hospitals is still

Table 11-2 Hospital Attributes That Attract Physicians

Attributes	Loadings[a]
Diagnostic and treatment attributes	
Radiology	.81
Lab services	.80
Test reporting	.78
Respiratory therapy facilities	.60
Nursing	.55
Convenience attributes	
Travel time from office	.90
Travel time from home	.84
Ease of making rounds	.55
Admitting and discharge attributes	
Admitting procedures	.81
Discharge procedures	.78
Communication attributes	
Accessibility of hospital administration	.93
Voice in policy making	.76
Surgical attributes	
Surgical facilities	.78
Anesthesia services	.73
Image attributes	
Patient referrals	.55
Staff prestige	.53
Hospital reputation	.49
Friendliness of personnel	.34
Appearance attributes	
Interior appearance	.74
Moderness	.46

[a]Loading refers to the correlations between the factor and the variable.

Source: Journal of Health Care Marketing, Vol. 7, No. 1, pp. 29–36, American Marketing Association, © March 1987.

controlled very much by doctors despite second-opinion programs, managed care plans, and more consumer involvement.

Physicians are health care's number one "consumers" when it comes to hospital services. Hospitals with expensive marketing and promotion programs aimed at the "retail" market of consumers are only going after 30 percent of the market. The success of acute inpatient care depends on the channeling of physician referrals to the hospital. Hospitals should adopt marketing plans that target physicians as well as potential patients.

Fewer than 10 percent of U.S. hospitals now have a marketing plan to market the hospital to their physicians, reports Holly King of the Kansas City office of Peat Marwick Main and Company (Coile 1988b). That oversight is being remedied. Physicians are becoming hospital marketing's first priority.

Hospitals are picking up the pace of physician marketing and doubling budgets, according to a recent survey of 300 executives by the Keckley Group for the AHA's Society for Healthcare Planning and Marketing (Perry 1988). The survey indicates that U.S. hospital marketing directors planned to increase their physician marketing budgets by 83 percent in 1988. The average expenditure was expected to be about $25,000 per hospital, ranging from $7,900 for small hospitals to $110,000 for major medical centers. Western hospitals of more than 150 beds were intending to spend most on physician marketing, according to the survey. In all hospitals, practice-building programs and physician referral services were the leading components. In small and midsize hospitals, physician recruitment was important; large hospitals emphasized physician office staff training. Such programs pay off: 29 percent of hospitals reported their programs were successful, 36 percent believed the money invested in physician marketing has brought a better return than consumer marketing, and 61 percent attested that physician marketing has improved their hospital's image.

Physician Market Plans

The key elements in a physician marketing plan include the following:

- A *medical staff audit* and a *practice analysis* of all hospital physicians are done to identify strengths and weaknesses as well as utilization and referral patterns on a department-by-department basis.
- *Market research* should investigate physician attitudes, expectations, and satisfaction with the hospital in such key dimensions as service, support, technical capacity and equipment, patient reporting, quality assurance, practice and marketing support, and physician involvement in decision making. Market research also needs to identify which physicians and specialties are of primary strategic importance and where the medical staff needs strengthening.
- A *physician development plan*, based on the physician life cycle, should be devised to assist young physicians in practice setup, established physicians in practice enhancement, and older physicians in preretirement planning. The development plan must be service-specific and include a work plan, a timetable, identified responsible staff, and a budget.

- A *physician development program* is needed to carry out the plan. It should be approved by the board and funded and staffed by the hospital. Its purpose is to build up the medical staff and support the practices of key physicians. The physician development program may involve a multi-million-dollar investment in computer networking, medical office buildings, joint ventures, or satellite ambulatory centers.
- A *physician liaison* needs to be put in charge of meeting the needs of the physicians on an ongoing basis. The liaison should be a problem solver who can cut through hospital bureaucracy and take care of a doctor's difficulties in 24–48 hours.
- *Communication* through a variety of formats is essential for continuously informing physicians of new hospital programs, technology and equipment, and policies and procedures that affect them.

PHYSICIAN INCENTIVES

To strengthen ties with key medical staff, hospitals are developing an array of incentives for doctors. Table 11-3 lists the top five services physicians would be interested in receiving from hospitals.

RECRUITING PHYSICIAN SUPERSTARS: HIGH RISK, HIGH REWARD!

What does the hospital industry have in common with the entertainment industry? Superstars! These high-visibility physicians can walk into any hospital and transform it into a medical center overnight. High-profile physician superstars are a magnet for referrals, research grants, ambitious protégés, and money. Hospitals who woo and win them can realize windfall profits and surging occupancies.

But the costs and the risks are high. Hospitals are accused of being like insurance companies and banks in having a low-risk business culture: process oriented and risk adverse. Not when it comes to competition for the nation's best doctors. Competing for top physicians is not for CEOs with a low stress tolerance. Be prepared to pay big money for new facilities, equipment, and staff. Everything must be first quality to please the physician stars, many of whom are prima donnas.

Take the example of cardiac surgeon Jerome Kay, M.D., the top heart surgeon at St. Vincent Medical Center in Los Angeles. With Dr. Kay, St. Vincent was one of the two leading heart surgery centers in southern California. Then Kay

Table 11-3 Top Five Services Physicians Want from Hospitals

	All M.D.s	Primary Care M.D.s	Specialists	Surgeons	Ob/Gyn M.D.s
1. Continuing medical education	57%	75%	50%	50%	59%
2. Physician referral service	46	43	45	49	58
3. Market research: patient referral and satisfaction	39	18	44	47	55
4. Malpractice insurance	35	37	31	31	64
5. Joint venture alternative delivery system	35	23	33	29	53

Source: Modern Healthcare, pp. 24–33, Crain Communications, Inc., © January 8, 1988.

was recruited away by 282-bed Good Samaritan to build its cardiology program into a regional referral center. Dr. Kay's departure threatened the viability of St. Vincent's open-heart program, which not only was the largest cardiac surgery program in California but accounted for 30 percent of the hospital's revenues.

In his first year with Good Samaritan, Dr. Kay did 400 open-heart procedures, boosting its volume to 875 admissions. Good Samaritan had been ranked 20th in the state in 1986. The hospital's operating revenues increased to $93.4 million in fiscal 1987, up 33 percent. Good Samaritan's average daily census increased by 36 patients to 232. By the first quarter of 1988, it had jumped to 245. Dr. Kay predicted his group will care for 1,200 patients in his second year at Good Samaritan.

For Good Samaritan, recruiting physician superstars was a way to quickly vault this midsize urban hospital into the top ranks of regional medical centers. John Westerman, Good Samaritan's president and CEO, had success in a similar effort to build up market share for the 678-bed Allegheny General Hospital in Pittsburgh before he was recruited by the Los Angeles hospital. The plan to build up the Heart Institute was intended to buy market share in a lucrative market. Good Samaritan had a $40 million "war chest," thanks to a huge bequest from a wealthy patient. The hospital is now working to enhance its reputation in obstetrics and pediatric surgery. A $1 million facility for artificial fertility treatment and research is giving Good Samaritan high visibility, part of its strategy for creating additional centers of excellence.

Good Samaritan's bold move to lure leading physicians away from competitors has created an unsettling precedent. Los Angeles area hospitals have reason to fear that a new "bidders war" could break out. At a time when more than half the hospitals in southern California expect to lose money, the potential for a medical superstar to make or break a hospital's fortunes is very high.

HOSPITAL CEO'S RULE NUMBER ONE: PLEASE THE MEDICAL STAFF

The secret to building a successful hospital is to build a successful medical staff. Staff members' loyalty and referrals will drive the hospital's future. Few hospitals can now take their doctors' loyalty for granted. Continuous hospital-physician communication is essential. Hospital executives cannot assume that their own medical staff members are well informed of all services the hospital currently offers, new technology or facilities, or the scope of consultation expertise available from other staff members.

Medical practice management consultant George Conomikes recommended in a recent commentary in *Modern Healthcare* that hospitals should conduct a continuous and targeted program of physician marketing (Conomikes 1988). Such a program might include:

- admissions and surgery scheduling
- advertising
- computer tie-ins
- health fairs
- joint ventures
- physician referral services
- practice management consulting
- practice management seminars
- public relations

For example, Southern Baptist Hospital in New Orleans recently implemented a physician development program with assistance from Peat Marwick (Perry 1988). The firm identified and analyzed the top physicians in New Orlean's two medical schools. The goal of hospital CEO Nelson Toebbe was to identify physicians with mature practices and concentrate on helping them. The cornerstone of the hospital's program was a comprehensive data base on the medical staff. Each profile included personal information such as age, sex, where the physician was trained, and board certification status. Practice information such as location, satellite offices, and hours was also included. Admission trends were monitored every three months. The hospital's efforts are paying off with improved referrals from its top admitters and incremental improvement in referrals from "semiloyal" physicians. Southern Baptist Hospital's investment in the physician development program was worthwhile. Similar programs are estimated to cost $200,000 to $300,000 per year.

STRATEGIC IMPLICATIONS FOR PHYSICIANS

1. *Now is the time for physicians with a significant hospital practice to choose their preferred hospital for long-term affiliation.* The advantages of selecting early include obtaining favored status and support.
2. *Physicians should become preferred providers.* Preferred physicians will be included in the hospital's contracts with insurance plans, HMOs, and PPOs. These contracts will provide a lifeline of physician referrals in the future. Physicians need to participate in as many managed care contracts as possible with the hospital to maximize their future referral potential. They must be centrally involved in all hospital contracting activities to ensure protection of their own interests.
3. *In the near future, physicians and hospitals will be asked to assume financial risks in managed care contracting.* This is the logical extension

of the gatekeeper concept that more than one-third of U.S. HMOs are trying. Risk-sharing contracts could cover as many as 15–25 percent of all insured patients by 1995. Early experience in Minnesota's Twin Cities suggests that the concept is workable but financial reserves must be adequate, physicians must be informed of the risk potential, and information systems must closely track physician performance.

STRATEGIC IMPLICATIONS FOR HOSPITALS

1. *Now is the time for selecting the cadre of physicians that the hospital will build its future around.* Perhaps 25–35 percent of the medical staff physicians have both the volume and loyalty to be part of this first circle. Physician selection criteria should include inpatient and ambulatory referrals, use of related hospital services, role in hospital centers of excellence, professional specialty, skills, age, location, type of practice (group or solo), credentials, participation in past hospital-physician ventures, and leadership capacity.

2. *For long-term loyalty, the hospital should map a campaign and invest strategically to enhance physician office practices.* More than any other incentive, practice support contributes directly to a physician's livelihood. Support programs include physician referral services, physician practice marketing, physician marketing tie-ins with hospital advertising, cross-selling referrals from hospital services to physicians, protocols to ensure the return of posthospitalization patients to the original referring physicians, and computerized physician networking.

3. *The hospital should experiment with a variety of incentives to gain and hold physician commitment.* Malpractice insurance may be one of the most important incentives for young physicians and for specialists such as anesthesiologists and obstetricians.

4. *Develop a medical staff marketing plan.* Since they are the most important customers of hospital services, the hospital needs a marketing strategy for its medical staff and outlying referral physicians. The goal of the physician marketing plan is to reinforce the value of the hospital to physicians by providing quality care and enhancing their practices. A professional sales force to call on physicians is being successfully employed by a number of hospitals.

BIBLIOGRAPHY

Barker, W. Daniel. 1987. "The Year 2000: A Look into the Future of Hospitals and Medical Staffs." *Journal of MAG* 76:556–60.

Berger, Sally. 1988. "Hospital Strengthens Ties to Doctors with Joint Venture." *Modern Healthcare*, 29 January.

Bloomfield, Randall D. 1988. "Hospital-Physician Relationships: A Changing Dynamic." *New York State Journal of Medicine* (January).

Bogdanich, Walt, and Michael Waldholz. 1989. "Warm Bodies: Hospitals That Need Patients Pay Bounties for Doctors' Referrals." *Wall Street Journal*, 27 February, 1.

Bulger, Robert T., and Karen C. Teitelbaum. 1988. "Addressing Operational Issues in Medical Practice Development." *Healthcare Financial Management* (July): 66–70.

Burda, David. 1988. "Hiring of Physician Executives on the Rise." *Modern Healthcare*, 8 April, 40.

Chapman, Thomas W., and Leo H. Mugmon. 1988. "Supporting Physicians in a Competitive Environment: One Hospital's Approach to Assist Private Practitioners." *Journal of Hospital Marketing* 2(1): 171–75.

Coile, Russell C., Jr. 1987. "The New Medicine." *Healthcare Forum Journal* (September–October): 14–17.

Coile, Russell C., Jr. 1988a. *Hospital Entrepreneur's Newsletter* 3 (February).

———. 1988b. *Hospital Strategy Report* 1 (November).

———. 1989. *Hospital Strategy Report* 1 (February).

Conomikes, George S. 1988. "Hospitals Should Adopt Marketing Plans that Target Both Physicians and Patients." *Modern Healthcare*, 15 January, 36.

de Lorrell, Walter, and Allen J. Budzichowski. 1988. "A Question of Altruism and Survival: Group Practices as Hospital Satellites." *Group Practice* (January–February): 60–61.

Denaro Dine, Deborah. 1988. "Joint Venture Exceeds Planners' Hopes." *Modern Healthcare*, 8 April, 50.

Droste, Therese. 1987a. "Physician Marketing Pays Off in Admissions." *Hospitals*, 5 October, 48–53.

———. 1987b. "1987: Physician Marketing Continues to Grow." *Hospitals*, 20 December, 28–29.

———. 1988a. "Physician Marketing Budgets to Grow in '88." *Hospitals*, 20 January, 32–34.

———. 1988b. "Practice Enhancement: What MDs Want." *Hospitals*, 20 March, 44.

———. 1988c. "FTC: Setting High Standards in Advertising." *Hospitals*, 20 April, 41–44.

Egdahl, Richard H., and Cynthia H. Taft. 1986. "Physicians and Hospitals: Competitors or Partners." In *The Corporation of Health Care Delivery*. Edited by Monica R. Dreuth. Chicago: American Hospital Publishing.

Green, Jane M. 1987. "The Role of Information Systems in the Hospital-Physician Relationship." *Topics in Health Care Financing* (Winter): 9–16.

Greene, Jay. 1988. "More Hospitals Contracting for Emergency Physicians." *Modern Healthcare*, 22 April, 31.

Holthaus, David. 1987. "Recruitment Schemes Face Legal Questions." *Hospitals*, 5 December, 54–58.

Kelsey, Ronn R. 1988. "Strategies in Physician Marketing: Clinical Data Base Marketing—New Way to Expand the Health Care Pie." *Hospital Strategy Report* 1 (November).

Koska, Mary T. 1988. "Low-Cost Strategies Aid Physician Bonding." *Hospitals*, 5 May, 60.

———. 1988. "JCAHO Survey: Interhospital Relationships Strong." *Hospitals*, 5 July, 54–56.

Larkin, Howard. 1988. "Do Physician-Managers Raise Hospital Costs?" *Hospitals*, 20 February, 68–69.

Lewitt, Suzanne M. 1982. *Physician Recruitment Strategies That Work*. Rockville, Md.: Aspen Publishers.

"Life with Physicians in the Relative Value Age." 1988. *Health Care Competition Week*, 28 November.

McDermott, Steve. 1988. "The New Hospital Challenge: Organizing and Managing Physician Organizations." *Health Care Management Review* 13 (Winter): 57–61.

Nelson, Susan. 1987. "Buying MD Practices: The Trend Continues." *Hospitals*, 20 July, 63.

Newald Martinsons, Jane. 1988. "What's the Top MD Recruitment Incentive?" *Hospitals*, 5 February, 69.

Nordstrom, Richard D., Devonne E. Horton, and Myron E. Hatcher. 1987. "How to Create a Marketing Strategy Based on Hospital Characteristics That Attract Physicians." *Journal of Health Care Marketing* 7 (March): 29–36.

Perry, Linda. 1988. "U.S. Hospitals Wooing Superstar Physicians." *Modern Healthcare*, 8 January, 24–33.

Powills, Suzanne. 1987a. "What Do Physicians Really Want from Hospitals?" *Hospitals*, 5 June, 46.

———. 1987b. "Segmenting the Physician Market: Some Guidelines." *Hospitals*, 5 June, 47.

———. 1987c. "Half of Physicians Say Ads Are Effective." *Hospitals*, 20 July, 40.

———. 1987d. "Hospital-Physician Link Generates $4 Million." *Hospitals*, 5 December, 66–67.

Sandrick, Karen. 1988. "Multis Putting More Effort into MD Relationships." *Hospitals*, 5 March, 70–71.

Sheldon, Alan. 1988. *Managing Doctors*. Homewood, Ill.: Dow Jones-Irwin.

Shortell, Stephen M. 1986. "New Models for Hospital-Physician Relations." In *The Corporation of Health Care Delivery*. Edited by Monica R. Dreuth. Chicago: American Hospital Publishing.

———. 1988. "The Medical Staff of the Future: Replanting the Garden." *New Frontiers of Health Care Management*.

Snook, I. Donald. 1987. *Building a Winning Medical Staff*. Chicago: American Hospital Publishing.

Sollins, Howard L. 1988. "Purchasing Physician Practices: Legal and Regulatory Concerns." *Healthcare Financial Management* (January): 56–63.

Speaker, Rick. 1987. "Hospital-Physician Bonding." *Computers in Healthcare* (October): 67–68.

Stromberg, Ross E. 1987. *Physician-Hospital Relationships in Today's Market-Driven Environment*. San Francisco: Epstein, Becker, Borsody, Stromberg and Green.

Super Palm, Kari. 1988. "Group Practices Mimic Venture Capital Firms Created by Hospitals, Physicians." *Modern Healthcare*, 26 February, 73.

Teitelbaum, Karen C., and Robert T. Bulger. 1988. "Strengthening Physician Bonds through Practice Development Planning." *Healthcare Financial Management* (May): 50–56.

Thomas, M. Carroll. 1987. "Joint Ventures: Who Knows What Evil Lurks . . ." *Medical Economics*, 30 March, 47–51.

Uhlar, Bob. 1987. "Sale/Lease-Back with Doctors Being Explored by Hospitals." *Hospitals*, 20 November, 44.

Waldholz, Michael, and Walt Bogdanich. 1989. "Doctor-owned Labs Earn Lavish Profits in a Captive Market." *Wall Street Journal*, 1 March, 1.

Wallace, Cynthia. 1987. "Physicians Leaving Their Practices for Hospital Jobs." *Modern Healthcare*, 8 May, 40–57.

Young, David W., and Richard B. Saltman. 1988. *The Hospital Power Equilibrium*. Baltimore: Johns Hopkins University Press.

Chapter 12

Medical Enterprise

We are involved in a health care revolution today. Some physicians will lead it. Some will be led, and some will sleep through it only to awaken and find themselves in financial trouble. One approach is sure to fail.
—Wayman R. Spence, *"Marketing Is Not a Question of Ethics—It Is a Question of Survival"*

Entrepreneurship will be the basis of tomorrow's hospital-physician relationships. In the next five years, hospitals will select first teams of preferred physicians, and doctors will make primary-hospital-affiliation decisions. Shared business experiences will be a major factor in these choices. *Healthcare Forum's* national panel predicted that hospitals may earn 30 percent of their revenues from noninpatient revenues. By 1995, the percentage will be closer to half.

The medical marketplace is just as entrepreneurial. Physicians are specializing in market-oriented niches, dispensing drugs in their offices, diversifying into laboratory and imaging centers, and building multisite practice networks through mergers and acquisitions. This is the new era of medical enterprise.

There is cause for mutual concern about competition. Doctors fear that hospitals will increase their share of ambulatory medicine at the expense of physician office practices. Hospitals do not know which doctors are truly loyal. Competition is the flip side of cooperation in medical enterprise. Although hospitals and doctors will collaborate, they will also compete across a broad array of medical businesses.

This competition will be healthy. In this "cooperate or compete" world, all parties will achieve new levels of respect. Forces bigger than hospitals or physicians are driving them together. Interdependence will be their shared future—but negotiated on a business basis.

217

JOINT VENTURES: QUESTIONS NEED ANSWERS

Achieving such an interdependent future may not be easy. The experience of hospitals and physicians in joint ventures has been no "rose garden." Following are some of the urgent questions hospitals and physicians are asking about the future of medical enterprise:

- What will be the driving forces motivating hospitals and doctors to collaborate or compete?
- Which diversified businesses hold most promise for joint ventures?
- What new organizational structures will successfully integrate financial interests and effective entrepreneurship?
- Given the history of joint ventures, what have hospitals and physicians learned about shared enterprises?
- What leadership skills and training are best suited to the management of joint ventures?

As the "business of caring" focuses intensely on the business aspect, answering these questions successfully may determine who will thrive and who will struggle to survive in the future health care marketplace.

DRIVING FORCES IN MEDICAL ENTERPRISE

A national survey in *Healthcare Forum* confirms that joint ventures are not a fad (Coile and Grossman 1987). Many powerful forces are driving higher levels of bonding between health facilities and their medical staff members:

1. *Declining Profitability.* Both hospitals and physicians are suffering income losses and shrinking net margins as their annual cost increases of 8–10 percent climb well above industrywide revenue gains of 4–5 percent for both medical and hospital care.
2. *Malpractice Crisis.* The malpractice situation is out of control and getting worse, as demonstrated by the situation of trauma and obstetric care in Florida. Hospitals and physicians will engage in joint risk management programs to reduce their malpractice exposure, and in the future they may share malpractice insurance costs under a hospital "blanket" liability policy or self-insurance program.
3. *Managed Care.* The most powerful force supporting hospital-physician relationships is economic risk sharing for managed care contracts. By the early 1990s, more than 75 percent of patients in most hospitals will be

covered by fixed-price contracts, including Medicare, HMOs, PPOs, and EPAs with major employers and third party administrators. An increasing number of these fixed-price agreements will bundle hospital and physician fees in a single reimbursement. The trend will be accelerated if DRGs known as "ambulatory visit groups" are extended to physicians by the federal government.

For hospitals and physicians, the choice of collaboration or competition is not an either-or situation. Some competition is inevitable. The tendency to collaborate is strongly rooted but has been buffeted by competitive forces in the past few years. More than ever, hospitals and physicians need to find common ground— shared medical enterprises that advance their mutual interests and bring benefits to the community in the form of new programs and services.

VENTURING: WHAT HOSPITALS AND PHYSICIANS HAVE LEARNED

Why do ventures succeed or fail? Reasons for success vary, but persistence, timing, innovation, flexibility, and leadership are important. More fundamentally, health care enterprises succeed or fail to the extent they have adequate capitalization and management expertise—just like other kinds of businesses.

In an article by Michael Costello (1986) in *Hospital and Health Services Administration*, health care ventures were analyzed for critical success factors. These were the key elements of entrepreneurial success for medical enterprises:

1. *Market Perspective*. Building any new business begins with customers and their defined needs. Health care enterprises started for defensive reasons (e.g., to defend inpatient market share) may miss important aspects of consumer wants. National Medical Enterprises sold its group of ambulatory care centers because they provided few inpatient referrals. The company chose instead to help the medical staff of its hospitals more effectively market their practices and channel patients to company facilities.
2. *Execution*. Venture capitalist Benjamin Rosen describes entrepreneurship as the "art of execution" (Costello 1986). Conceptualizing new ventures is much easier than successfully implementing them. Many medical enterprises have failed to meet timetables and thus drawn down scarce venture capital, postponed product introduction, and pushed back the break-even point. Costello (1986) notes that successful business plans may take 200–300 hours to prepare but are well worth the investment.
3. *Competitive Response*. All too frequently, hospitals underestimate how competitors will respond to a new medical enterprise. Some hospitals that

developed free-standing ambulatory care centers discovered that physicians could compete just by changing their office hours and increasing the size of their signs.

4. *Entrepreneurialism*. The final factor—the entrepreneurial mindset—is a subtle but significant factor. Entrepreneurs may find it difficult to thrive in a hospital's more bureaucratic corporate culture. A number of hospitals have created free-standing for-profit subsidiaries outside the traditional hospital organization and policies. Management studies suggest there may be an inherent conflict between the autonomy-seeking entrepreneur and any large organization. Managing entrepreneurial mavericks will be a challenge for health care executives.

WINNERS: JOINT VENTURES WITH PROMISE

Experiences with joint venturing vary widely. Across the nation, these are among the major categories of hospital-physician ventures that appear to be succeeding:

- Diagnostic *imaging centers* are among the most popular and profitable of joint ventures. Not all are local ventures. NMR Centers, of Newport Beach, California, has seven MRI facilities. NMR is the general partner and local physicians and hospitals are limited partners, and risk is spread evenly for the cost of the facility, equipment, and operation. Whereas some imaging centers are free-standing, others are hospital-based. In one Republic hospital, the imaging department's equipment is owned by an investor syndicate of 25 physicians, who each put up $5,000. The specialized cardiology diagnostic equipment is leased back to the hospital, which manages the facility.

- More hospitals are buying *lithotripters* through joint ventures. The cost is $1.5 to $2.5 million for equipment and facilities. Uro-Tech of Houston has set up eight lithotripter centers as joint ventures with local physicians and hospitals. Second-generation devices costing $400,000 to $800,000 should trigger a new round of lithotripter investment and venturing.

- *Independent practice associations* (IPAs) are the most popular of the alternative delivery systems. IPAs accounted for 61.7 percent of new HMOs formed and have a 38.6 percent market share of the 25 million Americans enrolled in HMOs, according to the mid-1987 HMO census conducted by InterStudy (1987), of Excelsior, Minnesota. Increasingly, physicians are taking the initiative in IPA formation. At St. Joseph's Hospital in Phoenix (632 beds), more than two hundred doctors invested $1,000 each in a new for-profit organization called St. Joseph's Physician Associates, then invited hospital executives to engage in joint ventures. The result is a full-fledged IPA capitalized with $300,000 from the physicians, the hospital, and the Fireman's Fund Insurance Company.

- Free-standing *cancer centers* are new but increasingly common medical enterprises. These facilities amount to minihospitals, with capital investments of $2.5 to $4 million for 5,000 to 10,000 square feet of advanced cancer diagnostic and treatment space. Treatment modalities run the gamut from ambulatory radiation to chemotherapy. Patients like state-of-the-art care available in nonhospital ambulatory settings. Early ventures, such as a free-standing center in Beckley, West Virginia, are experiencing return on investment of 20–30 percent.

- Physical *rehabilitation centers* are lower-cost ventures that require capitalization of $200,000 to $300,000, primarily for building and equipment costs. The Health Quest Group of South Bend, Indiana, is a for-profit firm that organizes rehabilitation center ventures. The number of limited partner physicians may be as few as five or six. Their referrals alone may be sufficient to generate $500,000 in annual gross revenues. All five Health Quest centers achieved profitability in their first year.

RISKY BUSINESS: VENTURES THAT FAILED

Joint venturing can be risky business! More than one venture has been a disappointment to its sponsors, and several have been financial flops.

- A *medical hotel* project of a large urban hospital in a southern metropolis was auctioned by its bank after the hotel failed to generate expected demand and revenues. The hospital was initially approached by a hotel developer with a turnkey project. The developer had worked with several other hospitals in medical hotel projects and had a formula approach. The hotel project fit with this hospital's concept of itself as a "dominant medical center" with a substantial referral business. Physician investors were limited partners. The hotel was built on the hospital campus. When demand failed to materialize at projected levels, the bank foreclosed the loan. This story may have a happy ending. The hospital was the only bidder at the bank auction. Under new loan terms, the hotel project may yet be viable. It gives the hospital and physicians an opportunity to reconceptualize new uses for the hotel space, such as an ambulatory substance abuse program with a residential component.

- *Ambulatory care centers* sponsored by two California nonprofit hospitals were market washouts for similar reasons: inadequate market research, high fixed operational costs, undercapitalization, high-cost locations, and too little marketing applied too late. Both experiences proved the market maxim that "lack of a product in a niche is no guarantee a profitable niche exists."

The two ambulatory centers intended to provide episodic care to insured customers with no regular source of care. The lack of market research on site location proved costly. Heavy traffic in the area never translated into demand for ambulatory care. Marketing consisted of putting up signs at the centers and distributing handbills to local employers. Full-time salaried physicians contributed to the high fixed overhead. Since all the physicians were young, none had an established practice to move to the new location. The convenience-care philosophy did not support the creation of a broad base of loyal customers and return business. The failures cost the health care systems and their limited partners millions in write-offs. One hospital lost $3.3 million. Compounding the error, the parent multihospital system, by creating ambulatory care competition for the medical staffs of its own member hospitals, stirred up local physician concern and opposition. Financial failure of the centers did little to assuage fears that the parent company might again intrude by attempting to create a local medical enterprise sometime in the future.

- *Diagnostic imaging centers* have not been all winners. Among the losers were two West Coast hospital sponsors and their physician partners. Medical staff commitment was the critical factor in both failures. In one situation, the hospital failed to provide the opportunity for limited partnership to the entire medical staff. When the limited number of shares were all subscribed by a medical staff faction, the hospital closed the partnership, effectively frustrating other doctors. They retaliated by sending MRI referrals to a competing hospital. The second case was similar. The hospital joint ventured the MRI project with an outside radiologist entrepreneur because the hospital's own radiologists were initially cool to the proposal. The radiology group then developed a competing imaging center, which garnered referrals through medical staff loyalty. The lesson of this experience is that medical support is critical to success. By joint venturing with an entrepreneur, the hospital saved time in market entry but cost the imaging facility the local medical support it needed to survive.

- *Medical practice acquisition* may be a loaded gun on the table of hospital-physician relationships. Acquiring a medical practice puts the hospital directly in the medical marketplace—as a competitor. When Sharp Hospitals, a two-hospital system in San Diego, acquired a 100-physician clinic, the medical staff revolted. In the brouhaha, the CEO and hospital administrator resigned and a member of the board was named as the new president. Now that the dust is settling, the hospital has moved to accommodate the dissident physicians while also supporting expansion of the medical clinic. The strategy is working, but hospital administration has learned there must be "no surprises" in medical staff relations.

REMOTE PRACTICE NETWORKS

The remote practice network (RPN) is an advanced response to the competitive health care marketplace of today and the managed care market of tomorrow. The hospital and physicians are linked electronically in a hub-and-spoke network, with computer terminals in the physicians' offices tied into the hospital's mainframe computer. Terminal and hookup costs may be donated by the hospital or shared with participating physicians.

The RPN concept was pioneered by the consulting firm of Magliaro and McHaney, based in San Diego, to electronically link hospitals and their medical staffs. The goal, for each hospital, is to achieve a powerful market position in the local medical service area and, by using several small multis and alliances, to control a larger medical service area.

Kalamazoo, Michigan, is a two-hospital town. Bronson and Borgess are two modern medical centers that compete across a broad range of services. The hospitals have a medical staff overlap of 75 percent and share radiology and pathology groups. In 1985 Borgess developed and installed an RPN. More than 100 physicians were linked into the network. Borgess issued a medical credit card to 75,000 preferred customers, providing instant identification in the office of any participating physician as well as in the hospital's various ambulatory and inpatient programs. In its first year, Borgess increased admissions by 3 percent and net revenues by 15 percent.

In Phoenix, Arizona, St. Joseph's Hospital and Medical Center developed a remote practice network that includes more than 300 physicians, several located outside the state. The RPN has helped maintain St. Joseph's market position and referral base despite a general decrease in admissions in the Phoenix area.

The purpose of establishing an RPN is nothing less than to attain market dominance. The hospital develops the network to include the 20–30 percent of the medical staff who provide 75–80 percent of the hospital's inpatient referrals. The RPN is more than a telecommunications network. It has both clinical and financial functions. It facilitates the easy transfer of data to and from each doctor's office. For example, specialized lab tests, including CAT scans, can be "read" remotely from each office. Admission procedures are simplified and admission is expedited.

Marketing is a central objective of creating an RPN. A detailed market research data base on the hospital's service area is compiled. The market data are then put to use by means of the latest in modern marketing methods, including direct mail and telemarketing. The sponsoring hospitals and physicians take new ventures and services to market jointly. Cataract surgery, obstetrics packages, cosmetic surgery, pain management programs, weight loss programs, and rehabilitation are among the range of programs that have been marketed by RPNs.

Organizing for managed care contracts is another major objective. The RPN provides easy electronic linkage for tracking and managing patients. It makes the hospital appear to managed care buyers as an attractive preferred provider.

Each physician and medical group is a venture partner in the network and contributes capital and commitment. Sharing the costs and benefits of the network strengthens the bonding between hospitals and the participating physicians. Jealousy on the part of nonparticipating physicians has generally not been a problem. The network is easily expandable if additional doctors and medical groups wish to join. The remote practice network is the perfect mechanism for the age of medical enterprise.

STRUCTURING JOINT HOSPITAL-PHYSICIAN VENTURES

Much has been learned about structuring hospital-physician joint ventures in the past five years. What was a highly experimental strategy is becoming "business as usual" in many hospitals. Yet joint ventures are still high risk, both as investments and in their potential to disrupt hospital–medical staff relationships.

Appropriate structuring of joint ventures can improve business prospects as well as build a foundation for positive relationships. It is not easy, as health care executives and physician participants in joint ventures can attest. Here are the most common kinds of hospital-physician ventures today:

- limited partnership syndicates
- sale and lease-back arrangements
- venture capital companies
- provider networks
- alternative delivery systems (ADSs)

MICRO AND MACRO VENTURES

Dale Rublee, of the AMA, and Bob Rosenfield, formerly with the law firm of Memel, Jacobs, Pierno, Gersh and Ellsworth of Los Angeles, make the distinction between *micro* and *macro* transactions (Rublee and Rosenfield 1987).

Micro joint ventures are asset transactions in which a small number of physicians invest in medical services rather than provide them. These activities are not significantly different from similar business ventures in the private sector.

The primary objective of micro ventures is to provide economic incentives to the investors. Secondary objectives include capital formation, preemption of competitor moves (including moves by medical staff), stimulation of hospital inpatient referrals, and closer bonding between hospitals and physicians. These joint ventures typically focus on a single specific project, such as an imaging center, medical office building, ambulatory surgery center, or reference laboratory. Few micro ventures require more than $2 to $5 million in hospital-physician capital, and many require much less.

Macro ventures have a broader scope and purpose than simply to respond incrementally to the "post-DRG" economics of health care. Profitability is still an objective but is often deferred in the interest of restructuring the local health care delivery system for the future. Macro ventures attempt what Rublee and Rosenfield refer to as a "systemic response," which is relatively complex and sophisticated. The risk is higher but macro ventures offer greater potential for physician involvement and control over the organization of health care.

ALTERNATIVE MODELS OF JOINT VENTURES

To advance the goals of medical enterprise, there is a spectrum of options for structuring hospital-physician joint ventures. The options are limited only by the imagination (and legal advice).

Limited Partnership Syndicates

Limited partnership syndication has been the most popular approach to structuring hospital-physician joint ventures. This type of syndication involves complex forms of legal organization that combine features of partnerships and corporations. A limited partnership has a general partner and at least one limited partner (more often there are many). The general partner has exclusive responsibility for management of the venture; the limited partners are simply investors and have no role in management. In return, the state statutes that regulate limited partnerships insulate the limited partners from the risks of the venture. The only money they put at risk is their defined investment or any notes or guarantees they have signed. Limited partners are not at risk for the venture's failure or any losses stemming from the venture that exceed its assets. Nor are limited partners at risk in the event the venture is sued and the judgment exceeds insurance coverage.

The limited partnership is considered a partnership for tax purposes, not a corporation. This is significant, because partnerships themselves are not taxable. If a limited partnership generates net income, it does not pay federal or state tax, as would a corporation. Instead, any income passes directly to the limited and general partners, who pay taxes on this income to the extent they have taxable personal income.

In a typical "micro" venture, physician investors contribute small amounts of capital, often less than $5,000, thereby purchasing units in the limited partnership. The investors are primarily motivated by the desire to acquire a significant return on investment (in the range of 15–20 percent cash on cash) and to achieve certain nonmonetary goals shared by the hospital and the participating doctors.

As the biggest player in joint venturing, the hospital often takes on the general partner responsibilities. The role of general partner can also be played by the hospital's parent corporation, a multihospital system, or a physician entrepreneur.

Before the recent tax reform legislation, limited partnerships had considerable appeal in their potential as tax shelters through depreciation, investment tax credits, and pass-through of operating losses to the individual investors. Since tax reform, limited partnerships have been reoriented to income and capital appreciation. This has cut down on joint ventures that were primarily attractive as tax shelters and had less potential to generate profits.

Sale and Lease-Back Arrangements

This model of medical enterprise is drawn right from the private sector. A sale and lease-back deal involves selling a hospital asset (e.g., a medical office building) to a group of investors, typically physicians. The hospital retains general partner status and manages the building. Constructing new facilities (e.g., free-standing diagnostic imaging centers) or purchasing capital equipment likewise uses outside capital provided by physician investors.

An "off-balance-sheet" strategy such as this keeps long-term debt off the hospital's statement of obligations. More important for the hospital, it provides more financial flexibility by protecting capital for other operating or investment opportunities. For the physicians, it provides a select investment option with limited risk and a reasonable to excellent rate of return. All parties gain from increased physician commitment, a critical success factor in virtually any medical enterprise.

Venture Capital Companies

The venture capital company is a for-profit business that pools investment resources from a large number of physicians. The venture capital pool has two advantages over project-specific ventures. First, the venture capital company is not limited to a specific project or the short-term goals of a small group of doctors. This is a midrange investment vehicle designed to meet the needs of a large number of physicians through collaboration with the hospital. Second, as Rublee and Rosenfield (1987) emphasize, the venture capital company has the resources and expertise to shape a coherent investment strategy and pursue it over time.

The venture capital company serves as a general partner in some transactions, as a limited partner in others, and as a lender in still others. Shares of stock are sold to physician investors, and the proceeds are utilized to finance a series of limited partnerships for specific projects. Physician investors may invest at several levels: in the diversified capital pool represented by the venture company as well as in limited partnership interests or other forms of securities sold in relation to particular projects.

Creating and managing a venture capital company is a sophisticated task that requires specialized venture capital expertise. Several multihospital alliances, including Voluntary Hospitals of America and American Healthcare Systems, have utilized venture capital companies, and others, are in the process of creating them. At the local level, hospitals such as Memorial Health System of South Bend, Indiana, have created venture capital funds with physician investment to pursue health-related projects.

The size of the venture capital company calls for sophisticated management, which greatly improves the chances of success. The venture capital pool can provide hospitals and physicians with the capital and the capacity to develop components of a continuum of care—from health promotion to home care. Likewise, the pool can finance development of a cluster of health-related programs and services. This "market management" approach links the hospital and physicians in an interlocking web of clinical and financial relationships.

Provider Networks

The provider network is a relatively simple organizational model. It can be organized as a for-profit or nonprofit corporation, although a tax exemption is unlikely. In the for-profit version, the provider network corporation sells securities to physicians to finance creation and marketing of the network. The network's customers are HMOs, PPOs, managed care insurance companies, health benefit trust funds, third party administrators, and self-insured employers.

The network is in reality a series of interlocking contracts whereby physicians and hospitals agree to provide services for a prenegotiated rate or at a discount from standard charges. Variations are endless. For example, Pacific Presbyterian Medical Group of San Francisco launched a "managed care independent practice association" in 1985. Its goal was to seek managed care contracts for its 208 physician members. With seed capital from the hospital, the IPA is now established and is part of a network providing managed care services. The IPA successfully competed for a CHAMPUS contract in northern California that could generate 90,000 patients, of which 15,000 would be in the hospital's San Francisco service area.

Managed care niches are being created by entrepreneurs. For example, in the past year, insurers have been contracting with new entrepreneurial networks focused on a specific condition or patient category, such as alcohol and drug abuse or Workers' Compensation.

Alternative Delivery Systems

The most complex and expensive form of hospital–physician joint venture is the ADS. These ventures go beyond provider networks in that they include risk sharing, case management, quality assurance, and other systems. Typical ADS joint ventures can cost their sponsors millions. A new HMO will require a minimum of $5 million in venture capital and may not reach profitability before 30,000 to 40,000 members are enrolled.

Other ADS ventures include PPOs, third party administrators, insurance companies, and speciality managed care plans (e.g., an alcohol and drug abuse plan). Despite a crowded and competitive marketplace, 99 new HMOs and an estimated 160 new PPOs were launched in 1986. Another 125 HMOs and at least 100 PPOs entered the field in 1987. Although the pace of HMO and PPO formation slowed in 1988–1989, acquistions and mergers continue to involve hospitals and health systems in developing ADS projects.

Some hospitals and physicians are getting outside help in ADS formation. Private Healthcare Systems (PHS) of Lexington, Massachusetts, launched a national PPO network with organizations in 40 major markets. PHS contracts with selected hospitals and physicians in each market area. The "customers" are 18 small and midsize insurance companies that have aligned with PHS and will use the local provider networks to design PPO options in their benefit packages. PHS itself is a joint venture of Great West Life Assurance Company, a Canadian company with U.S. headquarters in Englewood, Colorado, and several other companies, including the Health Data Institute, also in Lexington. Selected hospitals are invited to bid on a straight discount basis, and members of their medical staffs are recruited into the ventures. PHS is organizing or operating networks in Atlanta, Akron, Cincinnati, Chicago, Denver, Houston, Orlando, and a number of other U.S. markets.

Even with strong management and capitalization, ADSs are high-risk ventures. Several of the major for-profit health care management firms, including AMI, NME, and Whittaker have ended their HMO and insurance experiments after costly losses. Voluntary Hospitals of America lost more than $50 million in the Partners plan, a managed care joint venture with Aetna. ADS ventures are not for the timid, but the rewards may become too big to ignore as the managed care business grows.

INNOVATIVE VENTURES: FEE-FOR-SERVICE RESEARCH

Biotherapeutics, Inc.. is the first of a new wave of medical companies that will employ research techniques and experimental drugs in private patient care (Bylinsky 1987). Beginning in 1985, the company, which is based in Franklin, Tennessee, opened a private front in the war against cancer. By devising an experimental approach under FDA supervision, Biotherapeutics was able to launch a clinic specializing in advanced cancer therapy using Interleukin-2 (IL-2) treatments customized on a patient-by-patient basis. Already the company has won FDA blessing for its treatment approaches for kidney tumors and melanoma skin cancers. FDA action means that Blue Cross and other insurers are beginning to pay for the expensive laboratory procedures Biotherapeutics uses to tailor treatment to individual patients.

Biotherapeutics is now launching a licensing program that will make its treatments widely available in the United States and overseas. Its Biology Therapy Facilities are licensed to hospitals, allowing them to capture more cancer patients and reinforce their image as high-tech market leaders. In Newport Beach, California, Biotherapeutics sold a 20 percent share in the lab to Hoag Memorial Hospital for $300,000 and another 15 percent share to Hoag medical staff for $240,000. Biotherapeutics is the general partner and takes a 5 percent management fee. Other hospitals have signed up for Biology Therapy Facilities in La Jolla and Los Angeles, California; Plantation, Florida; and Nashville, Tennessee. The company had laboratories in more than 30 hospitals in 1988 and plans to expand into other markets to develop a national network of facilities by the early 1990s.

FDA approval given to Biotherapeutics for use of the potential wonder drug IL-2 was the breakthrough. At that point IL-2 was in use only in experimental trials at the National Institutes of Health. Biotherapeutics was founded by two prominent cancer researchers who left the National Cancer Institute to try a private approach to medical treatment and research.

By structuring its licensed labs as joint ventures with hospitals and physicians, Biotherapeutics could lock up a significant number of the nation's leading cancer centers and the 3,500 registered oncologists, giving it a substantial proprietary advantage. Biotherapeutics has no major competitors, although some hospital companies such as Humana are reportedly investigating the field. At least one private physician, Kenneth Alonso, of Atlanta, offers small-scale treatment with IL-2.

How big is the market for experimental therapies? That is highly speculative. It may have boom potential, but fee-for-service research is still very much an experiment. Biotherapeutics lost $8 million in its first three years but expects to reach profitability by the early 1990s. Biotherapeutics served about 800 patients in 1987 and aims for 80,000 by 1995. Securities analysts predict revenues could reach $200 to $385 million by 1992.

THE FUTURE OF MEDICAL ENTERPRISE

Hospitals and physicians will find the bonds that link them tightening in the months and years ahead. A report from the Health Care Advisory Board (1986), a market research firm in Washington, D.C., highlighted a study of 24 hospital-physician strategies. In-office computers and shared ventures will promote physician-hospital bonding, but those are only a few of the many medical enterprise alternatives. Some, like computers, have been well accepted; others, like office practice acquisitions, have experienced real resistance.

In the era of medical enterprise, the critical success factor for both hospitals and physicians will be a willingness to experiment with new methods of service delivery and reimbursement, reinforced by mutually designed systems and shared investments. There is no foolproof model, but remember the market advantage is always with the attackers!

CONCLUSION: A DOUBLE HELIX FUTURE

In the future hospitals and physicians can anticipate an increasing convergence of their clinical and economic interests. Their intertwining interests will resemble the double helix of molecular life as all parties become mutually interdependent in order to survive.

Hospitals and their medical staffs have a choice today. They can be forced together by ambulatory visit groups and bureaucratic medicine or they can step forward and develop shared medical enterprises. In other words, they can manage their own markets or wait to have competitors and outside forces manage them. This is the age of medical enterprise. As the Chinese philosopher Lao Tsu said, "Let a thousand flowers bloom."

STRATEGIC IMPLICATIONS FOR PHYSICIANS

1. *Physicians need to foster an entrepreneurial mindset.* This is the age of medical enterprise. The only way physicians and medical groups can beat

the pattern of declining reimbursement and increasing regulation is through investments. In a group practice, one partner should be designated and supported as the business developer on behalf of the group. Diversification and development are too important strategically to be left to chance.

2. *Every physician practice and medical group should have a long-range development plan for the growth of diversified practice revenues.* This strategic development plan should have a scope of at least five years. Potential development projects should include both independent ventures and joint ventures with preferred hospitals or local health systems. The goal should be to develop at least 25 percent additional revenues through diversification by the end of the five-year planning and development time-table.

3. *In support of its strategic development plan, each medical practice and group should set aside a venture capital fund to capitalize diversification activities.* Ideally, the budget set-aside should be at least 5–15 percent of annual revenues for investment in new technology, facilities, and services.

STRATEGIC IMPLICATIONS FOR HOSPITALS

1. *To achieve its goal of diversification, every hospital and health system should have a long-range (five-year) diversification and development plan.* The plan should be driven by the hospital's vision of its long-range future and should create the building blocks for a continuum of health and health-related services. A primary objective of the hospital's diversification plan should be the enhancement of the practices of the "first circle"—the key medical staff around which the organization will build its future.

2. *Hospitals should set a goal of 25–35 percent of revenues from nonpatient sources.* Hospitals should plan to get 25–35 percent of revenues from nonhospital sources by the end of a five-year period. Where diversification is already well underway, hospitals should aim for 30–40 percent by the end of five to seven years.

3. *Hospitals need a vice-president for corporate development.* A number of hospitals and health systems are reconceptualizing the functions of planning and marketing. Some have created a new position of vice-president for corporate development, based on the private sector model. This senior management position has primary responsibility for diversification and development. Compensation is highly results-driven, and bonuses may constitute 35–50 percent of total remuneration.

BIBLIOGRAPHY

"Ambulatory Care Joint Ventures Rise." 1986. *Hospitals*, 5 February, 59.

Anderson, Howard J. 1985. "Carle Using Branch Clinics to Expand Patient Base." *Modern Healthcare*, 2 August, 70.

Anderson, Maren D. and Peter D. Fox. 1987. "Lessons Learned from Medicaid Managed Care Approaches." *Health Affairs* (Fall): 71–85.

Barkholz, David. 1985. "Clinic Revives Downtown, Becomes Model for System." *Modern Healthcare*, 2 August, 72.

Brown, Montague. 1981. "Contract Management: Legal and Policy Implications." *Inquiry* 18 (Spring): 8–17.

Bylinsky, Gene. 1987. "The Anticancer Company Expands." *Fortune*, 23 November, 123–24.

Carter, Kim. 1987. "Spurred by Blue Shield Decision, Philadelphia Physicians Starting Lab." *Modern Healthcare*, 16 January, 52.

Coile, Russell C., Jr., and Randolph M. Grossman. 1987. "The New Medicine." *Healthcare Forum Journal* (September-October): 14–17.

———. 1988. "Tomorrow's Macrotrends." *Healthcare Forum Journal* (November-December): 50–53.

Costello, Michael M. 1986. "Caution: Business Opportunity Ahead." *Hospital and Health Services Administration* (November-December): 19–24.

Crane, Stephen C. 1986. "Issues and Trends in the Regulation of Officebased Clinical Laboratories." *Clinics in Laboratory Medicine* 6:369–86.

Feldstein, Paul. 1983. *Health Care Economics*. 2d ed. New York: Wiley Medical Publications.

Ferber, Stanley. 1986. "Will the In-Office Testing Boom Backfire?" *Medical Economics*, 28 April, 175–85.

Fine, Jennifer. 1986. "Joint Ventures Feeling Impact of Uncertainty over Tax Reform." *Modern Healthcare*, 4 July, 111–15.

Frederick, Larry. 1987. "Joint Ventures: The Hottest Game in Medicine." *Medical Economics*, 30 March, 40–45.

Free, Helen M., and Alfred H. Free. 1986. "Dry Chemistry: Its Expanded Role in Doctor's Office Testing." *Clinics in Laboratory Medicine* 6:267–71.

Gabel, Jon. 1987. "The Commercial Health Insurance Industry in Transition." *Health Affairs* (Fall): 46–60.

Health Care Advisory Board. 1986. *Physician Bonding: Overview of Strategies Coast to Coast*. Washington, D.C.: Health Care Advisory Board.

Herrell, John H. 1987. "The Multi-Regional Group Practice: A New Delivery Model." Paper delivered at a conference sponsored by Cain Brothers, Shattuck, Mass.

Hillman, Alan L., and J. Sanford Schwartz. 1986. "The Diffusion of MRI: Patterns of Siting and Ownership in an Era of Changing Incentives." *American Journal of Radiology* 146:963–69.

Huston, Phillips. 1987. "Joint Ventures: Choosing the Best Tax Strategy." *Medical Economics*, 30 March, 68–73.

Iezzoni, Lisa I. 1986. "The Impact of Reimbursement Changes on Doctor's Office Testing." *Clinics in Laboratory Medicine* 6:329–43.

InterStudy. 1987. *The InterStudy Edge*. Excelsior, Minn.: InterStudy. (Reported in *Medical Benefits*, 15 June 1987, 6.)

"Joint Ventures: A Go/No-Go Checklist." 1987. *Medical Economics*, 30 March, 74.

Jose, David E. 1986. "Antitrust and Joint Ventures." *Topics in Health Care Financing* 13 (Fall): 27–40.

Kirchner, Merian. 1987. "How Much Better Are Doctors in Groups Doing?" *Medical Economics*, 13 April, 226–47.

Laessig, Ronald H., Sharon S. Ehrmeyer, and David J. Hassemer. 1986. "Quality Control and Quality Assurance." *Clinics in Laboratory Medicine* 6:317–27.

Lutz, Sandy. 1987. "Marketing, Public Relations Are Keys to the Outpatient Surgery Business." *Modern Healthcare*, 13 February, 96–98.

Medical Executive Committee Reporter 2 (May-June 1987).

Moskowitz, Mark A. 1986. "Evaluating Doctor's Office Testing Patterns." *Clinics in Laboratory Medicine* 6:387–94.

Nash, David B. 1985. "Joint Ventures Popular." *Modern Healthcare*, 24 May, 82.

Needham, Cynthia A. 1986. "Rapid Methods in Microbiology for In-Office Testing." *Clinics in Laboratory Medicine* 6:291–304.

Ng, Ronald H. 1986, "Selecting Instrumentation for Physician's Office Testing." *Clinics in Laboratory Medicine* 6:305–15.

Owens, Arthur. 1986. "Earnings: Have They Flattened Out for Good?" *Medical Economics*, 8 September, 163–81.

———. 1987. "Doctors' Earnings: On the Rise Again." *Medical Economics*, 7 September, 212–37.

"Physician Involvement Helps Ventures Acheive Success." 1986. *Modern Healthcare*, 15 August, 38.

Reese Report 1 (March 1987).

Relman, Arnold S. 1987. "Dealing with Conflicts of Interest." *New England Journal of Medicine* 313:749–51.

Richman, Dan. 1985a. "Diverse Partners Join Hospitals in Ventures." *Modern Healthcare*, 24 May, 75–76.

———. 1985b. "Hospital-Staff Ventures Popular, but Critics Question Their Worth." *Modern Healthcare*, 24 May, 80–81.

———. 1985c. "Groups Hope Mergers Will Attract Business of Prepaid Health Plans." *Modern Healthcare*, 2 August, 67–68.

———. 1985d. "Cleveland Clinic Viewing Prepaid Plans, Risk Sharing." *Modern Healthcare*, 2 August, 74.

Riffer, Joyce. 1986. "New Tax Laws Won't Stop MOB Joint Ventures." *Hospitals*, 20 November, 76.

Rolph, Elizabeth S., Paul B. Ginsburg, and Susan D. Hosek. 1987. "The Regulation of Preferred Provider Arrangements." *Health Affairs* (Fall): 32–45.

Rublee, Dale A., and Robert H. Rosenfield. 1987. "Organizational Aspects of Physician Joint Ventures." *American Journal of Medicine* 82:518–24.

Sandrick, Karen. 1986a. "Group Practice: What's the Attraction?" *Hospitals*, 5 April, 46–50.

———. 1986b. "Joint Ventures: Why do 7 out of 10 Fail?" *Hospitals*, 20 December, 40–44.

Sax, Barry M. 1985. "HHS Begins to Monitor Recent Joint Ventures." *Hospitals*, 1 November, 87–90.

Shahoda, Teri. 1985. "Multis Look for Key to Success in Joint Ventures." *Hospitals*, 20 October, 38–39.

Spence, Wayman R. 1989. "Marketing Is Not a Question of Ethics—It Is a Question of Survival." *Practice Builders* (May): 1.

Statland, Bernard E. 1986. "The Role of the Hospital Laboratory and its Personnel in Doctor's Office Testing." *Clinics in Laboratory Medicine* 6:211–14.

Statland, Bernard E., and Mark A. Moskowitz. 1986. "Why Office Testing?" *Clinics in Laboratory Medicine* 6:205–10.

Stevens, Carol. 1987. "Joint Ventures: Don't Let the Law Take You by Surprise." *Medical Economics*, 30 March, 52–61.

Swett, Theresa F., and Dennis J. Conley. 1984. "Joint Ventures: The Theory and Practice." *Hospitals*, 1 May, 95–100.

"Tax-Exempt Debt, Joint Ventures Are Hospital Favorites." 1986. *Hospitals*, 5 July, 66.

Thomas, M. Carroll. 1987. "Joint Ventures: Who Knows What Evil Lurks . . ." *Medical Economics*, 30 March, 47–51.

Troyer, Glenn T. 1986. "Joint Venturing." *Topics in Health Care Financing* 13 (Fall): 1–12.

"Ventures Show Cooperation with MDs Up." 1985. *Hospitals*, 1 October, 37–39.

Wallace, Cynthia. 1986. "Groups' Advantages Luring More Physicians from Solo Practices." *Modern Healthcare*, 15 August, 58–62.

Western Network 6 (Fall 1987).

Wheeler, John R. C., Howard S. Zuckerman, and John Anderholdt. 1982. "How Management Contracts Can Affect Hospital Finances." *Inquiry* 18 (Summer): 160–166.

White, Elizabeth C. 1985. "Amenities Woo Patients to 'Designer' Hospital." *Modern Healthcare*, 2 August, 76–77.

Yanish, Donna. 1985. "Hospitals Warned of Hidden Costs in Joint Ventures with Physicians." *Modern Healthcare*, 11 October, 102.

Chapter 13

Physician Channeling

The greatest challenge for hospital strategists will be adapting to the retooling that will occur as private practice physicians are faced with challenging issues at the policy level . . . how to equitably offer economic incentives for specialists facing income shortfalls . . . how to efficiently carve out a slice of the strengthened primary care pie . . . how to negotiate deals with emerging megagroups.
—Paul Keckley, *"Life With Physicians in the Relative Value Age"*

Since physicians control an estimated 60–75 percent of all inpatient referrals, hospitals and health plans will increasingly engage in physician channeling to influence physician choices. In a period of declining inpatient revenues and increasing competition, hospitals must control market share through physicians. Channeling physician referrals can take many forms: providing incentives to physicians, engaging in joint ventures, and pursuing networking strategies (Exhibit 13-1).

There is considerable urgency for America's hospitals to increase admissions, even at the expense of their neighboring facilities. Hospital utilization shrank steadily from 1983 to 1988. This was a major shift in the use of hospital services that began before the passage of TEFRA and the change in 1983 to Medicare payment by DRG. Nationally, Americans consumed 1,214 hospital days per 1,000 population in 1981. That use rate plummeted over the next five years, averaging 5 percent fewer days each year in the process. Hospital admissions at the high point in 1981 reached 36,379,000. The nation has averaged nearly 1 million fewer inpatient admissions each year since.

The national decline in hospital days had been anticipated in California. According to the California Association of Hospitals and Health Systems, the state, which has the nation's largest HMO enrollment, was already experiencing in 1981 15.5 percent fewer hospital admissions per 1,000 population than the nation.

Exhibit 13-1 Physician Channeling: Hospital Strategies for Influencing Physician Choice on Inpatient Admission

Physician Incentives

Admitting privileges
Preferred surgical scheduling
Department chief appointment
HMO or PPO contracts
Medical continuing education
Physician practice subsidy
Teaching or research
Employment or contract
Recruitment of physician ''stars''
Medical executives

Joint Ventures

Diagnostic center
Ambulatory surgery center
Imaging center
HMO or PPO development
Health and fitness center
Medical office building
R & D venture fund
Rehabilitation center
Clinical institute
Insurance pool

Hospital-Physician Networking

Physician referral service (800 phone no.)
Remote practice network
Physician practice acquisition
Independent practice association
Physician service bureau
Hospital-based group practice
Research institute
Practice management services
Market-specialized clinical services
Risk management program

The gap had widened to 16.9 percent by 1985. U.S. hospital occupancy had fallen 11 percent in that five-year period, according to the AHA. The shrinking inpatient market has put increased pressure on every hospital to limit the damage and protect market share.

BONDING PHYSICIANS AND HOSPITALS

In the next decade, America's hospitals will pick their first team of physicians, a national panel of experts recently predicted for *Healthcare Forum* (Coile and Grossman 1987). Some hospitals will demand 100 percent commitment for inpatient referrals from their key admitters. The physicians will be "bonded" to their hospitals through a variety of incentives, joint ventures, and networking strategies.

The Privilege of Hospital Privileges

Soaring malpractice costs, the "glut" of physicians, and concerns about quality are driving hospitals to be more restrictive in granting and renewing medical staff privileges. A growing number of hospitals are tightening medical staff bylaws and staff admission criteria. Renewal of privileges is no longer automatic. More hospitals are putting conditions on surgical and other privileges and compelling recertification for specialized procedures.

An article in the *Medical Executive Committee Reporter* was headlined "Should You Shrink Your Medical Staff?" (Lang 1988). The newsletter is published for hospital medical executives by the National Health Foundation, a nonprofit arm of the Hospital Council of Southern California. The article directly confronts the problem of physician loyalty and commitment. A minimum of one admission per month is listed in many hospital medical staff bylaws as the requirement for maintaining "active" status. With such a meager requirement, a physician could maintain active standing at five or six hospitals and make a commitment to none. Some hospitals have raised the ante. Three admissions per month is not an unreasonable standard for maintaining active status on the medical staff, recommends Dr. Daniel Lang, editor of the *Medical Executive Committee Reporter*. Some recognition for consultation, outpatient activity, or chairing of significant committees can be granted to accommodate special circumstances. The tightening of active status may lose a few patients from physicians with marginal commitments, but it will channel more admissions from committed active members of the medical staff.

COMPUTERIZED PHYSICIAN REFERRAL SERVICES

In today's highly mobile society, just finding a physician is no simple matter. New computerized physician referral services that establish the physician-patient link are winning consumers and providing physicians with new clients.

The Health-Finder system pioneered by Scripps Memorial Hospital of La Jolla, California, was launched in mid-1985. The system takes customer information on desired physician specialty, location, hours of service, and insurance coverage and within seconds matches the customer with a doctor. The caller is then transferred directly by telephone to the physician's office. All this is accomplished with a single call.

Health Match, a computerized referral system created by Baxter Healthcare Corporation, based in Deerfield, Illinois, has been installed in more than 100 hospitals. The system is typically marketed by local hospitals utilizing a toll-free telephone number. Hospitals that have installed Health Match experience 30 calls a day or more. One South Florida hospital received more than 3,000 calls in a month.

For physicians, computerized referral services are a welcome source of new patients. More than 60 percent of the calls result in direct appointments. Most customers are not using the services to switch doctors: Over 95 percent of those who seek help from a computerized referral system have no regular physician.

Hospitals can utilize data from the referral services for a variety of marketing efforts. The referral systems generate mailing lists and regular reports by zip code. Each new customer of a referral service receives a computer-generated follow-up letter within days of the call to check that the physician appointment was made and that service was satisfactory. Referral service callers are a ready-made source of customers for other hospital marketing initiatives, such as educational and weight loss programs and health promotion services.

Ask-A-Nurse is an innovative spinoff of the original physician referral service concept. Referral Systems Group, a subsidiary of the Adventist West system in Roseville, California, developed a series of standardized responses to frequently asked health questions and put a nurse at the computer of its physician referral service. The service immediately attracted a tremendous number of callers, and Referral Systems Group has since marketed the Ask-A-Nurse system to more than 100 hospitals nationwide. One Ask-A-Nurse service drew 5,000 phone calls in a single month. Forty percent of the calls are for information only, but at least 40 percent of the Ask-A-Nurse callers make physician appointments.

RESTRUCTURING THE HOSPITAL-PHYSICIAN RELATIONSHIP

The next three to five years will bring major changes in physician-hospital relationships. The days of the voluntary medical staff may be numbered. What will replace it? A physicians union? Unlikely—the number of physicians aligned with unions is fewer than 2,500 nationally. More likely are new business relationships between hospitals and medical groups.

Scenario for the Future: Dissolve the Medical Staff

Picture this scenario in the mid-1990s:

> The medical staff of the average community hospital has been dis-
> solved. Instead, many hospitals have entered into a series of contracts
> with medical groups to operate the hospitals' clinical departments. The
> medical staffs are not "closed" because the hospitals put the depart-
> ments out to competitive bidding every two or three years. Physician
> groups compete for hospital affiliation on the basis of price, quality,
> and performance. The doctors are at risk under fixed-price contracts
> for services—not just pathology or radiology but intensive care, the
> nursery, and all clinical departments. The number of nongroup phy-
> sicians has fallen to less than 10 percent of all physicians. The non-
> aligned physicians are either "superstars" whose talents are so in
> demand they hold privileges at several competing hospitals or "lone
> wolves" who subsist on the few remaining fee-for-service patients or
> who work for a temporary-physician personnel agency.

Sound far-fetched? Yes, but it could happen. One major factor is the physician
surplus. Nearly 100,000 more doctors will be in practice in the 1990s. Only
31.5 percent of the young physicians under 40 are going into solo medical practice
(Jolly 1988). The rest are joining physician groups or HMOs.

Strategic Hospital Relationships with Physician Groups

The shifting economics of medicine is altering hospital-physician relationships,
basically by replacing individual physicians with medical groups in bargaining
situations. A growing number of physicians are accepting that groups are essential
in negotiated relationships.

It is a "buyers' market," observes Ronald P. Kaufman, vice-president for
medical affairs at 551-bed George Washington University Medical Center in
Washington, D.C. (Coile 1988a). Buyers such as insurance companies and HMOs
are negotiating with physicians on the basis of price. Although a single physician
has no bargaining power, a group of physicians can effectively negotiate with
clout, Dr. Kaufman believes.

"The day of the solo practitioner is gone," laments William S. Weil, M.D.,
chairman of the Los Angeles County Medical Association, in an interview with
Modern Healthcare (Burda 1988). Dr. Weil left private practice a year ago to
join CIGNA Healthplans of California as chairman of the HMO's department
of family practice.

Group practices have grown at an annual rate of 9.5 percent from 1980 to 1984, according to the AMA. The growth continues—from 10,762 groups in 1980 to 16,294 in 1986. The size of groups is climbing, too. Single specialty groups averaged just under six members in 1984, up from slightly over four in 1980; multispecialty group membership climbed from 15 to 27 physicians in the same period.

For many doctors, the rationale for joining groups is simple: earning power. Doctors in medical partnerships and groups on average earn more than solo practitioners. Doctors in solo private practice grossed 17 percent less than their group counterparts, according to a 1987 survey of physician incomes by *Medical Economics*. Worse yet, the median income of sole practitioners was 27 percent below the median income of group physicians (Owens 1988).

PHYSICIAN CONTRACTS

The competitive marketplace is forcing changes in hospital-physician contracting. Among the beneficiaries will be contract management firms. Hospitals are turning to outside management firms to provide physicians for emergency rooms, ambulatory care centers, and urgent care centers. Higher premiums for malpractice insurance and the growth of ambulatory care are driving forces in physician contracting. Hospitals not only want competent physicians but are paying for risk management, billing, and administration.

For example, the Fischer Mangold Group of Pleasanton, California, has 33 contracts with hospitals for the provision of emergency services. The emergency rooms of these hospitals have from 24,000 to 60,000 visits annually. Physicians are paid on a fee-for-service basis, with Fischer Mangold providing management services for fees of $3,000 to $58,000 per year. Coastal Emergency Services of Durham, North Carolina, has 160 hospital emergency room contracts, with 20 hospital customers added in the past year. Coastal's contracts range from $50,000 for emergency departments with 5,000 annual visits to more than $1 million for those with 100,000 visits.

In the laboratory and x-ray departments, traditional relationships and unwritten agreements are rapidly being replaced with formal contracts. The terms of a growing number of hospital contracts include a fee to the pathologist or radiologist for department management and administrative services. Hospitals like Rose Medical Center in Denver are revising their radiology contracts and asking their radiologists to accept Medicare assignment as payment in full.

Some physicians fear a loss of control in the shift to formal contracting and are hiring business consultants and attorneys to assist in negotiations. A typical firm is Medical Business Consultants of Wheeling, Illinois. The consulting group charges $85 to $110 per hour and reviews hospital contracts for a fee of $1,000 to $2,000.

HOSPITAL-BASED PHYSICIAN PRACTICES

All but two states prohibit "corporate medicine," the direct provision of health care services by a corporation. In real life, these laws and prohibitions are largely ignored. Physicians fear a future in which doctors, like pharmacists, would work for wages in hospital chains. That is an unlikely future for most physicians and hospitals. For the next decade ahead, hospitals will work intensely to capture the hearts and minds of key medical staff.

A small but growing number of hospitals are developing hospital-based group practices to staff the hospital's ambulatory care services and satellite centers. The creation of hospital-based groups may pose the danger of competition for other members of the medical staff. Hospitals are acquiring physician practices and sometimes relocating them for strategic purposes at satellite clinics or well-sited medical office buildings. Practice acquistions and mergers are widespread, but the number of physician practices involved is unknown. The annual percentage may be as high as 1–3 percent of solo practices and small groups if acquisitions and mergers initiated by hospitals and by larger medical groups are included.

Hospital-based medical groups typically contract with a hospital's parent corporation or a physician service bureau subsidiary to avoid direct conflicts of interest. Hospital-based groups can provide a cadre of physicians for managed care contracting and channel referrals to specialists on the hospital's medical staff.

JOINT VENTURES

Hospitals today are experimenting with new clinical and business relationships to strengthen physician loyalty—and to gain the inpatient referrals. This is the era of medical enterprise (see Chapter 12). Although not all physicians are responding enthusiastically, economic pressures are driving doctors into the arms of their hospitals. Some physicians are concerned about the potential conflicts of interest in joint ventures. In an article in *Medical Economics* entitled "Joint Ventures: Who Knows What Evil Lurks . . .," author M. Carroll Thomas urged doctors to take a "hard look at potential ethical quandaries" that may arise from their participation in hospital-physician ventures (Thomas 1987).

Fiscal Crunch Provides Opportunity

The reduction of Medicare fees to hospitals under prospective payment has hit hard at laboratory services. Some hospitals and physicians have taken advantage of the payment squeeze to consolidate laboratory services in new hospital-physician joint ventures. Miami Valley Hospital of Dayton, Ohio, has entered into a three-way partnership with the hospital's pathologists and an outside firm, International Clinical Laboratories. The purpose of the partnership is to create a regional laboratory (CompuNet Clinical Laboratories) that will serve physician offices, group practices, and other hospitals. This is potentially a win-win situation for the hospital and the pathologists. The hospital will save $150,000 to $200,000 annually because it will no longer be operating a full-time laboratory, and the pathologists will gain new revenues from the expanded outpatient services.

Restructuring and consolidating hospital-based programs is a strategic response to the decline of inpatient reimbursement, the need for cost containment, and the shift to ambulatory care. The Alta Bates Corporation, a multihospital system based in Berkeley, California, is saving $750,000 to $1 million annually through personnel cutbacks and group purchasing after consolidating the laboratories of its two Bay Area hospitals. In a similar situation in Waterloo, Iowa, the consolidated lab of Schoitz Medical Center and St. Francis Hospital is expanding reference and ambulatory services and providing new revenues to its pathologists.

PHYSICIAN EXECUTIVES

Placing physicians in key management positions signals the return of an old trend. Fifty years ago, before the rise of professional training in hospital management, many hospitals were headed by physician administrators. Now the trend has returned, driven by the need to strengthen physician loyalty and provide a medical perspective in hospital management. Mark Doyne, M.D. (1987), chronicled the rise of the physician executive in *Healthcare Forum Journal*. The last decade has witnessed an explosive growth in the numbers of physicians entering the executive suite. The American Academy of Medical Directors grew from 64 members in 1975 to nearly 3,000 by mid-1987, and the membership is increasing at a rate of about 100 per month.

The Physician Executive Management Center, a physician-executive counseling and recruitment firm, recently surveyed more than 2,200 physician executives. Of the 1,000 who responded, 208 are in senior medical management positions on a full-time basis. Forty-five percent continue to practice, but most spend fewer than one day a week with patients. A study by Witt Associates, a recruitment firm based in Oakbrook, Illinois, reveals that 86 percent of physician executives are board certified, 5 percent hold another professional degree (e.g., M.B.A., Ph.D.), and 97 percent are male (Burda 1988).

As described in the cover story of the May 8, 1987, issue of *Modern Healthcare*, physician executives like Robert B. Klint, M.D., CEO of 393-bed Swedish American Hospital in Rockford, Illinois, are heading up some of America's premier hospitals and health systems. Bruce Spivey, M.D., of San Francisco's Pacific Presbyterian Medical Center, shares credit for his hospital's financial turnaround with the medical staff. Their loyalty kept the hospital viable when it appeared headed into bankruptcy in the mid-1970s. The hospital has since made a substantial recovery, turning a $5.2 million operating profit on revenues of $108.6 million in 1986.

Physician executives work in hospitals of under 100 beds and in megafacilities of 1,000 beds. Most are found in hospitals of between 100 and 349 beds. Salaries range from an average of $106,964 in facilities under 100 beds to an average of $135,600 in hospitals over 1,000 beds. Additional perks and benefits can add $20,000 to $30,000 per year to total compensation.

Job descriptions for medical executives are changing. In the past, physician executives focused on clinically oriented tasks, such as credentials and staff hiring. In the future, more management responsibilities will be added, giving the physician executive more participation in finance, strategy, and operational management decision making. For example, Dr. Mark Doyne has both strategic planning and physician liaison responsibilities as senior vice-president of corporate development at 670-bed Baptist Hospital in Nashville, Tennessee.

PHYSICIAN NETWORKS

Networks provide one of the most promising strategies for physician channeling. In the modern era, the term *network* is both verb and noun. For the purpose of tying physicians more closely to hospitals, networks are loosely structured organizations built by interweaving clinical and economic relationships. Physician networks, which can take multiple forms, include computer communication networks, independent practice associations, and satellite clinic "feeder" networks.

Computer Communication Networks

Computer-based networks bring the 21st-century medicine into the 20th century. Taking advantage of telecommunications and the proliferation of microcomputers, hospitals are extending electronic links into the offices of their medical staff.

Remote practice networks were conceptualized by the San Diego–based firm of Magliaro and McHaney as a way to promote bonding between a hospital and its key admitters. The Borgess Medical Center in Kalamazoo, Michigan, was the first hospital to fully implement the computer communications concept, which it did in 1985. The hospital created a for-profit subsidiary to lease minicomputers and place them in the offices of 110 primary care physicians. Borgess, a 462-bed facility, relies on tertiary care for 80 percent of its patient volume. Selection of participating doctors was done carefully. Market research determined which zip code areas had preferred patients and relatively low numbers of practicing doctors. Physicians were chosen for the network practice in the preferred areas, including the 100 doctors responsible for 80 percent of the hospital's admissions. The network facilitates admission directly from the doctors' offices by means of electronic preregistration and allows the doctors to monitor their patients from their offices. Regionwide distribution of a medical credit card to 75,000 residents provided instant consumer recognition in any of the doctors' offices. Initial capitalization was $1.5 million—for system design, computer leasing, and staff support. Did it work? And how! Borgess inpatient admissions have increased 10 percent, and the hospital credits 100–200 patients each month to the network.

AnnsonLink is a hospital–medical office computer communications system developed by the Baxter Healthcare Corporation. The November 1986 issue of *Physicians and Computers* profiles both AnnsonLink and the companion IBM software, Doctor's Office Management (DOM), which is authored by Annson. St. Lukes Samaritan Health Care in Milwaukee is an early adopter of the AnnsonLink system. Using the Annson software link, St. Lukes physicians can access patient care data directly from the hospital's mainframe information system. Doctors can automatically integrate (or download) that information into the DOM practice management and word processing systems in their office computers. Specifically, doctors can preadmit patients, obtain lab and radiology results immediately, conduct "electronic rounds" and check on the status of each hospitalized patient, obtain medical transcriptions, and review medications. The system was an immediate success with the four initial physician groups, and it has been provided to other medical staff. In nearby Chicago, Baxter is testing AnnsonLink's impact on admissions by comparing two matched groups of physicians. At the Little Company of Mary hospital, 40 physicians participating in the AnnsonLink system have been matched with 40 nonlinked physicians. The results have been most favorable. The AnnsonLink physicians admitted 30 percent more patients and generated $4.7 million in revenues, and the system achieved a 95 percent satisfaction rating from the participating doctors.

Independent Practice Networks

IPAs are increasing faster than other HMOs. According to InterStudy of Excelsior, Minnesota, the IPA continues to be the most common model type. Of plans three years old or younger, 78 percent are IPAs, and these have already captured 38 percent of the national IPA enrollment.

IPAs cost less to start than staff or group models. More hospitals and physicians are joint venturing IPA-type plans, despite the fact that, according to some experts, the market is saturated. New HMO startups have slowed from the 1985–1986 record pace (99 HMOs entered the market in 1986). In the first quarter of 1988 only 13 new plans were formed, compared with 34 in the first quarter of 1987, according to InterStudy. Many of the new plans are for-profit. If current trends continue, more than half of all HMO enrollees will be members of for-profit plans. Of plans three years or younger, 79 percent chose for-profit status. Many new IPA plans are also not seeking federal qualification. This provides them with more market flexibility and the ability to sell to employers and major buyers who demand rates based on experience rating, not community-rated premiums.

HMO enrollment topped 32 million in 1988, and HMOs are becoming a significant source of inpatients for America's hospitals. HMOs and managed care contracts may channel 50 percent of hospital admissions annually by 1992.

HMO physicians channel patients to hospitals. In Boston, the Harvard Community Health Plan joined forces with Brigham and Women's Hospital, which could generate up to $110 million in additional revenues to the hospital over a five-year period. Harvard chose to send the bulk of its inpatients to Brigham in exchange for a discount from the hospital.

Control of an HMO increases control of patients and market share. In the Bay Area, a group of hospitals purchased publicly held Bay Pacific Corporation. The purchase, in mid-1987, gives the hospitals control of the 67,000-enrollee plan and lets them expand into new markets. The local hospitals joined forces to protect themselves and their physicians. They feared a buyout of Bay Pacific by an outside firm.

Feeder Networks

Branch satellite clinics can be used to create feeder networks for hospitals and HMOs. The Carle Clinic in Urbana, Illinois, has established a network of seven satellite clinics to increase referrals to the main clinic and to the Carle Foundation Hospital next door. The network enhances marketing of the HMO owned by the clinic. Both the clinic and hospital operate under the same brand name, which is used extensively in marketing campaigns. The nonprofit Carle Foundation

Hospital owns and operates the hospital and builds clinic facilities that it leases to the Carle Clinic Association, which is owned by member physicians. The hospital and clinic share a number of services. The 170-physician medical group was formed in 1931 on the Mayo Clinic model by two physicians trained at the Rochester facility. The network-model HMO is nonprofit and federally qualified. HMO enrollment has jumped by 30,000 since 1985 and totalled nearly 70,000 by 1988. In response, the 50-member Christie Clinic in Champaign launched a major building campaign and affiliated with Mercy Hospital in Urbana to better compete with Carle. Market leader Carle is convinced that networking is the wave of the future. Now other HMOs in the Champaign-Urbana region must play catchup.

MARKETING AND INCENTIVES FOR PHYSICIANS CHANNEL REFERRALS

Malpractice insurance is the amenity most desired by physicians. In a study for *Health Care Competition Week* by the Nashville-based Keckley Group, doctors ranked malpractice insurance in the top five services in which physicians said they were "very interested" (Keckley 1988). Not surprisingly, Ob/Gyns and other physicians expressed greatest interest in subsidized malpractice coverage (64 percent and 39 percent respectively). Fewer specialists and surgeons felt the need for assistance on malpractice insurance; only 31 percent of each group were "very interested." Not many physicians receive any help with malpractice coverage from their hospitals. The survey of 300 doctors revealed that only 5 percent were already receiving medical malpractice insurance from their hospitals.

Physician catalogs can increase physician referrals from community primary care physicians to hospital specialists. Catalogs enhance physician-to-physician referrals by creating awareness of staff skills and special expertise. The University of Alabama Medical Center in Birmingham sent a catalog highlighting information about staff doctors and surgeons to primary care physicians in its service area. The catalog strategy helped boost the hospital's market share ranking from seventh to first in the region.

Other hospitals, like Parkview Episcopal in Pueblo, Colorado, take the catalog strategy a step further by using a unique doctor-to-doctor marketing effort. Parkview's program is enhanced by a peer-enforced "re-referral" program to ensure that referring physicians will not lose patients to specialists. Primary care physicians can refer patients to hospital specialists confident in the hospital's guarantee of re-referral back to the original physicians when the specialized treatment is complete.

Telemarketing and physician referral tracking systems use computers to locate an appropriate doctor and book an appointment while the caller is on the line. The Profiles program developed by Atlanta's Medi-Marketing Agency is a plastic surgery program in which promotion is linked with physician referral. Regional advertising draws the calls to trained telemarketing operators, who make appointments with participating physicians. A tracking system monitors each step from appointment to postdischarge follow-up. Republic Health Corporation, one of the most innovative companies in health care marketing, franchises programs to hospitals nationwide, such as its cataract surgery program Gift of Sight. Republic's marketing and computerized tracking system, the Profiles program, channels patients to participating physicians and hospitals.

CONCLUSION: WHAT'S NEXT IN PHYSICIAN CHANNELING?

Hospital efforts to influence physician commitment and admissions are stepping up. More innovation and activity can be expected by hospitals in physician channeling in the next three to five years. The following developments should be expected:

- an increase in group practice acquisitions
- HMO and PPO joint contracts with selected medical groups
- increased volume requirements for active staff status
- tighter medical staff credentials processes
- more physician executives in line management positions
- integration of case management and quality assurance programs
- more physicians on boards of trustees

To be the dominant medical center in any health care market requires effective physician channeling strategies. In tomorrow's competitive health care marketplace, gaining and retaining market leader status will increasingly depend on physician loyalty and referrals.

STRATEGIC IMPLICATIONS FOR PHYSICIANS

1. *During the next five years, many physicians will be forced to choose a primary-affiliation hospital.* The time is now for strategic deal making. Those physicians who take advantage of this opportunity early will be in the best position to benefit from the relationship with their preferred hospital.

2. *Doctors should expect hospitals and boards to impose higher volume requirements for active medical staff status in the near future.* Setting higher requirements will be part of a strategy to increase the level of physician commitment and referrals. Some flexibility is appropriate in the case of primary care physicians and specialists whose practices involve few inpatient referrals and in the case of physicians who give extra time as a result of chairing medical staff or hospital committees, for example.

3. *Better hospitals will begin to raise the threshold criteria for hospital privileges.* Hospitals will take this step to enhance their image and to lock in doctors with preferred skills and credentials. Some hospitals may impose a new standard: All physicians must be board certified or eligible for certification. Those who were only eligible would have to become certified with a limited period.

4. *More physicians will be seen in the executive suites of America's hospitals and health systems.* One way hospitals can gain and hold the commitment of physicians is to ensure that medical judgment plays a role in every senior management decision. The rise of medical executives is both symbolic and real. Medical executives know the base business of medical care better than any lay administrator and can gain the respect of the medical community more readily. In some marketplaces and for some hospitals, hiring medical executives will be an important strategy for image enhancement and for increasing referrals from area physicians.

STRATEGIC IMPLICATIONS FOR HOSPITALS

1. *Hospitals will continue to buy and affiliate with physician practices.* The acquisitions will move from the defensive mode (e.g., purchasing practices of retiring physicians to protect referral patterns) to the offensive mode (e.g., purchasing practices for their strategic locations or importance to a hospital's centers of excellence).

2. *There are many strategies available to hospitals for influencing physician choice.* Incentives are a tricky business in health care—for professional, ethical, and legal reasons. State laws against inurement have been reinforced by a Medicare prohibition against incentive policies or arrangements that directly benefit referring physicians. Hospital-physician joint ventures must avoid violating antitrust provisions.

3. *Experimentation will continue to realign the basic hospital-physician relationship.* In tomorrow's dynamic health care enterprise, hospitals and physicians will create new ventures and develop new clinical and business relationships. Innovators always have the tactical advantage over market followers. The medical community is demonstrating a substantial interest

in restructuring the hospital-physician relationship. Physician channeling has arrived.

4. *Computer networking is an important step toward the effective channeling of physician referrals.* When combined with joint hospital-physician marketing efforts, remote practice networks can increase the practices of participating doctors by 10–15 percent and augment hospital inpatient admissions by 3–5 percent or more. In the future, with increasingly sophisticated information systems and software, much more can be done to clinically and economically integrate the practices of physicians and their preferred hospitals. Integration might include the use of sophisticated on-line patient monitoring from bedside computers, centralized patient data bases, consumer "smart cards" that are essentially pocket medical records, remote telecommunications access for consultation, and automated physician services billing (with centralized collections and expedited payment).

BIBLIOGRAPHY

Barker, W. Daniel. 1987. "The Year 2000: A Look into the Future of Hospitals and Medical Staffs." *Journal of MAG* 76:556–60.

Berger, Sally. 1988. "Hospital Strengthens Ties to Doctors with Joint Venture." *Modern Healthcare* 29 January.

Bloomfield, Randall D. 1988. "Hospital-Physician Relationships: A Changing Dynamic." *New York State Journal of Medicine* (January).

Bogdanich, Walt, and Michael Waldholz. 1989. "Warm Bodies: Hospitals That Need Patients Pay Bounties for Doctors' Referrals." *Wall Street Journal*, 27 February, 1.

Bulger, Robert T., and Karen C. Teitelbaum. 1988. "Addressing Operational Issues in Medical Practice Development." *Healthcare Financial Management* (July): 66–70.

Burda, David. 1988. "Hiring of Physician Executives on the Rise." *Modern Healthcare*, 8 April, 40.

Chapman, Thomas W., and Leo H. Mugmon. 1988. "Supporting Physicians in a Competitive Environment: One Hospital's Approach to Assist Private Practitioners." *Journal of Hospital Marketing* 2(1): 171–75.

Coile, Russell C., Jr., and Randolph M. Grossman. 1987. "The New Medicine." Healthcare Forum Journal (September–October): 14–17.

Coile, Russell C., Jr. 1988a. *Hospital Entrepreneurs' Newsletter* 3 (February).

———. 1988b. *Hospital Strategy Report* 1 (November).

———. 1989. *Hospital Strategy Report* 1 (February).

Conomikes, George S. 1988. "Hospitals Should Adopt Marketing Plans That Target Both Physicians and Patients." *Modern Healthcare*, 15 January, 36.

de Lorrell, Walter, and Allen J. Budzichowski. 1988. "A Question of Altruism and Survival: Group Practices as Hospital Satellites." *Group Practice* (January-February): 60–61.

Denaro Dine, Deborah. 1988. "Joint Venture Exceeds Planners' Hopes." *Modern Healthcare*, 8 April, 50.

Doyne, Mark. 1987. "Physicians As Managers." *Healthcare Forum Journal* (September–October): 11–13.

Droste, Therese. 1987a. "Physician Marketing Pays Off in Admissions." *Hospitals*, 5 October, 48–53.

———. 1987b. "1987: Physician Marketing Continues to Grow." *Hospitals*, 20 December, 28–29.

———. 1988a. "Physician Marketing Budgets to Grow in '88." *Hospitals*, 20 January, 32–34.

———. 1988b. "Practice Enhancement: What MDs Want." *Hospitals*, 20 March, 44.

———. 1988c. "FTC: Setting High Standards in Advertising." *Hospitals*, 20 April, 41–44.

Egdahl, Richard H., and Cynthia H. Taft. 1986. "Physicians and Hospitals: Competitors or Partners." In *The Corporation of Health Care Delivery*. Edited by Monica R. Dreuth. Chicago: American Hospital Publishing.

Green, Jane M. 1987. "The Role of Information Systems in the Hospital-Physician Relationship." *Topics in Health Care Financing* (Winter): 9–16.

Greene, Jay. 1988. "More Hospitals Contracting for Emergency Physicians." *Modern Healthcare*, 22 April, 31.

Holthaus, David. 1987. "Recruitment Schemes Face Legal Questions." *Hospitals*, 5 December, 54–58.

Jolly, Paul. 1988. "Medical Education in the United States, 1960–1987." *Health Affairs* (September): 144–57.

Keckley, Paul. 1988. "Life with Physicians in the Relative Value Age." *Health Care Competition Week*, 28 November, 1–4.

Kelsey, Ronn R. 1988. "Strategies in Physician Marketing: Clinical Data Base Marketing—New Way to Expand the Health Care Pie." *Hospital Strategy Report* 1 (November).

Koska, Mary T. 1988. "JCAHO Survey: Interhospital Relationships Strong." *Hospitals*, 5 July, 54–56.

Koska, Mary T. 1988. "Low-Cost Strategies Aid Physician Bonding." *Hospitals*, 5 May, 60.

Lang, Daniel. 1988. "Should You Shrink Your Medical Staff?" *Medical Executive Committee Reporter* (May–June): 1–2.

Larkin, Howard. 1988. "Do Physician-Managers Raise Hospital Costs?" *Hospitals*, 20 February, 68–69.

Lewitt, Suzanne M. 1982. *Physician Recruitment Strategies That Work*. Rockville, Md.: Aspen Publishers.

McDermott, Steve. 1988. "The New Hospital Challenge: Organizing and Managing Physician Organizations." *Health Care Management Review* 13 (Winter): 57–61.

Nelson, Susan. 1987. "Buying MD Practices: The Trend Continues." *Hospital*, 20 July, 63.

Newald Martinsons, Jane. 1988. "What's the Top MD Recruitment Incentive?" *Hospitals*, 5 February, 69.

Nordstrom, Richard D., Devonne E. Horton, and Myron E. Hatcher. 1987. "How to Create a Marketing Strategy Based on Hospital Characteristics That Attract Physicians." *Journal of Health Care Marketing* 7 (March): 29–36.

Owens, Arthur. 1988. "How Much Did Your Earnings Grow Last Year?" *Medical Economics*, 5 September, 59–180.

Perry, Linda. 1988. "U.S. Hospitals Wooing Superstar Physicians." *Modern Healthcare*, 8 January, 24–33.

Powills, Suzanne. 1987a. "What Do Physicians Really Want from Hospitals?" *Hospitals*, 5 June, 46.

———. 1987b. "Segmenting the Physician Market: Some Guidelines." *Hospitals*, 5 June, 47.

———. 1987c. "Half of Physicians Say Ads Are Effective." *Hospitals*, 20 July, 40.

———. 1987d. "Hospital-Physician Link Generates $4 Million." *Hospitals*, 5 December, 66–67.

Sandrick, Karen. 1988. "Multis Putting More Effect into MD Relationships." *Hospitals*, 5 March, 70–71.

Sheldon, Alan. 1988. *Managing Doctors*. Homewood, Ill.: Dow Jones-Irwin.

Shortell, Stephen M. 1986. "New Models for Hospital-Physician Relations." In *The Corporation of Health Care Delivery*. Edited by Monica R. Dreuth. Chicago: American Hospital Publishing.

Snook, I. Donald. 1987. *Building a Winning Medical Staff*. Chicago: American Hospital Publishing.

Sollins, Howard L. 1988. "Purchasing Physician Practices: Legal and Regulatory Concerns." *Healthcare Financial Management* (January): 56–63.

Speaker, Rick. 1987. "Hospital-Physician Bonding." *Computers in Healthcare* (October): 67–68.

Stromberg, Ross E. 1987. "Physician-Hospital Relationships in Today's Market-Driven Environment." San Francisco: Epstein, Becker, Borsody, Stromberg and Green.

Super Palm, Kari. 1988. "Group Practices Mimic Venture Capital Firms Created by Hospitals, Physicians." *Modern Healthcare*, 26 February, 73.

Teitelbaum, Karen C., and Robert T. Bulger. 1988. "Strengthening Physician Bonds through Practice Development Planning." *Healthcare Financial Management* (May): 50–56.

Thomas, M. Carroll. 1987. "Joint Ventures: Who Knows What Evil Lurks . . ." *Medical Economics*, 30 March, 47–51.

Uhlar, Bob. 1987. "Sale/Lease-Back with Doctors Being Explored by Hospitals." *Hospitals*, 20 November, 44.

Waldholz, Michael, and Walt Bogdanich. 1989. "Doctor-owned Labs Earn Lavish Profits in a Captive Market." *Wall Street Journal*, 1 March, 1.

Wallace, Cynthia. 1987. "Physicians Leaving Their Practices for Hospital Jobs." *Modern Healthcare*, 8 May, 40–57.

Young, David W., and Richard B. Saltman. 1987. *The Hospital Power Equilibrium*: Baltimore: Johns Hopkins University Press.

Chapter 14

Restructuring Hospital-Physician Relations

There is a need for an integrated response by physicians and hospitals to alternative delivery system developments and selective contracting pressures and opportunities. There is a need for an integrated response by hospitals and physicians to economic joint venturing opportunities, where physicians and hospitals can joint plan a diversification strategy and where the arrangement can be structured so that both hospitals and physicians have an equity participation opportunity.
—Ross E. Stromberg, *Physician-Hospital Relationships in Today's Market-Driven Environment*

TIME FOR A "NEW DEAL"

The integration of medical care and hospital care is inevitable. Hospitals and physicians will integrate clinically and economically under pressure from government, insurance plans, and consumers. The result will be a new kind of hospital-physician organization that gives doctors substantially more power than they have under the medical staff model. The price of power will be a new kind of contract that binds the doctor to the hospital exclusively. The result will be a "new deal" for hospitals and physicians.

Integration could create a win-win situation. Both physicians and hospitals may get from the revision of their traditionally ambiguous relationship what they have long sought:

- *Hospitals* want the 100 percent loyalty and commitment of the medical staff—which means 100 percent of the physicians' inpatient admissions and a significant share of the physicians' out-of-office referrals for specialized services such as lab and x-ray.

253

- *Physicians* want from hospitals a substantial share of decision-making power over key factors such as the budget, facilities, and staffing and any strategies that affect their clinical and financial interests.

Medical Staff Relationships Must Change

A new deal is not merely important, it is imperative. The question is not whether hospitals and their physicians will change but how soon and in what ways. Stephen Shortell, in a long article in *Frontiers of Health Services Management* (1988), identifies six driving forces that he believes will impel development of a new pattern of relationships between America's health institutions and the medical community (Figure 14-1).

The impact of these forces can be seen in the rising tension between hospitals and their doctors. The old mechanisms are simply inadequate to deal with the complexities of modern health care delivery. Too many aspects of the hospital-physician relationship are based on trust and are not holding up under pressure. The "rules of the game" played by hospitals and physicians are frequently unwritten, and all parties must rely on voluntary suasion and consensual decision making.

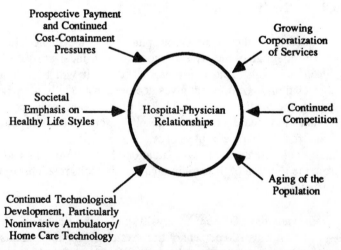

Figure 14-1 Forces Shaping the Future Delivery of Health Care. *Source*: Reprinted from *Hospital Strategy Report*, Vol. 1, No. 4, p. 2, Aspen Publishers, Inc., © February 1989.

Don't send for the attorneys yet. The point is not that all aspects of the hospital-doctor relationship must be codified in a legal contract but the entire structure needs strengthening. Just as important, new mechanisms more flexible than the medical staff bylaws are needed to adapt to the market in innovative ways.

NEW DESIGNS FOR HOSPITAL GOVERNANCE

The best and brightest of America's health care organizations are actively experimenting with restructuring the hospital-physician relationship. The "three-legged stool" consisting of the board, the administration, and the medical staff is rapidly becoming obsolete.

Shortell suggests there are three models for the hospital-medical staff relationship: (1) the independent corporate model; (2) the divisional model, and (3) the parallel model. And there are variations on these. Below are descriptions of a number of alternative models for the hospital-physician relationship, models that may reshape hospital governance in the 1990s.

Incorporated Medical Staff Model

In this model, the medical staff becomes an independent legal entity that negotiates with the hospital for professional services in exchange for the hospital's clinical and administrative support (Figure 14-2).

Sound far-fetched? Hardly. This is the relationship common to many staff model HMOs, like the Kaiser Foundation Health Plan and the Kaiser Permanente Medical Group. Incorporating the medical staff drastically reduces the control traditionally possessed by the board of trustees. No longer are medical staff bylaws subject to the approval of the trustees. Hospitals could insist that certain policies and procedures be in place for quality assurance, but this would be defined and negotiated contractually. Independence places the responsibility en-

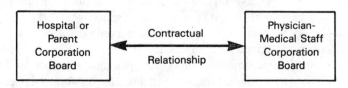

Figure 14-2 Incorporated Medical Staff Model. *Source*: Reprinted from *Hospital Strategy Report*, Vol. 1, No. 4, p. 3, Aspen Publishers, Inc., © February 1989.

tirely with the medical staff for credentialing, quality assurance, peer review, and self-governance. The downside of separate legal status includes the difficulties posed for hospital-based physicians such as radiologists. As a result of these difficulties, only community physicians might decide to incorporate separately. Incorporation may also limit the ability of doctors to obtain malpractice insurance at favorable or subsidized rates through the hospital.

Hospitals would lose a measure of control over the medical staff if the doctors incorporated separately. Separate incorporation runs counter to the general trend toward greater integration of medical staff and hospitals. Integration is an attempt to overcome the traditional dual lines of authority, and the incorporated medical staff model has the potential to accentuate the differences between management and medical staff and to stimulate divisiveness. In HMOs, that tendency is countered by the sharing of responsibility and rewards for efficient patient care management. Under managed care, both the hospital and physicians receive economic rewards if they keep costs below the HMO premium revenues. As managed care becomes increasingly widespread in the 1990s, the independent corporate model may become more common.

Experience with the incorporated medical staff model suggests that it can promote risk sharing and joint ventures. With the traditional bonds broken, both sides can be innovative in structuring new arrangements. However, independence does little to strengthen trust and bonding, relying as it does on contractual mechanisms to resolve differences. More importantly, it takes physicians out of the hospital's decision-making process and limits them to the role of vendor.

Service Line Management Model

When a hospital reorganizes around service line clusters, one result is the creation of a number of mini–medical staffs aligned with the hospital's market-based structure. This form of organization uses a market orientation to subdivide the overall medical staff into semiautonomous groupings of physicians who serve the same patient base (Figure 14-3). The service line management model in hospitals is inspired by industry's product line management approach, which organizes work units into divisions based on product or customer groupings.

Each service line subunit or division has its own management and support functions, including activities such as nursing, marketing, finance, quality assurance, or human resources. The service line approach integrates the administration and clinical management aspects better than most other models. In this model, collaboration between management and medicine occurs at the operational level—in the day-to-day decision making. Chiefs of clinical services are service line managers, which increases their marketing and customer orientation and

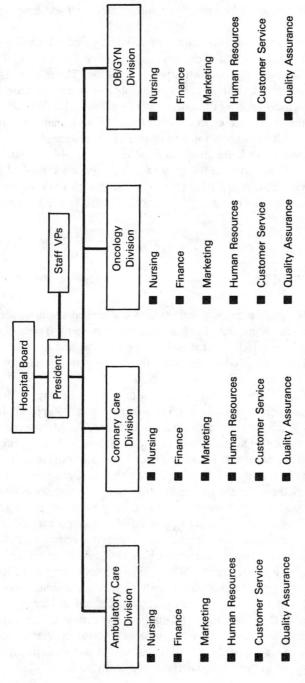

Figure 14-3 Service Line Management Model. *Source:* Adapted from *Hospital Strategy Report*, Vol. 1, No. 4, p. 3, Aspen Publishers, Inc., © February 1989.

consolidates their operational control over both clinical and administrative support activities.

In a service line approach, managing for efficiency and effectiveness takes place on a smaller scale and more directly. Each service line has a high degree of autonomy and can develop its own esprit and culture. The model has limits: Service line management reduces central control, and it can increase internal competition and cause an overall lack of strategic direction. The sum of the whole can lack the coherence of the parts. Further, not all managers are comfortable with the multirelationship nature of matrix management.

Although not widespread, the model is used in such notable hospitals as the Johns Hopkins Medical Center in Baltimore and Rush-Presbyterian-St.Lukes' in Chicago. A service line management approach seems to fit academic health centers, which have higher percentages of hospital-based specialists and of full-time clinical service chiefs.

Partnership Model

Some hospitals that find medical staff bylaws too limited a vehicle for change are creating "parallel organizations," as Shortell calls them. These new "offshore" corporations are independent of both the hospital and the medical staff (Figure 14-4). They can conduct certain activities that the formal governance and medical staff structures do not handle well.

Because hospitals share power equitably with their physicians in these new organizations, they represent a new form of partnership. Often physician investors are given a 49 percent ownership share or a straight 50-50 partnership. This is in contrast to the typical hospital board, which averages 3–4 physician trustees among 18–25 board members. Instead of such limited physician participation, hospitals are openly sharing power in these new partnership organizations.

The purpose of the partnership organization is to face strategic issues in a united way. The partnership corporation—and there may be several aligned with one hospital—conducts activities on a joint basis. Common examples include HMOs, or IPAs, preferred provider networks, imaging center joint ventures, and real estate partnerships for projects such as medical office buildings.

The advantages of a partnership corporation include not having to work through the medical staff and governance structures when making decisions. The decision chain in hospitals is ponderous and slow on both the board and the medical staff sides. With a parallel organization, all this can be avoided. The partnership corporation is small and highly flexible, able to respond efficiently to market opportunities and to react quickly if need be. Boards of partnership corporations, like corporate boards in private industry, are typically small.

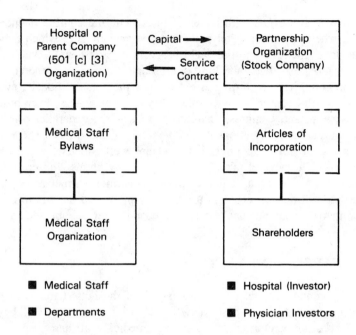

Figure 14-4 Hospital-Physician Partnership Model. *Source*: Reprinted from *Hospital Strategy Report*, Vol. 1, No. 4, p. 4, Aspen Publishers, Inc., © February 1989.

For the physicians as well, one perceived advantage is the avoidance of the medical staff structure and internal politics. More importantly, physicians have a much stronger role in the management of partnership corporations. In some cases, creating a corporation allows an "end run" that bypasses physician traditionalists who control the upper echelon of medical staff leadership. A partnership corporation can involve younger members of the medical staff years before they would have ascended the medical staff seniority ladder.

A second-generation partnership model is now being developed. The new model uses a single governance structure and capitalization to manage multiple projects. At this early stage of development, the best thing about partnership corporations is that there are few prototypical examples. The organizations are quite innovative, and a number of variations are being tested, including venture capital companies, limited partnerships, and stock companies. Structure, participation, management, location, range of activities, capitalization, control, and staffing are all in the experimental stage. Most partnership models have set limited goals, are staffed part time by hospital employees, and have initiated only a few projects. It is still an open question in what areas hospital-physician collaboration will work—or will not.

Congress is concerned with issues of inurement and conflict of interest, for example, when physicians refer patients to organizations in which they have a financial investment. Some political observers believe new legislation will be enacted by Congress that could limit or eliminate partnership corporations. Such legislation could have a chilling effect on new partnership models, even if not all forms of joint ventures, e.g., ambulatory surgery centers, were prohibited.

If they withstand Congressional scrutiny, will these parallel organizations become the parent corporations of the hospitals of the future? They do give a greater share of power to physicians and are well suited to a managed care environment. The general takeover of hospitals by partnership corporations is possible—but not in the near future. In the meantime, partnership corporations provide a transitional mechanism to allow hospitals and doctors to collaborate in adapting to the changing health care market and to new reimbursement patterns.

"NEW WAVE" JOINT VENTURES

Creating venture capital companies is one of the hottest trends in hospital-physician joint venturing. These "new wave" joint ventures go well beyond the one-deal-at-a-time venturing by the average medical staff and hospital.

Pioneered in 1985 by Torrance Memorial Hospital in Torrance, California, the concept is inspired by high-tech venture capital firms responsible for many private sector start ups. Memorial's president, George Graham, evolved the concept of a venture capital firm as a vehicle to align and expand several out-patient activities established by the hospital in conjunction with its physicians.

The Memorial venture is owned equally by a holding company for the hospital and 150 members of the hospital's medical staff. Capitalized initially with $3.5 million, the venture company made $2 million on revenues of $11.5 million in 1987. Memorial executives credit the venture with increasing physician commitment and boosting the hospital's market share from 37 percent to 42 percent. The Los Angeles office of the Chicago law firm McDermott, Will and Emery assisted with legal documents for the innovative corporation.

In Urbana, Illinois, the 483-bed Carle Foundation Hospital and the Carle Clinic, a 190-member group practice, have created a venture capital company that is intended to strengthen the ties between the hospital and the physicians (Figure 14-5). As recently reported in *Modern Healthcare*, Carle's venture capital company is designed as a master limited partnership (Super Palm 1988). Sixty-five percent of ownership is held by the hospital and 35 percent by the clinic. Initial capitalization was $3 million.

One goal of the venture capital company is to expand the hospital and clinic's market referral area. An existing remote clinic is being expanded and a new one is being built in Champaign County. Construction funding is being provided by

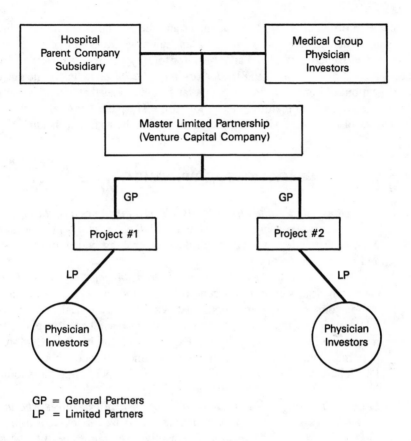

Figure 14-5 A Master Limited Partnership Venture Capital Company

the hospital. The venture capital company will lease the facility from the hospital, from which it will obtain management and support services via a service contract. Other projects include a retail pharmacy company, a home health care agency, and an industrial rehabilitation company. Percentages of ownership in these businesses vary. Profits from the ventures will be distributed to the owners of the venture capital company (Super Palm 1988).

LOOKING FORWARD: RESTRUCTURING THE PARTNERSHIP

Physicians and hospital executives must forget what they were taught in medical school and health care management school, namely that the physician is an obstacle to efficient hospital management and the administrator an impediment to quality medicine. In the words of Dan Lang, M.D., editor of the *Medical Staff Executive Reporter*, "the administrator [or physician] is neither your friend nor your enemy" (Coile 1988). Doctors must be *partners* in the health care organizations of tomorrow. Partnerships can be built today that will lay a platform for future success. Remember this simple truth: Hospitals can replace their key executives a lot more easily than they can replace their key physicians.

STRATEGIC IMPLICATIONS FOR PHYSICIANS

1. *Physicians will demand higher levels of control in future hospital-physician relationships.* To achieve better balance in these relationships, physicians must be better represented on all decision-making bodies of the hospital and parent corporation.
2. *Now is the time to invest in hospital-physician joint ventures.* Today's entrepreneurial ventures between doctors and hospitals are more than just a fad. Joint ventures are bonds that will cement clinical and economic relationships in the future. Hospitals will put a safety net in place under most ventures to insure physicians against catastrophic losses. More importantly, joint ventures are symbolic investments in a collaborative future. Physicians' loyalty will be determined in part by their willingness to invest in the future side by side with their hospital.
3. *Each medical staff must create a cadre of medical executives who understand the economic and management issues as well as clinical aspects of today's health care.* Medical staff executive committees need to act more like corporate committees managing a complex organization. Seek hospital subsidies for management training for interested physicians, and use continuing education programs to strengthen leadership capacity.

STRATEGIC IMPLICATIONS FOR HOSPITALS

1. *To gain and maintain physician loyalty, hospitals must open up the hospital governance structure and share power more broadly with physicians.* Doctors constitute at least one-third of the trustees of all hospitals. This includes doctors in hospital-based practices and also community physicians. In the governance of joint ventures, hospitals should aim for a 50-50 sharing of power and capitalization. At the program and service level, medical service chiefs should be given more authority. Some hospitals are using full-time clinical chiefs as service line managers.

2. *All hospitals over 300 beds should have a vice-president for medical affairs.*
It is past time for physicians to take on positions of authority in the hospital
executive suite. Ideally, the position of vice-president for medical affairs
would be filled by a management-trained physician from the growing cadre
of medical executives. The vice-president should not simply be a liaison
between management and staff. Instead, he or she should have a portfolio
of responsibilities, including quality assurance, utilization review, licensure
and accreditation, and what is coming to be called "outcomes management" (measuring and monitoring clinical outcomes of the hospital's care).
The vice-president for medical affairs would also play a key role in strategy
formulation, contracting, marketing, and planning and work closely with
nursing in managing patient care activities.

3. *This is a time for experimentation in hospital-physician relationships.* There
are many ways to bond hospitals and physicians more effectively. New
partnerships and relationships are being invented by hospitals in all parts
of the country. Tomorrow's relationships will involve risk and reward
sharing, new types of joint ventures, and new legal arrangements.

BIBLIOGRAPHY

Barker, W. Daniel. 1987. "The Year 2000: A Look into the Future of Hospitals and Medical Staffs."
Journal of MAG, 76:556–60.

Berger, Sally. 1988. "Hospital Strengthens Ties to Doctors with Joint Venture." *Modern Healthcare*,
29 January.

Bloomfield, Randall D. 1988. "Hospital-Physician Relationships: A Changing Dynamic." *New York
State Journal of Medicine* (January).

Bogdanich, Walt, and Michael Waldholz. 1989. "Warm Bodies: Hospitals That Need Patients Pay
Bounties for Doctors' Referrals." *Wall Street Journal*, 27 February, 1.

Bulger, Robert T, and Karen C. Teitelbaum. 1988. "Addressing Operational Issues in Medical
Practice Development." *Healthcare Financial Management* (July): 66–70.

Burda, David. 1988. "Hiring of Physician Executives on the Rise." *Modern Healthcare*,
8 April, 40.

Chapman, Thomas W., and Leo H. Mugmon. 1988. "Supporting Physicians in a Competitive
Environment: One Hospital's Approach to Assist Private Practitioners." *Journal of Hospital
Marketing* 2(1): 171–75.

Coile, Russell C., Jr. 1988a. *Hospital Entrepreneurs' Newsletter* 3 (February).

———. 1988b. *Hospital Strategy Report* 1 (November).

———. 1989. *Hospital Strategy Report* 1 (February).

Conomikes, George S. 1988. "Hospitals Should Adopt Marketing Plans That Target Both Physicians
and Patients." *Modern Healthcare*, 15 January, 36.

de Lorrell, Walter, and Allen J. Budzichowski. 1988. "A Question of Altruism and Survival: Group
Practices as Hospital Satellites." *Group Practice* (January-February): 60–61.

Denaro Dine, Deborah. 1988. "Joint Venture Exceeds Planners' Hopes." *Modern Healthcare*,
8 April, 50.

Droste, Therese. 1987a. "Physician Marketing Pays Off in Admissions." *Hospitals*, 5 October, 48–53.

———. 1987b. "1987: Physician Marketing Continues to Grow." *Hospitals*, 20 December, 28–29.

———. 1988a. "Physician Marketing Budgets to Grow in '88." *Hospitals*, 20 January, 32–34.

———. 1988b. "Practice Enhancement: What MDs Want." *Hospitals*, 20 March, 44.

———. 1988c. "FTC: Setting High Standards in Advertising." *Hospitals*, 20 April, 41–44.

Egdahl, Richard H., and Cynthia H. Taft. 1986. "Physicians and Hospitals: Competitors or Partners." In *The Corporatization of Health Care Delivery*. Edited by Monica R. Dreuth. Chicago: American Hospital Publishing.

Green, Jane M. 1987. "The Role of Information Systems in the Hospital-Physician Relationship." *Topics in Health Care Financing* (Winter): 9–16.

Greene, Jay. 1988. "More Hospitals Contracting for Emergency Physicians." *Modern Healthcare*, 22 April, 31.

Holthaus, David. 1987. "Recruitment Schemes Face Legal Questions." *Hospitals*, 5 December, 54–58.

Keckley, Paul. 1988. "Life with Physicians in the Relative Value Age." *Health Care Competition Week*, 28 November.

Kelsey, Ronn R. 1988. "Strategies in Physician Marketing: Clinical Data Base Marketing—New Ways to Expand the Health Care Pie." *Hospital Strategy Report* 1 (November).

Koska, Mary T. 1988. "JCAHO Survey: Interhospital Relationships Strong." *Hospitals*, 5 July, 54–56.

Koska, Mary T. 1988. "Low-Cost Strategies Aid Physician Bonding." *Hospitals*, 5 May, 60.

Larkin, Howard. 1988. "Do Physician-Managers Raise Hospital Costs?" *Hospitals*, 20 February, 68–69.

Lewitt, Suzanne M. 1982. *Physician Recruitment Strategies That Work*. Rockville, Md.: Aspen Publishers.

McDermott, Steve. 1988. "The New Hospital Challenge: Organizing and Managing Physician Organizations." *Health Care Management Review* 13 (Winter): 57–61.

Nelson, Susan. 1987. "Buying MD Practices: The Trend Continues." *Hospitals*, 20 July, 63.

Newald Martinsons, Jane. 1988. "What's the Top MD Recruitment Incentive?" *Hospitals*, 5 February, 69.

Nordstrom, Richard D., Devonne E. Horton, and Myron E. Hatcher. 1987. "How to Create a Marketing Strategy Based on Hospital Characteristics that Attract Physicians." *Journal of Health Care Marketing* 7 (March): 29–36.

Perry, Linda. 1988. "U.S. Hospitals Wooing Superstar Physicians." *Modern Healthcare*, 8 January, 24–33.

———. 1987a. "What Do Physicians Really Want from Hospitals?" *Hospitals*, 5 June, 46.

———. 1987b. "Segmenting the Physician Market: Some Guidelines." *Hospitals*, 5 June, 47.

———. 1987c. "Half of Physicians Say Ads Are Effective." *Hospitals*, 20 July, 40.

———. 1987d. "Hospital-Physician Link Generates $4 Million." *Hospitals*, 5 December, 66–67.

Sandrick, Karen. 1988. "Multis Putting More Effort into MD Relationships." *Hospitals*, 5 March, 70–71.

Sheldon, Alan. 1988. *Managing Doctors*. Homewood, Ill.: Dow Jones-Irwin.

Shortell, Stephen M. 1985. "Medical Staff of the Future: Replanting the Garden." *Frontiers of Health Services Management* 1 (February): 3–48.

Shortell, Stephen M. 1986. "New Models for Hospital-Physician Relations." In *The Corporatization of Health Care Delivery*. Edited by Monica R. Dreuth. Chicago: American Hospital Publishing.

Snook, I. Donald. 1987. *Building a Winning Medical Staff*. Chicago: American Hospital Publishing.

Sollins, Howard L. 1988. "Purchasing Physician Practices: Legal and Regulatory Concerns." *Healthcare Financial Management* (January): 56–63.

Speaker, Rick. 1987. "Hospital-Physician Bonding." *Computers in Healthcare* (October): 67–68.

Stromberg, Ross E. 1987. "Physician-Hospital Relationships in Today's Market-Driven Environment." San Francisco: Epstein, Becker, Borsody, Stromberg and Green.

Super Palm, Kari. 1988. "Group Practices Mimic Venture Capital Firms Created by Hospitals, Physicians." *Modern Healthcare*, 26 February, 73.

Teitelbaum, Karen C., and Robert T. Bulger. 1988. "Strengthening Physician Bonds through Practice Development Planning." *Healthcare Financial Management* (May): 50–56.

Thomas, M. Carroll. 1987. "Joint Ventures: Who Knows What Evil Lurks . . ." *Medical Economics*, 30 March, 47–51.

Uhlar, Bob. 1987. "Sale/Lease-back with Doctors Being Explored by Hospitals." *Hospitals*, 20 November, 44.

Waldholz, Michael, and Walt Bogdanich. 1989. "Doctor-owned Labs Earn Lavish Profits in a Captive Market." *Wall Street Journal*, 1 March, 1.

Wallace, Cynthia. 1987. "Physicians Leaving Their Practices for Hospital Jobs." *Modern Healthcare*, 8 May, 40–57.

Young, David W., and Richard B. Saltman. 1988. *The Hospital Power Equilibrium*. Baltimore: Johns Hopkins University Press.

Chapter 15

Service Management

This is truly the Age of Service. . . . Too many executives and managers think of service workers as unimportant and replaceable. But in reality, the service people are the most important ones in the organization. Without them there is no product, no sale, and no profit. Indeed, they are the product. Service is, and should be, a high calling.

— J.W. Marriott, Jr., President, Marriott Corporation

THE AGE OF SERVICE

In the future, America's to hospitals will compete with respect to physicians and two factors: *quality* and *service*. Price will not be a significant factor, since price levels have been reset by the market and there is little price difference between hospitals.

Satisfying customers is the essence of quality medicine. Service management is the strategic path to success in the future. There are really three groups of consumers whose expectations must be met:

1. *The General Public*. This group is composed of all members of the community served by the health organization. Depending on the markets reached by some hospitals and specialized services, this may vary from the adjacent zip code areas to multistate regions. The "general public" really consists of many small minipublics—segments of consumers who must be satisfied one episode of care at a time.

2. *The Physician Market*. Physicians, as brokers and agents for patients, constitute a second group of consumers for the hospital or health organization. Like "Morris the cat", physicians are finicky about quality and service, both for themselves and for their patients.

3. *Major Purchasers*. These "carload customers" (e.g., insurance companies, HMOs, and employers) buy health care in volume. Major buyers are becoming

increasingly sophisticated consumers and now use large data bases and expert consultants to identify exactly which providers should be "preferred."

USING SERVICE TO CREATE A COMPETITIVE ADVANTAGE

Most hospitals now have full-time marketing directors. Spending for marketing and advertising soared in the 1980s and has become a permanent line-item in hospital budgets. Having gotten the attention of consumers, hospitals must now deliver on the expectations that their marketing created!

Service is the next strategic initiative for market-oriented hospitals and health systems. A growing number of hospitals are adding consumer relations staff to coordinate their service management programs. "Guest relations" training is widespread. Customer service guru Kristine Peterson of Laventhol and Horwath estimates that as many as 4,000 hospitals have given their employees training in guest relations and customer service (Peterson 1988). The attention paid to consumer comfort and convenience has resulted in better signage, warmer food, and quicker service times. Now hospitals are searching for ways to institutionalize the service orientation at all levels of the organization.

Is consumer-driven health care just another fad? Customer service experts warn that most of the changes to date have been cosmetic. Hospitals still need to dig deeper and try harder—a tough assignment for the 1990s, when hospital profit margins will reach all-time lows and nursing shortages will push staff to the limit.

Today's health institutions can be classified by where they fall on the spectrum of service (Table 15-1). The differences between the three levels are essentially a matter of staff attitude. When staff care about customers, it shows in the details of their attitudes and their caring—the "50,000 moments of truth" service management consultant Karl Albrecht (1988) describes in his new book *At America's Service*. Most of these moments take place out of sight of direct supervision. Hospitals can manage them only by influencing the values and attitudes of employees, who will make or break the health organization's reputation for service the countless times each day they are in contact with a patient, visitor, or guest.

THE "MAUVING OF AMERICA"

In this age of the consumer, America's hospitals and physicians have been working hard to change their image. Just look at the hospital lobbies and physician waiting rooms in New York City and Los Angeles and lots of smaller towns in between—they have all been redone in shades of pink, gray, and green. Gone are the rows of plastic chairs, grim tile floors, and general hubbub. Instead,

Table 15-1 The Spectrum of Service

Dimension	Level I	Level II	Level III
Staff attitude	Bureaucratic	Polite	Empathetic
Noise level	Highly disruptive	Moderately noisy	Low and unobtrusive
Privacy	None	Staff knock first	Staff respect privacy
Continuity of care	On your own	Assistance to next point of care	Case management
Information	Patient told need-to-know information only	Staff responsive to questions	Informed patient
Amenities	Spartan or institutional environment	Comfortable surroundings	Caring environment
Service time	Long wait and late service	Moderate wait	Brief and punctual service
CEO commitment	Promote theme of month	Minimize complaints	Give high priority to service
Customer impact	Disgruntled ex-customers	Reasonably satisfied	Repeat business and loyal customers

Source: Reprinted from *Hospital Entrepreneurs' Newsletter*, Vol. 4, No. 2, p. 2, Aspen Publishers, Inc., © July 1988.

plush carpeting lowers noise levels and groupings of well-padded furniture invite repose.

In trying to become consumer driven, hospitals are mimicking fine hotels. They are attempting to provide tasteful surroundings, more attentive staff, and lower noise levels. The interior designers are waging war on institutional environments, prettifying bare institutional corridors with carpeting and hanging art prints on freshly papered walls. Patient rooms have been repainted and then newly curtained with color-coordinated fabrics. Physician waiting rooms are changing as well. Gone are fish tanks and copies of *Readers Digest*; instead there are designer sofas and *Architectural Digest*. This is a good start but only a beginning.

PLANETREE: THE NEW INDUSTRY STANDARD FOR SATISFYING CONSUMERS

The "hospital" of the future is here: a 13-bed med-surg unit called *Planetree* in San Francisco's Pacific Presbyterian Medical Center. This customer-centered unit is setting a new industry standard for patient satisfaction and quality care.

Planetree is a model and a symbol. Medicine's earliest beginnings were under the plane tree where Hippocrates taught the first principles of health care. Two and a half centuries later, the plane tree is the emblem of one of the most successful models in consumer-centered health care.

The "High Touch" That "High-Tech" Medicine Needs

The goals of the Planetree board are simple but sweeping in their reach: to *humanize* health services, to provide consumers with *access to information*, and to *empower* consumers to take charge of their own health.

Planetree is dedicated to the new paradigm of health. The basic idea is to treat the whole person and to actively involve the patient in the healing process. Planetree hopes to provide a working model that demonstrates how to translate "new age" values into marketing and clinical successes.

Will Mainstream Medicine Accept Consumerism?

Is Planetree a unique phenomenon, something only acceptable in trendy California? A good question, and it will be put to the test in the coming year when Planetree installs a program in an East Coast teaching hospital.

A better question for now is, Does it work? Early results of this pilot project already demonstrate that it does. The Planetree unit consistently runs at 85 percent occupancy and has a waiting list. More than 300 Pacific Presbyterian doctors have voluntarily affiliated with the unit for patient referrals, up from an initial 75. The unit has handled every type of med-surg case, and with no more nursing staff than comparable units.

To test its theories, Planetree is now the subject of a rigorous three-year evaluation by the University of Washington under a grant from the Kaiser Foundation. The evaluation will analyze factors such as patient satisfaction, cost, staffing, utilization, and the ultimate quality indicator—patient outcome. Patients are randomly assigned to Planetree and other med-surg units for research comparisons.

Starting a Revolution for Health Consumers

Standing behind Planetree are Angelica Thierot and a small group of prominent San Franciscans who leveraged their social clout to create a new movement in consumer-centered health care. Today Planetree has been featured in dozens of journal articles. Executive director Robin Orr is an international spokesperson for consumer-centered health care, and hundreds of hospitals have visited the model unit and resource center.

Gaining acceptance wasn't easy, but Thierot, a high-energy persuader, was successful in convincing the Pacific Presbyterian Medical Center to provide space for the Planetree Resource Center, a library for health care consumers, in 1983. Two years later, the hospital provided a 13-bed med-surg unit for an experiment in consumer-centered inpatient care.

Instrumental in Planetree's model hospital project was architect Rosalind Lindheim of the University of California. Her pioneering design for a children's hospital 30 years ago revolutionized hospital architecture. Lindheim's central tenet is that health institutions should be designed to suit the consumers, not the doctors and nursing staff. The mauving of American hospitals may have prettified the institutional environment, but it did little to change basic hospital design. Lindheim and the Planetree board had a different notion of how hospitals should be planned, namely, to best serve the most important users: the patients and their families.

Planetree's Principles of Consumer-Centered Care

The principles of Planetree's philosophy are deceptively simple, as in the case of all good movements (Exhibit 15-1). Planetree is an attitude, not a place. The concepts and philosophy could be adapted to and implemented in any patient care program, from critical care to home care. If the Planetree board is successful, their philosophy will become the new standard for health care.

Planetree Looks Different—And It Is!

Turn in from the busy corridor and the difference is immediately obvious. It's like entering a Japanese garden. There is a sense of tranquility on the Planetree unit, due to the soft lighting, muted colors, oak trim, art prints on the walls, and quiet carpeting. Patient rooms look like hotel suites, with chintz curtains and designer bedding. This is the hospital unit patients have been dreaming about!

The first thing visitors notice on the Planetree unit is the lack of a prominent nursing station. Planetree did away with that fortress of hospital bureaucracy and instead gave nurses and physicians small writing desks for note writing. The philosophical and architectural center of the unit is a family room for patients and visitors, which is well stocked with books and has a TV and VCR. A small kitchen for patients rounds out the homey design. The kitchen has a microwave

Exhibit 15-1 The Planetree Philosophy of Consumer-Centered Care

- *Informed Consumers.* Information is the baseline of the Planetree program. At first, the unit had a full-time health educator. Now the nursing staff provide the education.
- *Volunteer Staff.* The nursing staff on Planetree are self-selected nurses who share the program's philosophy. Their holistic concern is the linchpin that makes Planetree work case by case.
- *Consumer-centered Environment.* Colors, lighting, carpeting, fabrics, furniture, and the absence of sharp corners exemplify the Planetree commitment to creating a warm, nurturing environment.
- *Open records.* Consumers can read their own medical records and can add "patient notes" about their feelings and responses.
- *Family Involvement.* Visiting hours are at the patient's discretion. In-room sleeping chairs let family stay near. Personal caregivers—relatives and friends—are encouraged and trained to participate in patient care during and after hospitalization.
- *Physician Commitment.* To admit patients to the Planetree unit, physicians must sign a statement of principles to show their acceptance of the Planetree philosophy.
- *Body-Mind Connection.* The Planetree concern is for the whole person. The latest addition to the Planetree staff is a part-time masseuse who adds a therapeutic touch to the high-tech medicine.

and refrigerator for "midnight snacks" and to allow a change from institutional cooking.

If visitors sense something else is missing on this hospital unit, they're right— institutional *clutter.* Supply carts and trash containers have been skillfully integrated into wood cabinets and closets. Give credit to architect Lindheim and the Planetree board, who fought fire marshals and state bureaucrats to create a consumer-sensitive environment.

Next Step: A National Movement

The Planetree concept is on a roll. Already San Jose Hospital is creating a Planetree unit, and dozens of other hospitals are interested in a Planetree franchise. That still leaves more than 5,000 community hospitals to go!

What's next for this concept in consumer-centered care? At a recent strategy session, the Planetree board identified other settings and services that need this approach, including

- emergency rooms
- critical care units

- physician offices
- medical office buildings
- public health clinics
- mental health hospitals
- teaching hospitals
- rural hospitals
- for-profit hospitals
- HMOs
- home care

For the future, what Planetree wants is not just followers and imitators but innovators and friendly competitors who share its concern and create new models of service and settings that put consumers first. Planetree's 13-bed med-surg unit may be the conceptual model for a new generation of health care organizations dedicated to satisfying consumers.

SERVICE MANAGEMENT: FROM PHILOSOPHY TO PROGRAM

Health care is a service industry—intimate, hands-on, person-to-person service. But as Theodore Levitt, editor of *Harvard Business Review* (1983), reminds us, "There are no such things as service industries. There are only industries whose service components are greater or less than those of other industries. Everybody is in service."

Service management is more than an attitude or a "management trend of the month." Two of America's service management gurus are Karl Albrecht of Albrecht and Associates in La Jolla, California, and Ron Zemke of Performance Resources Associates in Minneapolis, Minnesota. The two collaborated on the best seller *Service America!*, published in 1985, and both have new books: Karl Albrecht's *At America's Service* (1988) and Ron Zemke's *The Service Edge* (1989).

The Service Edge

Ron Zemke's search for the best service companies in America led to dozens of Fortune 500 and midsize firms. The result is profiled in *The Service Edge: 101 Companies That Profit from Customer Care* (1989). Some familiar names top the list: Disney, Marriott, Federal Express, L. L. Bean, and Nordstrom. Others are known only within their industry niche, such as Southern New England

Telephone and Stop'n Chek. In the area of health care, three hospitals were selected: Riverside Methodist in Columbus, Ohio, Beth Israel in Boston, and the Mayo Clinic in Rochester, Minnesota.

Personal leadership is one of the hallmarks of Zemke's customer-driven companies. Riverside's Eric Chapman III periodically takes off his pinstripe suit and works alongside his employees in the dishroom, laboratory, and x-ray department. He spent several shifts as a patient escort and encouraged his vice-presidents to follow his example and get closer to customers by pushing wheelchairs. The Elizabeth Blackwell Center, designed for women, was named after America's first woman physician. The center was the outcome of meetings and focus groups involving more than 500 Columbus-area women. Riverside's employee uniforms were designed by Ann Stevens, a nursing manager in the hospital. Riverside's concern for its customers does not end with discharge. Patient relations representatives make 3,500 annual calls and home visits to former patients.

Beth Israel Hospital is one of the major teaching facilities for the Harvard Medical School. It has a national reputation for excellence, not for teaching or research, although it does both well, but for inpatient nursing. The concept of primary care nursing was developed at Beth Israel in 1975. Three years before, Beth Israel was the first hospital in the nation with a statement on the rights of patients. The basis of primary care nursing is individualized patient management. Each admission is assigned a primary nurse who manages the stay of care from intake to discharge. So much care planning and decision making was decentralized that the hospital eliminated two layers of nursing management.

At the famed Mayo Clinic, one of the principal rules is that there is no rule for how long a physician should spend with a patient. Every doctor on the medical staff is available for consultation. Since all physicians are salaried, there is no economic incentive to see more patients to boost income. Mayo uses the primary physician concept. The primary physician responsible for a Mayo physical takes overall responsibility for coordinating needed care. Patients respond to the personalized attention; waiting lists are weeks long, sometimes months. Mayo's staff morale is excellent. Turnover is less than 2 percent. Mayo's success is being extended to new satellite clinics in Phoenix and in Jacksonville, Florida. Patients of these clinics will still get the Mayo treatment. Mayo specialists conduct clinical consultations via telecommunications.

Albrecht on Service

Karl Albrecht's *At America's Service*, published in 1988, is the sequel to *Service America!* Since the first book's publication, hospital interest in service has grown from a trickle to a torrent. As many as four thousand hospitals have engaged in guest relations training. Many hospital executives and marketers bought copies of Albrecht's first book. Many health care managers are now asking, Is customer service just a hula-hoop—another fad that will disappear when top executives grab the next theme of the month? (Peterson 1988).

Their fears are reasonable. Customer service could be a casualty of the current wave of budget cuts and nursing shortages. Hospitals that shortchange service because they "can't afford to provide extra service" miss the point. Customer service is not a matter of hiring an extra employee or putting up a plaque in the lobby. Rather, it is a matter of instilling an attitude about serving people in employees throughout the organization—from the CEO to the security guard in the remote parking lot.

The Service 500

Service is big business. More than three-fourths of all jobs created in the last decade have been in service industries (Preskett 1986). A majority of new businesses are service or service-related. While the Fortune 500 companies shed 2.5 million jobs in the past ten years, the economy added 8 million new jobs, most of them in the service sector. To track the growth of the powerful service side of the economy, *Fortune* magazine created the "Service 500." The numbers tell an interesting story. While the 500 largest manufacturing companies experienced an aggregate decline in profits of 6.6 percent in 1986, the Service 500 boosted their profits by 8 percent.

If Albrecht is right, the "service revolution" in American business is well underway and gathering steam. Many companies are trying to lift their volume and profitability by becoming more effective at delivering service products. More advertising campaigns are zeroing in on service as the competitive factor. Hospitals, hotel chains, financial services companies, banks, and telecommunications companies are trying to position themselves competitively on the basis of service quality. Many companies are spending heavily to provide better consumer service, like Sprint's billion-dollar investment in fiber-optic cables so consumers can "hear a pin drop" from coast to coast.

Lessons Learned

Since the publication of *Service America!*, Albrecht and Zemke have consulted extensively with Santa Monica Hospital Medical Center in Los Angeles and with dozens of other businesses and industries. Here are ten lessons distilled from that experience:

1. Service has more economic impact than was thought and is worse than was imagined.

2. Most service organizations are in a defensive mode with respect to service.
3. Management must see the profit impact of service in order to take it seriously.
4. The longer people are in the service business, the greater the odds they don't understand their customers.
5. A service product is profoundly different from a physical product.
6. Managers do not control the quality of service products.
7. Service improvement starts at the top; managers must "walk the talk."
8. Management practice will have to evolve from a manufacturing orientation to a "moments of truth" orientation to meet the demands of competition.
9. Its employees are a company's first market; it has to sell them on a service idea or it will never sell the service to its customers.
10. Systems are often the enemies of service.

Service Management Equals Corporate Culture

Service management, according to Albrecht's definition, is a total organizational approach that makes service quality, as perceived by customers, the primary driving force of the business. Under the service management philosophy, the whole organization should act like one big customer service department.

Managing the "moments of truth" is the essence of the service management concept. Each day, a hospital may experience 50,000 such moments when a customer's expectations meet the service reality. Moments of truth are just as likely to occur in the parking lot as the critical care unit. It is at such moments that the hospital (or any organization) shows whether it really cares about customers. Producing and delivering a service is a fundamentally human process, and it usually occurs beyond the range of direct supervision. The moments of service provision can only be "managed" by influencing the hearts and minds of front-line employees. Their actions telegraph the message of quality and caring. When mistakes happen or employees don't care, a bad impression remains with the customers. Their dissatisfaction will be hard to erase.

Customers are in the center of the "service triangle," Albrecht's concept of the interplay of three key elements that together compose service management (Figure 15-1). The three elements are as follows:

- *A Well-Conceived Service Strategy.* An organizational plan for satisfying customers should be conceived and developed (unit by unit) by front-line employees who will carry out the strategy.
- *Consumer-Oriented Front-Line Employees.* Service quality depends on the one-to-one relationships between consumers and providers. The moments

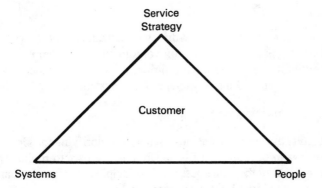

Figure 15-1 The Service Triangle. *Source*: © 1984 Karl Albrecht. Reprinted by permission.

of truth occur when service employees come face to face with consumers and meet (or exceed) their expectations.

- *Consumer-friendly Systems.* The delivery system that backs up the service employee is designed for the convenience of the customer, not the service provider. The facilities, procedures, and communications should all reinforce this message: "We're here to serve your needs."

Blunders, Pitfalls, and What Doesn't Work

Service management is a "transformational concept" that turns the organizational pyramid upside down and places the customer on top. Service management requires more than the creation of a customer service department or the installment of a concierge in the lobby. Albrecht believes that frequently the main obstacle is a lack of top management commitment to quality service, not calloused behavior by front-line troops. Motivating and training the employees is easy (look how many hospitals have conducted guest relations training). The hard part is overcoming barriers to change and then sustaining the commitment to 24-hour-a-day, 365-day-a-year service.

Common Blunders

For any hospital that has launched a guest relations or customer service program, these "blunders" will have a familiar ring: misreading the customer, lack of a clear business focus, mixed messages to the employees, brass bands and lapel buttons, smile training, one more program, and so on.

Common Pitfalls

The road to becoming a consumer-driven organization is beset with problems: culture and climate problems, quality of work life problems, employee cynicism, executive credibility, organizational arthritis, middle management inertia, misaligned incentives, and taking advantage of the system.

General Motors Management Doesn't Work for Service

Albrecht faults the Harvard Business School for glorifying the General Motors authority-based approach, which fits square employees into round job descriptions, and for teaching the "one best way" principles of scientific management. The problems engendered by this approach include management neuroses, lack of motivation, low productivity, poor performance, unions, and the "failure of MBO" (management by objective).

HOW TO IMPLEMENT A SERVICE MANAGEMENT PROGRAM

Albrecht's second book on service management reflects his accumulated experience at Santa Monica Hospital and dozens of other firms. It is essentially a more complete and detailed presentation of the ideas sketched in *Service America!* Service management programs should be put into place using five phases of implementation.

Phase 1: Understanding the Customers

The foundation of any effective service management strategy is a well-developed understanding of the customers. Consumer perception research is essential to check assumptions (often erroneous) about what consumers want. Research on employee attitudes is essential for managing feelings and attitudes. Finally, measuring service levels and satisfaction provides a standard against which to measure program effectiveness.

Phase 2: Clarifying the Service Strategy

What is a service strategy? In the simplest possible terms, the service strategy answers this question: Why should consumers choose us? The service strategy is the plan by which every unit of the organization—from Admitting to the Business Office and every service stop in between—seeks to satisfy consumer expectations regarding service. In the health field, a service strategy also attempts to create a "zero defects" process of medical care that results in the best possible recovery outcome. At Santa Monica Hospital, each unit developed its own strategy after assessing problems and barriers to high consumer satisfaction. The strategy was then incorporated into the unit's annual objectives and budget.

Phase 3: Educating the Organization

Formulating the best service strategy will be an academic exercise without commitment. The value of consumer service must be sold—from the top to the bottom of the organizational chain of command. Albrecht advocates "wall-to-wall" training of every employee. At Santa Monica Hospital, 1,500 employees were put through the program.

Phase 4: Implementing Grass-Roots Improvements

Implementation is where promise meets performance. Albrecht recommends planting many seeds. He suggests using service quality task forces (with middle managers in charge). When Albrecht talks about "Application Labs" and "Service (SQ) Circles," he means pilot projects and pushing responsibility down to the unit level. Redesigning service systems is a "bottom-up effort to reform the endless layers of process and protocol that impede customer service."

Phase 5: Making the Program Permanent

Without structural changes in the organizational culture (and budget), service will be just another theme of the month. Managers must "walk the talk" and systems must support service as the first priority. Employee selection needs more attention, and so do performance incentives. To ensure service comes first, managers must track success in satisfying consumers and improving profitability. It's not as elusive as many fear. Simple systems for measurement and feedback create a continuous information flow to let management know where service is high—or failing.

EXECUTIVE EVANGELISM

If there is one factor which determines whether a service orientation flourishes or flounders, it is executive commitment. Service-driven organizations are led by executives whose commitment to service is often obsessive. They are compulsive about the details (as Einstein said, "God is in the details"). These committed executives, the Bill Marriotts and Walt Disneys, understand that success is never final.

Service is a minute-by-minute challenge, but it does pay off. Albrecht suggests that only 10–15 percent of firms in any industrial sector even *attempt* to provide high-quality service. The firms that do also charge premium prices, but customers seldom complain. They know that the company stands behind what it sells. When Mercedes gets a service call, they will send a technician hundreds of miles for road service and provide a "loaner" if the car needs overnight attention. Think of the last time your organization went that far to serve a patient or family member. Imagine it making a similar effort every time there was an extraordinary problem. That kind of dedication and effort is the hallmark of businesses—and hospitals—that are putting themselves "at America's service."

SERVICE FIRST! IT PAYS

Health care is at the center of the transformation of American enterprise. This transformation is as profound as the decline of agriculture and the rise of industry in the 19th century. Service is the new tractor that is pulling the GNP forward at stable rates of 2–4 percent annual growth. The transition from an economy based on manufacturing to one based on service is one of the most important trends in American life, not to mention the American business world.

It hasn't been easy. Even the experts have a hard time defining quality. Service quality is a slippery concept that has defied standardization and measurement. The essence of quality service is still an elusive intangible that consumers describe best when they don't get it!

If health care can satisfy its customers, a 15 percent share of the GNP may be a low guess. Health care is well positioned for the future. The service component of American business has been remarkably recession resistant. The health care economy grew at a rate of 8–10 percent in 1987–1989, twice the increase in the GNP. Much of the service industry's profitability in the past five years has come from the declining dollar, lower interest rates, and cheap oil. The challenge for the future, Albrecht and Zemke suggest, is to create customer value through superior service. Profitability will come from the combination of reasonably efficient service combined with higher volume and prices. Superior service organizations in all industry sectors can and do charge above-market rates without dampening demand. Clifford and Cavanagh's 1988 study of 750 midsize, high-growth companies, *Winning Performance: How America's Midsize High-Growth Companies Succeed*, demonstrated that only 4 percent of these very successful firms were low-price leaders. Hospitals charging higher rates for "premium service" options have encountered virtually no consumer resistance.

Forget lower prices as a major factor in health care consumption for the next three years. A new "floor" for hospital and physician service prices has been set by government and managed care buyers. Prices are essentially equal among competitors. Now the competition shifts to quality—both consumer satisfaction and technical quality. All health care consumers, from carload customers like Medicare to individual patients, will select their preferred providers based on quality. That is both a challenge and an opportunity to fulfill the high promise implied in health care's definition of service: patient care.

STRATEGIC IMPLICATIONS FOR PHYSICIANS

1. *Service management will invade physician offices.* The concepts of managed customer service are needed as much in physician offices as in hospital emergency rooms. Consulting services are commercially available to help physicians assess patient satisfaction and develop a service improvement plan. A number of hospitals offer education or consultation services at no cost to medical staff.
2. *Hospitals will encourage service-oriented doctors.* As part of their own service management program, many hospitals are actively involving medical staff and soliciting voluntary participation in service improvement programs. Although some doctors will resist the "charm school" approach, such participation will be a significant factor as hospitals align with preferred physicians for managed care contracting and hospital-physician ventures.
3. *Quality assurance includes customer satisfaction.* Physicians with a gruff bedside manner can expect to hear from the hospital's medical director on the style as well as the clinical content of their patient care.

STRATEGIC IMPLICATIONS FOR HOSPITALS

1. *All of the experience of customer relations shows that a commitment to service management must start at the executive level.* More important than slogans and communications are the lessons of behavior. The CEO and senior managers must "walk the talk" of customer-first service if the message is to be accepted throughout the organization.
2. *Service management requires bottom-up planning.* It needs to be planned (and executed) in the front lines, not back in the corporate office. A

participative approach to planning and training is essential for the spread of customer service attitudes.

3. *One of the most effective mechanisms for developing service strategies is the use of quality circles.* Work teams at the unit level meet to identify service barriers, then develop an action plan. Management must respond with resources and a commitment to carrying out the recommendations of the employees. Quality circles need to meet periodically to monitor progress, resolve problems, and identify new barriers to optimum service.

4. *Hospitals need to devise ways of measuring and rewarding superior service.* They should establish a base line of patient satisfaction in every unit, then continually sample patient attitudes. The satisfaction surveys can be used to monitor progress and problems. Those departments and service units that are providing high-level service should be rewarded with team bonuses. Customer satisfaction should be included in employee and managerial performance appraisals. Department managers and service unit supervisors should be assessed on the customer satisfaction ratings of their service and be compensated accordingly.

BIBLIOGRAPHY

Albrecht, Karl. 1988. *At America's Service*. Homewood, Ill.: Dow Jones-Irwin.

Albrecht, Karl, and Ron Zemke. 1985. *Service America!*. Homewood, Ill.: Dow Jones-Irwin.

Clifford, Donald K., and Richard C. Cavanagh. 1988. *Winning Performance: How America's Midsize High-Growth Companies Succeed*. New York: Bantam Books.

Heskett, James L. 1986. *Managing in the Service Economy*. Boston, Mass: Harvard Business School Press.

Jenna, Judith K. 1986. "Toward the Patient-Driven Hospital." (Parts One and Two.) *Healthcare Forum Journal*, 29:52–59.

Levitt, Theodore. 1983. *The Marketing Imagination*. New York: Free Press.

Peterson, Kristine. 1988. "Guest Relations: Substance or Fluff?" *Healthcare Forum Journal* (March–April): 23–26.

Rice, Alan. 1987. "PLM in Action." *Healthcare Forum Journal* (January–February): 29–28.

Ruffner, John. 1986. "Product-Line Management." *Healthcare Forum Journal* (September–October): 11–15.

Senna, Craig. 1988. "Consumer Clout: Healthcare Customers Take Control." *Healthcare Forum Journal* (March–April): 10–20.

Zemke, Ron. 1989. *The Service Edge: 101 Companies that Profit from Customer Care*. New York: New American Library.

Chapter 16

Contract Management

We see a very definite trend of hospitals looking at contract management as an important way to respond to prospective pricing and competitive pressures. More hospitals feel contract management allows them to provide the broadest range of services with a minimum administrative burden.
—Ernest A. Bates, *"Services for Hire"*

Build or buy? When it comes to diversification, enterprising hospitals have the same choices as any business developer—to build new programs or products from internal resources or buy from outside contractors. With increasing frequency, health care organizations are contracting with outside firms that specialize in the management of administrative support or clinical services. The trend is presenting new opportunities for physicians and new companies, and all indicators signal growth ahead.

Health care is being reshaped by a wave of new entrepreneurs who provide contract management services, install and run franchise programs, and license hospitals to use brand names and generic advertising. In return, enterprising hospitals and physicians with innovative programs are licensing or franchising them to other hospitals outside their market area, like "You're Becoming", Republic's plastic surgery program. Multihospital systems are developing pilot programs and trying to market them nationally.

The trend toward contract management is widespread and growing. By 1988, 1,997 facilities, more than one-third of America's hospitals, contracted for a wide array of administrative, support, clinical, and service functions in this multi-billion-dollar industry (Exhibit 16-1). Every type of hospital is involved in contract management today—small and large, rural and urban, public and private. Contract management services are provided in inpatient, ambulatory, home care, and extended care settings. Once thought of as the suppliers of food service and cleaning personnel, contract management firms now provide physicians, hospital administrators, financial officers, information systems specialists, biomedical

Exhibit 16-1 Growth Markets for Contract Management Services

Established Contract Management Services	Emerging Contract Management Services
Full-service management	Task-oriented management
Bundled management services	Unbundled management services
Department management	Department management
Housekeeping	Physical therapy
Food service	Gourmet food service
Laundry	Rehabilitation
Plant maintenance	Risk management
Biomedical engineering	Information systems
Pharmacy	High-tech home health
Emergency	Obstetrics
EEGs	Mobile diagnostic imaging

engineers, and virtually every other type of personnel. Contract management is a growing and dynamic sector of health care and is wide open to enterprise.

Hospitals may be both buyers and sellers of contract management services in the future. Enterprising hospitals and their medical staff are discovering niches overlooked by major national contract firms. Hospitals seeking to strengthen market share are creating networks of community and rural hospitals and providing joint purchasing and contract management services to promote referrals. To bring in new revenues, innovative hospitals are creating "boutique" products and services, which are often highly focused on a particular disease or customer segment. Successful products are being franchised and licensed to out-of-area hospitals for management fees and royalties.

HOSPITAL MANAGEMENT CONTRACTING

A new boom for hospital management contracting is on the horizon. What are the driving forces? Money and market share! Financial experts predict that America's hospitals will be pressed against the financial wall in the next three years (Newald 1987). The reasons: increasing financial pressure from declining inpatient utilization, a squeeze on capital payments by Medicare, and a rising percentage of patients covered by fixed-priced contracts with managed care buyers.

In this bear market for hospitals, prospects are bullish for expansion of contract management. In a recent survey of contract management by *Modern Healthcare*

(Wallace 1988) the following firms anticipated new growth in full-service contract management:

- Brim and Associates, the contract management subsidiary of NME (which has 47 hospitals and 5,300 beds), expects at least 10 percent growth in the year ahead.
- HCA, one of the largest hospital-management firms, expects to sign 30–40 new full-service contracts this year (it currently manages 225 facilities).
- Hospital Management Professionals, of Brentwood, Tennessee, plans to add a hospital per month to its portfolio of 46 facilities in the East, South, and Midwest. It experienced a 48 percent increase in hospital management contracts in 1986.
- HealthOne of Minneapolis manages 13 hospitals, mostly smaller facilities, and anticipates future growth through developing regional hub-and-spoke networks in which small rural facilities link themselves to tertiary medical centers.
- Sisters of Mercy Health Corporation of Farmington Hills, Michigan, contract manages a dozen hospitals in the Midwest and is well positioned to link smaller hospitals to its larger hospitals to strengthen clinical ties and management resources.

Increases in full-service management contracts will not be limited to investor-owned firms. HealthOne and Sisters of Mercy, for example, are nonprofit hospital companies

REGIONAL HEALTH SYSTEMS

Contracting is a mechanism for developing regional health systems. Virginia Mason Medical Center of Seattle, Washington, is solidifying its position as one of the Northwest's premier tertiary care hospitals. In 1973 the medical center founded the Health Services Consortium, a 17-hospital network. All are community or rural hospitals within 200 miles of Seattle. The affiliation is strengthened by Virginia Mason's tie with Amerinet, a national shared-purchasing organization. Virginia Mason's local affiliates can contract for group purchasing, consulting, practice management, and continuing medical education. Virginia Mason is planning for a managed care future. A for-profit HMO, Northwest MedCenters, will give the medical center a managed care product that could be offered statewide through the Consortium network.

Voluntary Hospitals of America (VHA) actively supports development of regional multihospital "clusters" linked to its 99 shareholder hospitals. The alliance has grown from 30 hospitals to 791 hospitals in 48 states (with more than 200,000 beds). Nonshareholder hospitals have access to VHA group purchasing and contract management services. VHA has sold most of the subsidiaries of the alliance's development arm, VHA Enterprises, which operated 13 for-profit businesses. Its most profitable venture was Behavioral Medical Care, which developed and managed inpatient chemical dependency and acute psychiatric programs in 37 VHA hospitals. Partners, VHA's managed care joint venture with Aetna, is one of the health industry's largest experiments in developing a national managed care product. Partners now operates 18 HMOs and 37 PPOs in 67 markets but has yet to turn a profit. VHA clusters have shared investments at the local level, (e.g., mobile imaging units, HMOs, and physician referral services).

DEPARTMENTAL MANAGEMENT CONTRACTING

Mounting financial pressures from prospective payment systems (PPSs) are motivating hospitals to take a fresh look at contracting for management of hospital departments, both support and clinical (Lutz 1988b).

Housekeeping is the most popular contract service. Nearly 2,000 hospitals contract with outside vendors for cleaning services, and the number is growing. Illinois-based ServiceMaster is the largest housekeeping service vendor, with 1,500 hospitals under contract in 1988, followed by United Healthserve, ARA, Marriott, and others.

Food service is the second most frequently contracted function. ARA, the food service vendor for the 1984 Olympics, is also the food service contractor for more than 250 of America's hospitals. ARA competes for hospital food service business by offering a guaranteed rate for services. Because of the financial pressures on hospitals, nearly 60 percent of ARA's food service contracts now include price caps. ARA was leapfrogged as the market leader in food service contracting when fifth-ranked Marriott purchased third-ranked Saga in 1986, making Marriott the largest purveyor of hospital food in the nation.

Laundry service has been another profitable niche for contract management. ServiceMaster is the largest vendor of laundry services, but other companies are finding opportunities in the steam-and-starch niche. Foussard Associates of St. Paul saw its hospital laundry management business double in the first year after prospective payment was implemented, and it now has more than 50 hospital clients.

Multidepartment management contracts offer to hospital buyers the "one-vendor" advantages of negotiability and accountability. ServiceMaster Industries of Downers Grove, Illinois, is the giant of the contract management industry, providing services to nearly 25 percent of America's hospitals. ServiceMaster has experienced strong growth in its six departmental contracting lines of busi-

ness: housekeeping, plant operations and maintenance, laundry, materials management, biomedical and clinical equipment maintenance, and food services. It
has signed multiyear master contracts with alliances, including VHA in Dallas,
Consolidated Catholic Healthcare in Chicago, and SunHealth of Charlotte, North
Carolina. The SunHealth deal, one of the largest of its kind, could be worth
$100 million in revenues to ServiceMaster.

CLINICAL SERVICE MANAGEMENT

Contract management of clinical services is gaining popularity (Lutz 1988b).
Hundreds of U.S. hospitals now contract the management of clinical departments
to outside firms. Managed services include cardiopulmonary diagnostics, home
IV nutrition, nursing, pharmacy, and physical and respiratory therapy. There
are nearly 20 clinical services now available from contract firms.

Emergency services are the most often contracted clinical services. By 1988,
698 hospitals contracted out the management and staffing of their emergency
rooms, a gain of 18.3 percent for the emergency room contract firms from the
preceding year. A half dozen major firms dominate the field, including Spectrum
Emergency Care, a subsidiary of ARA, Emergency Medical Services of Plantation, Florida, and California Emergency Physicians of Oakland, California.
Urgency care centers are also a prime target for contract management. Many
hospitals have experienced low profitability in their ambulatory care centers,
suggesting a need for outside management (Lutz 1988a). HealthStop Medical
Management of Wellsley, Massachusetts, may have a winning formula. HealthStop
joint ventures its free-standing primary care centers with local physicians and
hospitals. Through an aggressive strategy of construction and acquisition, HealthStop
built a network of more than three dozen primary care centers around the Boston
metropolitan area. HealthStop also purchased 34 MedFirst centers from Humana
in the Chicago area after Humana was unable to make them profitable. HealthStop
believes equity participation from local hospitals and physicians increases customer acceptance and brings the primary care centers into mainstream medicine.

Departmental contracting is definitely on the upswing. Horizon Health Management Company, a subsidiary of Dallas-based Republic Health Systems, now
manages 40 psychiatric, chemical dependency, and eating disorders units, and
it began to manage diabetes units in 1987. Horizon is one of more than 80 firms
that responded to a recent survey by *Modern Healthcare* on contract management
services.

Entrepreneurs are discovering tomorrow's niches. The Diabetes Institute of
America, based in Glendale, California, experienced promising results from its
first diabetes unit (located in 171-bed Downey Community Hospital in Downey,
California). Such specialized units help a community hospital achieve market

differentiation, which is especially important in intensely competitive market-places like Los Angeles. Diabetes is a "magnet" program for hospitals. Diabetics are four times as likely to be hospitalized as the average adult.

CONTRACTING OUT: WHAT HOSPITALS WANT

Management expertise is the number one reason why hospitals choose to enter into full-service contract management agreements. A study of 1,100 board members of the 170 hospitals managed by HCA provides some insight into why hospitals contract for management services. The study was conducted for HCA by a research team from the Leonard Davis Institute of Health Economics at the University of Pennsylvania (Newald 1987).

Key findings from the study shed light on why hospitals enter management contract agreements:

- Small hospitals typically cite declining patient census, inadequate marketing, and decreasing revenues as prime factors that drive their contracting decision.
- Larger hospitals focus more on issues of administrative concern: physician-administration conflict, unsatisfactory management performance, rising expenses, and retiring administrators.
- Public hospitals are especially sensitive to issues of community relations, accreditation, plant and equipment, as well as administrative concerns such as cost containment and labor relations.
- Medical staff issues are a key factor in the contracting decision. Many managed hospitals cite hospital-physician relations and the need for physician recruitment as motivating factors in contracting for outside management expertise.
- A declining market share can prompt a decision to bring in an outside management firm with marketing expertise.

FRANCHISES AND LICENSES

No discussion of contract management and licensing agreements would be complete without an examination of the franchise. If the industrial corporation was the major organizational innovation of the 19th century, the franchise may be the organizational innovation of the 20th.

Few concepts have had such an impact on American society as franchising, and the trend is sweeping worldwide. In every town there is a new growth area commonly called the "fast-food strip." In reality, this is franchisors row, an array of many small businesses that share a common form of ownership and a common market need to be located near or on major auto routes. The development of franchised businesses has refashioned small towns and set the pattern for suburban sprawl. Across the interstate highway network, franchised gas stations and fast-food outlets service the immediate needs of America's motorists.

Franchising has not fared well in the health industry in the past. Health care's self-concept has been that it provides custom, not production line, services. That was then, and this is now! In the days before DRGs and the Joint Commission, uniqueness may have been the rule, but the unique is giving way to the systematic. Many health needs are commonplace, patterns of practice and quality standards are well developed, advanced technologies are widely available, and standardized support systems are in place.

The stage has been set for franchising. All that is needed are the entrepreneurs. Physicians and hospitals exploring new business forms and relationships would do well to consider one of the most pervasive business structures invented in this century: the franchise.

Franchises are more than roadside empires of fast food or no-wait medical care. Health care entrepreneurs are beginning to see the possibilities of franchising and licensing products and programs. One of franchising's pioneers in the health field, Republic Health Corporation, now has 120 licenses for its six "branded" services, including "Gift of Sight" (cataract surgery) and "You're Becoming" (cosmetic surgery). Bethesda Hospitals in Cincinnati has 49 licenses in 32 sites for its two occupational health and employment assistance programs ("Share and Concern"). St. Anthony's Hospital in St. Petersburg, Florida, has licensed 20 hospitals to utilize its "Pregnagym" program. Phoenix Memorial Hospital has already licensed 16 of its "Easy Street" simulated environments for rehabilitation patients since launching a national marketing effort in March 1986.

Franchises and licenses to operate programs are similar in many respects. Typically, franchises provide more control over use of franchise registered trademarks as well as extensive training and control over operations. Licenses often involve one-time fees for the use of trademarks, program materials, and generic advertising.

The advantages of franchises and licenses are easy market entry, brand name identification, established systems, training programs, generic advertising, and business and market plans. When timing is a factor in establishing market position—especially with new services—then franchises and licenses can help hospital entrepreneurs move quickly into the market.

"HOLLOW HOSPITALS": THE ULTIMATE MANAGEMENT CONTRACT

Where is contract management leading? Hospitals may find themselves adopting the private business sector concept of the hollow corporation. With this business strategy, a firm perhaps owns no facilities or distribution outlets but contracts out for many aspects of the enterprise, retaining control through a series of interlocking agreements with outside suppliers and sellers.

To illustrate, much of the microcomputer "clone" business is controlled by hollow corporations that neither manufacture nor sell the products directly. These corporations buy the components through original equipment makers, pay assemblers to put the computers together, and make arrangements with wholesalers and mail order houses to sell the products to consumers.

In the health care analog, the board of a "hollow hospital" would contract out for full-service management as well as a wide array of clinical services. Management firms would be at risk for capital and meeting performance objectives set out in the contract. Administrative, operational, and clinical services would be managed by contractors. Would the board contract for a medical staff? Probably not, but the hospital's medical director would be a contract employee, like all of senior management. Even marketing and public relations would be conducted by contracted firms. And the patients? Naturally, they would come from managed care contracts. This picture of tomorrow's hospital is not unrealistic. The future of contract management is about to arrive.

NEW VENTURES: INNOVATIONS IN CONTRACT MANAGEMENT

Innovation abounds in the field of contracting for management of clinical departments. Here are five niches that hold out promise for new ventures.

Freestanding ambulatory surgery centers (ASCs) will flourish under the new Medicare rules. These rules are due to the 1986 Omnibus Budget Reconciliation Act, which mandated the creation of a prospective pricing system for selected ambulatory surgery procedures. The modified payment policies reimburse hospitals for ambulatory care based on a blend of ASC rates and hospital rates or the lower amount of a hospital's customary charges. Free-standing ASCs will benefit from the new policies. With their lower overhead, free-standing ASC costs are typically well under those of hospital-based ASCs. To sweeten the incentives for ASCs, HCFA granted an 18.7 percent increase for Medicare outpatient reimbursement as of July 1, 1987, the first raise in five years. In April 1987, HCFA doubled the number of surgical procedures covered by Medicare outpatient payment, from 100 to nearly 200. This provides ASCs with an opportunity to expand their market base. There are incentives for physicians to shift to ASCs. When a physician performs one of the approved surgical procedures in an ASC or hospital outpatient department and accepts assignment for it, Medicare will pay 100 percent of "reasonable charges" instead of the usual 80 percent. Ambulatory surgery is booming. Nearly 1 million procedures were performed in 529 outpatient surgery centers in 1986, according to SMG Marketing Group in Chicago (Henderson 1987). SMG forecasts an increase to 829 centers and 1.9 million procedures by 1990.

Emergency departments will be a hot spot for contract management services, according to a market forecast by Frost and Sullivan (Newald 1987). The marketing firm projects a five-year growth chart for contracted emergency department management services, with annual revenues rising from $115 million in 1984 to $179 million in 1990. Larger hospitals are contracting out this critical service to gain better quality assurance, risk management, and marketing and a systems approach to physician management. Beneficiaries should be companies like Spectrum Emergency Care of St. Louis, which has 415 emergency department contracts, and Coastal Emergency Services, based in Durham, North Carolina, which has over 200 contracts.

Obstetric services that deliver babies for indigent mothers may be a growth niche of the future. Florida is a bellwether state. Soaring malpractice costs are driving Florida obstetricians out of business. Hardest hit have been obstetric services for the poor and for Medicaid beneficiaries. Watch for new entrepreneurs and enterprising contract management firms that will see Medicaid obstetrics as a market opportunity.

Home care joint ventures can be win-win development projects for competing community hospitals. In several cases, hospitals in the same medical market area have contracted with management firms such as ServiceMaster to develop joint home care programs. ServiceMaster developed four multihospital joint ventures in home care in 1986, setting a promising precedent for the future. In the multiple joint ventures, the hospitals typically own shares totaling 80 percent; ServiceMaster owns the other 20 percent and acts as the managing partner. Hospital partners are experiencing 4 percent profitability. The partners share overhead expenses, marketing costs, billing, and management services.

Child and adolescent psychiatry services are booming. To illustrate, three years ago one of every four patients treated at the 41 free-standing psychiatric hospitals owned by HCA was a child or adolescent. Today, the ratio is one patient in two, including patients being treated for chemical dependency problems. Managing psychiatry programs in general acute hospitals has been a growth business for contract management firms. Mental Health Management of McLean, Virginia, manages 85 hospital inpatient psychiatric programs. The aging of the population offers new opportunities for "geropsych" services, despite limited Medicare benefits and reimbursement. Management contractors such as Mental

Health Management are developing specialized programs for the elderly and are experiencing favorable market responses and 90 percent occupancy rates.

VENTURE MANAGEMENT: MAKING THE DECISION TO BUILD OR TO BUY

Whether to create or purchase a product or service is one of the classic business quandaries. The ultimate decision often rests on factors other than cost, including psychological factors.

As management contracts grow in popularity, many hospitals and medical staffs will face the "build or buy" decision. Decision makers should consider a broad array of quantitative and qualitative factors. Both kinds of factors can be weighted, scored, and ranked, as shown in Exhibit 16-2.

In the decision process, explicit criteria should be used. By applying these criteria, the management, the medical staff, and the board will be able to weigh and rank the options and thereby determine whether to build internal capacity or contract with an outside firm. Here are sample criteria for the build or buy decision:

- *Operating Cost.* Simply stated, which alternative offers the lowest cost of operation per unit of service or product. These estimates should accurately reflect hospital overhead in considering the build option and include some leeway for inflation and contingency costs in the contractor's prices.
- *Capital Needs.* New or expanded services will require capital for development and for subsidizing operations until the ventures reach the break-

Exhibit 16-2 Build or Buy Decision Matrix

Decision Factors	Weight	Alternatives		Ranking
		Option 1	Option 2	
Operating cost				
Capital needs				
Expertise				
Product quality				
Medical Staff				
Risk				
Market entry				
Community image				
Buyer value				
Competitor impact				
Related synergy				

even point. Capital sources and requirements for all options should be considered. Outside contractors may bring new capital to the venture. Alternatively, the build option offers investment opportunities to medical staff and other insiders that may enhance their commitment.

- *Expertise*. One of the most frequent reasons for selecting outside contract management firms is to obtain scarce and valuable expertise. This criterion should be heavily weighted. Many hospital ventures have failed to meet expectations for lack of expertise. By the time the hospital educated itself in the new field, it had already exhausted its venture capital or failed to match competitor performance. The contractor's experience is worth a fee, and the less knowledge the hospital has about the field in which it hopes to venture, the more valuable that expertise should be considered.

- *Product Quality*. The quality of a new service or product is both a symbolic and a real decision factor. The underlying concern is often control. The key criterion is whether the outside contractor or the internal development alternative can provide quality that meets board and management expectations. Both options will have advantages. An outside firm will have an established track record of buyer satisfaction and product defects, whereas internal operations can be monitored intensively.

- *Medical Staff*. One of the major criteria in any program development decision is the impact on the medical staff. The medical staff should be considered a resource for internal development. The build option, however, carries the risk of alienating medical staff who are not participants in the venture. Outside contractors must be acceptable to the hospital's medical staff or they will fail to win loyalty and referrals. This is a sensitive area, and medical staff reaction may be based on history of previous ventures and have little to do with the present one.

- *Risk*. In all new ventures there is risk. When considering whether to build or buy, determine how much risk the hospital can or would be prudent to assume. Financial, legal, malpractice, and image risks are among the most important to consider. Outside firms can share risk or guarantee to limit the hospital's liability to a negotiated level. When moving into a new service, check with other clients of potential outside firms on the terms of and their experience with risk-sharing arrangements.

- *Market Entry*. When facing an opportunity to gain market leadership or a desired market position, the criterion of market entry may weigh heavily. Selecting an experienced contractor with an established package of services can assist a hospital to move expeditiously into a new product line. "Ramping up" can be accomplished in weeks or months rather than years. A quick market entry can also hasten the achievement of the financial objectives of breaking even and eventually making a profit. When time is a less critical factor, the speed or ease of market entry may be offset by other decision criteria.

- *Buyer Value.* A major question to be asked is which decision alternative would bring greatest value to the buyer. Michael Porter (1985), business guru from the Harvard Business School, advances the theory that the "value chain" should be a strategic business criterion. The buyer's value chain is simply the set of factors that will achieve the buyer's objectives: lower costs, improved performance, superior quality, reduced downtime, ease of operations, convenience of distribution, and so on. The buyers of hospital products or services whose value chains must be considered may include major purchasers such as employers or insurance companies, the medical staff (as brokers of hospital services), and the consuming public.

- *Competitor Impact.* In launching a new product or service, the hospital's objective may be to expand its market share, take share away from a particular competitor, achieve a significant or perceived advantage over competitors, or shift the hospital's reputation and ranking in comparison with competitors. The element of surprise (a "preemptive strike") may be achieved by use of an experienced outside contractor with a market-ready program. Acquisition of new technology or establishment of new distribution outlets may affect the relative market positions of the hospital and its competitors. Generic advertising, trademarks, and brand names that a contractor brings may help the hospital to establish (or change) its market reputation vis-à-vis the competition. Alternatively, when competing with another hospital using an outside firm, the "home-grown" option may resonate well with the community and medical staff.

- *Related Synergy.* Few business decisions for today's hospitals are simple. Factor in the complexity and look for "synergy" in making the build or buy choice. Choosing an outside firm may bring expertise and capacity that could be used for other activities and ventures. The freeing up of internal capital by selecting an outside vendor might be another synergistic result. If the hospital chooses to develop a new product or service internally, it may find the product or service has franchising or licensing potential. Or the new internal capacity in one product line (e.g., home care) may facilitate development of a related service (e.g., durable medical equipment).

LOOKING FORWARD: FUTURE TRENDS IN CONTRACT MANAGEMENT

What is the future outlook for contract management? Here are the major trends which will shape this health industry sector in the next five years (see Exhibit 16-3).

Exhibit 16-3 Megatrends in Contract Management, 1990–1995

1. Growth will be experienced in administrative, support and clinical contracting.
2. A market shift from small to large hospitals and from rural to urban hospitals will occur.
3. Task-oriented contracts will be available for hospitals that don't want full-service management agreements.
4. Full-service firms will develop unbundling flexibility in order to sell desired services such as joint purchasing.
5. Capital for working funds and development will be an important component of many contract management agreements.
6. Turnaround management of ailing hospitals will increase.
7. Risk sharing by contract management firms will demonstrate commitment.
8. Consolidation and market shakeout can be expected as growth attracts undercapitalized entrepreneurs.
9. Market volatility will increase as hospital finances worsen.
10. Volume deals will increase between multihospital buyers and large contract management vendors.

Growth. Look for growth in this sector of the industry. In the future, the hospital without outside management contracting may be the exception. Contract management services will be the direct beneficiary of the "pincers" that will squeeze hospitals in the future—the need to reduce costs and increase revenues.

Shifting Markets. Who will need contract management services? The trends of the past may be reversing. Anticipate that in the next one to three years larger hospitals in urban areas may seek full-service management contracts as financial pressures mount. Historically, full-service management contracts have been sought primarily by small and rural hospitals, whereas larger facilities in metropolitan areas have limited outside contracting to departmental management. In the future, smaller facilities may seek competitive advantages through hiring outside contractors specializing in services such as rehabilitation or chemical dependency to assist in the startup of new clinical services or the expansion of existing business lines. Small and rural hospitals may also try to reduce costs by contracting for the management of high-cost but essential services such as emergency rooms and critical care units.

Task-Oriented Contracts. A growing number of hospital management contracts are task-specific, (i.e., they are intended to achieve particular purposes). Under these management agreements, the outside firm tackles objectives such as reducing accounts receivable, training middle management, and developing business plans for product lines. Instead of supplying the administrator and chief financial officer, the contract management company works for the existing management team. Task-oriented agreements will range from months to years under a broad but defined charter.

Unbundling Flexibility. The market for contract services can grow more rapidly if the major hospital management firms relax their "full-service only" policies. Increased flexibility would permit clients to access desired services such as joint purchasing. Client hospitals would then be able to contract only for needed management, support, or clinical expertise. If the major firms will not increase their flexibility and unbundle desired services, watch for entrepreneurs to fill these niches (including some who jump ship from major management firms that won't bend to market demand).

Capital. At the foundation of many future management contracts will be capital. The need for working capital is likely to increase with the ratcheting down of Medicare capital payments and elimination of period interim payments. Access to development capital for facility improvements or service upgrading will be a major factor in the contract decision. Contract management firms with capital to invest in financially vulnerable hospitals will have a major market advantage.

Turnaround Management. Predictions of financial turmoil for America's hospitals abound. In this bear market, the need for experienced turnaround management firms should grow. Outside firms will need skills in more than cost reduction. Strategic planning, service development, physician relations, team and culture building, and marketing and sales will all be needed from contract management vendors.

Risk Sharing. As this field becomes more competitive, contract management companies will take on more financial risk as a cost of doing business and a demonstration of long-term commitment to their client hospitals.

Consolidation and Market Shakeout. Some acquisition and consolidation among contract management firms can be expected as this industry sector grows and matures. Doing business will carry more risk. Small firms that aggressively take on "problem hospitals" may run up real losses and be driven from the field. Some nonprofit multihospital systems with only a few management agreements may discover this "sideline" needs more expertise and capital and divest their contract services.

Market Volatility. The contract management field can anticipate an increased rate of change in the future health care market. Knowing when to get out of some contract management businesses will be as important as when to enter them. Not all niches will be profitable. Already, inpatient psychiatric, rehabilitation, and chemical dependency services are showing signs of market saturation and will be vulnerable to market shifts as buyers switch to ambulatory programs and cut back inpatient stays.

Volume Deals. ServiceMaster's agreement with SunHealth is a signal of a new era of bigger deals between major contract management firms and hospital groups. Multihospital systems and alliances will seek master contract agreements to gain lower prices and special incentives from contract management companies. Use of outside firms to manage clinical services can also provide the multihospital systems with needed services and thus make them competitive for HMO and PPO contracts with regional or statewide buyers.

STRATEGIC IMPLICATIONS FOR PHYSICIANS

1. *The management of hospital departments is a promising niche for physicians.* Any new service added by a hospital, such as psychiatry or substance abuse, is a prime target for clinical management contracting.

2. *Physicians may be hired by hospitals as full-time department chiefs under contracts.* Physician managers will be given time-limited contracts with performance clauses—like the contracts given to NFL football coaches. And like their coaching counterparts, physicians with a "winning record" of volume and profitability will get bonuses and have their contracts renewed.

3. *Exclusive contracts will become more common.* Laboratory and radiology are typically managed under exclusive contracts with a preferred medical group. Add anesthesiology and emergency care as services for which exclusive arrangements are becoming the standard. Most likely to be contracted out are those departments where existing medical staff are not well established or where there are only a limited number of specialists, such as psychiatry, substance abuse, or renal dialysis. In the future, the trend may grow to include cardiac surgery, critical care, and other subspecialties such as neonatology.

4. *One of the most desired professionals of the future will be the management-trained physician.* Doctors with proven management track records will form their own contract management firms to oversee clinical departments.

5. *The basic concept of a medical group is being altered by contract management companies.* National firms are being established that utilize physician managers and cadres of clinicians who work under contract. Most contract management firms have a small circle of partners, and the majority of the doctors are simply contract employees who receive bonuses but lack access to equity participation. Many physicians fear a future in which they work for a megahospital or governmental bureaucracy. This is a low-probability scenario. More likely is that many salaried physicians will work for other doctors in clinical departments managed under contract by large physician-owned companies.

STRATEGIC IMPLICATIONS FOR HOSPITALS

1. *Hollow hospitals may be just over the horizon.* By 1995 more than 75 percent of all hospitals will use contract management services in clinical departments. The trend is powerful and widespread. Although the early development of contract medicine has been in smaller hospitals, it is quickly spreading to hospitals of all types and locations. Eventually some hospitals may contract out virtually all services to a full service management firm.

2. *The vice-president for professional services may be a lawyer.* As contract medicine becomes pervasive, hospitals may need a full-time legal counsel to handle contracting for the many departments that are being managed by outside firms or medical groups. Hospitals and physicians will negotiate on an arms-length business basis for the management of clinical departments. These agreements will become increasingly specific in terms of performance, reimbursement, and mutual expectations.

3. *Managed care and risk sharing are both growing factors in the medical marketplace.* One of the advantages of contract medicine is the potential for risk sharing. To stimulate a high level of clinical and financial performance, the outside firm or physician group will be put at financial risk. In a managed care environment, an increasing number of HMOs will insist that hospitals and medical staff take a share of financial risk in exchange for volume guarantees—or simply as a condition of participation in the HMO networks. Risk sharing agreements will be especially prevalent in "single-business HMOs," which focus on a speciality niche such as mental health or substance abuse.

4. *Outside contract management firms can bring fresh capital to revitalize an existing hospital service or to capitalize a new one.* This is a frequent reason for bringing in an outside firm, particularly among hospitals that have limited access to capital. Hundreds of small and rural facilities have been rebuilt using outside funding provided by contract management companies. This trend is spreading to clinical departmental contracting. Capital can be used for remodeling, capital equipment, and even construction of new specialized facilities (e.g., a rehabilitation hospital, a free-standing cancer center, or an imaging facility).

BIBLIOGRAPHY

Alexander, Jeffrey A., and Bonnie L. Lewis. 1984. "The Financial Characteristics of Hospitals under For-Profit and Nonprofit Contract Management." *Inquiry* 21 (Fall): 230–42.

———. 1984. "Hospital Contract Management: A Descriptive Profile." *Health Services Research* 19 (October): 461–77.

Alexander, Jeffrey A., and Thomas G. Rundall. 1985. "Public Hospitals under Contract Management: An Assessment of Operating Performance." *Medical Care* 23 (March): 209–19.

Anderson, Howard J. 1987. "Convenience Clinic Franchise Gives Not-for-Profits a Tool to Draw Patients." *Modern Healthcare*.

———. 1985. "Hospitals' Eating Disorders Units Fill Empty Beds with Paying Patients." *Modern Healthcare*, 25 October, 62–66.

———. 1986a. "Hospitals Will Form New Links with Alternative Site Providers." *Modern Healthcare*, 3 January.

———. 1986b. "Ambulatory Care Centers Offer Broader Range of Health Services." *Modern Healthcare*, 6 June.

———. 1986c. "Home Care Providers' Business Expanded Rapidly during 1985." *Modern Healthcare*, 6 June.

———. 1986d. "ServiceMaster to Expand Home Care through Joint Ventures with Hospitals." *Modern Healthcare*, 1 August, 46.

———. 1986e. "Large Hospitals Hiring Contract Managers to Reduce Expenses." *Modern Healthcare*, 29 August, 48–64.

———. 1986f. "Rehabilitation Services Market Offers Development Opportunities." *Modern Healthcare*, 10 October, 59–62.

Baldwin, Mark F. 1988. "Private Groups Seek Status in Certifying Process." *Modern Healthcare*.

Barkholz, David. 1985a. "MHM Has Agreement with the Sun Groups." *Modern Healthcare*, 4 January.

———. 1985b. "HCA's Hospital 'Clusters' Will Centralize Management." *Modern Healthcare*, 6 December.

———. 1989. "Use of Managed Insurance Plans Will Rise to Stem Decline in Profits." *Modern Healthcare*.

Bell, Clark W. 1987. "Hospital Systems Report 47.1% Drop in Profits Last Year." *Modern Healthcare*, 5 June, 37–58.

Biggs, Errol L., John E. Kralewski, and Gordon D. Brown. 1980. "A Comparison of Contract-Managed and Traditionally Managed Nonprofit Hospitals." *Medical Care* 18:585–96.

Brown, Montague, and William H. Money. 1976. "Contract Management: Is It for Your Hospital?" *Trustee* 29 (February).

Carter, Kim. 1986. "Reimbursement Cuts May Slow Steady Growth of Dialysis Chains." *Modern Healthcare*, 6 June.

"Contracting Hikes Occupancy in Psych Units: Study." 1985. *Hospitals*, 1 May, 60–62.

Droste, Therese. 1987. "Freestandings Bound to Gain under New PPS Plan." *Hospitals*, 5 July, 60–61.

Fackelmann, Kathy A. 1985. "Analysts Predict a Bright Future for the Psychiatric Care Industry." *Modern Healthcare*, 10 May, 55–57.

Fine, Jennifer. 1986. "Vision Center Chains Add Outlets, Develop Marketing Strategies.' *Modern Healthcare*, 6 June.

Graham, Judith. 1985. "Corporately Managed Healthcare Will Dominate 1990s, Experts Say." *Modern Healthcare*, 11 October, 34.

Henderson, John A. 1986. "Surgery Center Growth Slows, More Procedures Done." *Modern Healthcare*, 6 June.

———. 1987. "Cost Containment, Hospital Competition Aren't Limiting Surgery Center Expansion." *Modern Healthcare*, 5 June, 148–54.

"Inpatient Chemical Dependency Program Costs Lower Than Residential Programs: Twin Cities." 1985. *Hospitals*, 1 May, 63.

Jensen, Joyce, and Bill Jackson. 1985. "Consumers Prefer Same-Day Surgery to Inpatient Care for Minor Procedures." *Modern Healthcare*, 10 May, 76–78.

Jensen, Joyce, and Ned Miklovic. 1985. "Eighty-Three Percent of Hospitals Reporting Increased Outpatient Use." *Modern Healthcare*, 25 October, 86–88.

———. 1985. "Physical Therapy Most Popular Service in Growing Rehabilitation Marketplace." *Modern Healthcare*, 22 November, 56–59.

Johnson, Donald E. L. 1985a. "HCA, American Agree to Form $8.5 Billion Giant." *Modern Healthcare*, 12 April, 16–22.

———. 1985b. "Investor-owned Chains Continue Expansion, 1985 Survey Shows." *Modern Healthcare*, 7 June, 75–90.

———. 1985c. "Hospitals Pay about $700 Million for Consulting Services in 1984." *Modern Healthcare*, 16 August, 50–57.

———. 1985d. "More Hospitals, Nursing Homes Try to Cut Costs with Contracts." *Modern Healthcare*, 30 August, 50–68.

———. 1986. "Hospital Chains Are Searching for Good Acquisitions, Mergers." *Modern Healthcare*, 6 June.

Kahn, Lynn. 1984. "Departmental Contract Management Up as Much as 162 Percent." *Hospitals*, (February): 62–64.

Kralewski, John E., et al. "Effects of Contract Management on Hospital Performance." *Health Services Research*, 19:479–97.

Lutz, Sandy. 1987a. "Outpatient Surgery Centers Slated for Growth as Fees, Demand Increase." *Modern Healthcare*, 16 January, 54.

———. 1987b. "Not-for-Profit Hospital Systems Lead Growth in Ambulatory Care Industry." *Modern Healthcare*, 5 June, 138–44.

———. 1988a. "For-Profit Chains Retreat from the Ambulatory Business, Not-for-Profits Fill the Void." *Modern Healthcare*, 3 June, 74–80.

———. 1988b. "Services for Hire." *Modern Healthcare*, 12 August, 31–48.

McCormick, Brian. 1988. "Alcohol Centers Now Treating 'Food Addicts.' " *Hospitals*.

Moore, W. Barry. 1985. "CEOs Plan to Expand Home Health, Outpatient Services." *Hospitals*, 1 January, 74–77.

Morgenson, Gretchen. 1987. "Harsh Reality." *Forbes*, 15 June, 48.

Newald, Jane. 1986. "Hospitals Show 'Business Smarts' by Diversifying." *Hospitals*, 20 December, 60.

———. 1987. "What's Ahead for the Full-Service Contract Management Industry?" *Hospitals*, 20 May, 70–76.

Porter, Michael. 1985. *Competitive Advantage*. New York: The Free Press.

Powills, Suzanne. 1988. "Consumers Snub Freestanding Surgical Centers." *Hospitals*.

Punch, Linda. 1985. "Ambulatory Care Industry Has Financial Growth Pains." *Modern Healthcare*, 12 April.

Richman, Dan. 1985. "System Expanding to Vertical Integration." *Modern Healthcare*, 10 May.

Riffer, Joyce. 1986. "Can Surgicenters Stand Alone." *Hospitals*, 20 July, 44–48.

———. 1988. "Units Focus on Unique Care Needs of Adolescents." *Hospitals*.

Rundall, Thomas G., and Wendy K. Lambert. 1984. "The Private Management of Public Hospitals." *Health Services Research*, 19:519–44.

Sabatino, Frank. 1985. "Contracts for Clinical Services Rising." *Hospitals*, 16 September, 94–97.

Shahoda, Teri. 1988. "Specialty Services Boost Psych Providers." *Hospitals.*

Siegner, Catherine A. 1985a. "Large Multihospital Chains Divesting Financially Troubled Rural Hospitals." *Modern Healthcare*, 11 October, 104.

———. 1985b. "Outside Management Firm Puts Ailing Hospital on the Right Track." *Modern Healthcare*, 6 December.

Super, Kari. 1987. "Product Developers and Providers View the Benefits of Franchises and Licenses." *Modern Healthcare*, 10 April, 60–62.

Tatge, Mark. 1985. "HMOs Seeking Benefit Packages for Psychiatric, Substance Abuse." *Modern Healthcare*, 10 May, 60.

Wallace, Cynthia. 1985a. "Cocaine Addicts Seeking Care at Hospitals and Other Facilities." *Modern Healthcare*, 10 May.

———. 1985b. "More Rural Hospitals Are Affiliating with the Larger Healthcare Systems." *Modern Healthcare*, 24 May, 70–72.

———. 1988. "Hospitals, Physicians Seeking Ventures with Surgery Centers." *Modern Healthcare.*

———. 1986. "Psychiatric Management Firms Capitalize on Growing Market." *Modern Healthcare*, 10 October, 68–70.

———. 1987a. "Investor-owned Hospital Chains Streamlining Existing Operations." *Modern Healthcare*, 2 January, 47–48.

———. 1987b. "Psychiatric Hospital Industry Still Growing, but Rate of Expansion Slower Than Last Year." *Modern Healthcare*, 5 June, 92–98.

Chapter 17

Strategic Deal Making

Because he understands the full range of alternatives that lie before him and constantly weighs the costs and benefits of each one, the true strategic thinker can respond flexibly to the inevitable changes in the situation that confronts the company. And it is that flexibility which, in turn, increases the chances of success.

—Kenichi Ohmae, *The Mind of the Strategist*

Enterprise in health care has just entered a new and more sophisticated era. The deals may be fewer and the pace less frenzied, but hospitals and physicians are making better choices of products, markets, and venture partners. The success rate is beginning to rise, and profitability should soon rise as well.

In the first wave of diversification and venturing, the boldest hospital and physician entrepreneurs inspired a movement and set the pace. Enterprise in health care needed a publicist—and found one. Under editor Phil Newbold, now CEO of Memorial Health System in South Bend, Indiana, the *Hospital Entrepreneurs' Newsletter* was established to chronicle the successes and failures experienced by health care organizations across the nation.

With little preparation, America's hospitals launched a broad array of new ventures in collaboration with their medical staff. Many ventures fell victim to the classic failure factors of any new business: undercapitalization, limited market research, and excess competition. Other new programs and products thrived and marketed their success nationally (e.g., Carondelet Rehabilitation Centers, a spinoff of Carondelet Health Care, a Catholic hospital system based in Culver City, California).

ENTERPRISE IS DRIVING HEALTH CARE

Fundamental changes are sweeping health care. They are driven by competition and entrepreneurship. Today, diversification is making a significant contribution

303

to physician incomes and hospital bottom lines. Numerous health care executives report their noninpatient activities are contributing 15–25 percent of total revenues.

Becoming a Multihealth Corporation

When does a multihospital system become a multi*health* company? One nonprofit system, UniHealth America (formerly the Lutheran Hospital Society of Southern California), pulls in more than 50 percent of revenues and profits from nonhospital product lines. Entrepreneurship made the difference. UniHealth operates highly successful for-profit HMOs and PPOs built from scratch.

The entire health care industry is entrepreneurial, not just hospitals. Entrepreneurs are probing every profitable market segment and product line and inventing new ones. Every hospital can expect outside competition to target its best profit centers. Entrepreneurs will try to do it better (quality) or cheaper (discounting), market it to a specialized set of buyers (niche seeking), or package the product with related services (bundling).

The Second Wave of Entrepreneurship

Deal making has developed a base of experience and expertise. Entrepreneurism in health care is better targeted, disciplined, capitalized, and supported. New ventures are strategically chosen. This is the second wave of health care enterprise. Many of the pioneers of hospital entrepreneurism are gone. They have been promoted to senior management posts when they were successful and cycled into other careers when they failed. Since the original entrepreneurs often lacked training or experience in managing new ventures, they had to learn how to succeed in a hurry. As one CEO bluntly stated, "It's sink, swim or get out of the pool!" (Coile 1987).

Today, deal making and venturing in health care organizations are high-priority activities and involve major capital investments. As the deals get bigger and more strategically significant, the CEO and the chief of the medical staff are now the "entrepreneurs." The ventures management team is often the senior management group, and for assistance it draws upon an experienced set of attorneys, market analysts, appraisers, and financial advisors.

INNOVATION: THE ATTACKER'S ADVANTAGE

In any industry, the competitive advantage always lies with the innovator—the attacker. The defending technology or business concept must protect its profits from the innovator with the better mousetrap. This is the message of Richard Foster (1986), senior vice-president for technology at McKinsey and Company. The way to gain market leadership is with a better idea.

In the private sector, the lessons abound. Look how compact discs are taking market share from cassette tapes. The same thing happened in the case of surgery (the wave of ambulatory surgery centers) and is about to in cardiac bypass surgery (balloon angioplasty and the new cardiac surgical lasers).

In health care, innovation is the strategic imperative no hospital can ignore. This is why Michael Porter's *Competitive Strategy* (1980) and *Competitive Advantage* (1985) became "must reading" for everyone in the executive suite. In this new high-risk environment, health care executives and physicians need to learn a new set of skills—those required for identifying and developing a worthwhile investment through strategic deal making and diversification.

STRATEGIC DEAL MAKING

The most important phase of managing new ventures is *deal selection*. This is preventive business medicine. Of course, any new venture should "pencil out" (i.e., demonstrate its potential to meet financial objectives). More fundamentally, the selection of ventures should be strategic. The chosen venture should align with the long-range plans and mission of the health care organization.

Strategic deal making is the investigation and implementation of those new ventures that advance the long-term market objectives of the firm. Doug Collier, senior business consultant with the Denver office of Ernst and Whinney, articulated the strategic deal making concept in a recent conference on R & D in health care sponsored by AMI's Presbyterian-St. Lukes Medical Center. Called in to review more than a dozen potential acquisitions of physician practices by Western hospitals, the consulting firm recognized the need for more strategy in selecting and structuring new ventures.

The Test of Strategic Fit

Deal making is much more than a determination of financial feasibility. Both buyers and sellers have strategic objectives. The best deals will enhance the long-range interests of all parties. Buyers are concerned that any deal they make will

- promote their business mission
- meet their profit criteria

- generate sufficient cash flow
- generate goodwill
- benefit important stakeholders
- provide an easy market entry for the new business
- put the new business in a competitive market position
- fit well with the portfolio of related products and services
- result in high-value use of investment capital
- build organizational capacity through the addition of new staff and programs
- position them to take advantage of future market trends
- fit with the image and culture of their organization

Sellers are concerned that any deal they make will

- be terminated satisfactorily
- be at (or above) the market price
- include acceptable terms of payment
- generate goodwill
- benefit owners and shareholders
- result in a timely market exit for the business being sold
- enhance the market position of the remaining businesses
- strengthen the portfolio of remaining products
- provide a smooth transition for existing staff and programs
- position them to take advantage of future market trends

The test of strategic fit—not short-term profitability—should be paramount. Many ventures have the potential to break even or be profitable. The question every health care entrepreneur must ask is, Will this venture be to the long-term advantage of the organization?

DECISION SCREENS

To determine strategic fit, there are a number of criteria that can be applied in the decision-making process. The quality of the decisions will be highly dependent on the quality of the criteria. There is no magic formula from business to guide health care entrepreneurs in making decisions. Every industry, every market, and every product is unique.

For health care organizations, there are a number of generic decision screens:

- financial performance
- indirect financial benefits
- marketing
- utilization
- resources
- product maturity
- medical staff
- strategic significance
- ethics

Use these decision criteria as a point of departure for setting the organization's own objectives and decision rules. The criteria should be refined by senior management and marketing staff so that they are aligned with the strategic goals and plans. Some hospitals have developed a diversification plan that articulates long-range goals for business development and new revenues. These goals and objectives should drive the criteria for venture selection.

There are nine sets of criteria for evaluating the strategic potential of new business ventures in health care. These may be weighted and ranked using a decision matrix like the one shown in Exhibit 17-1. For each set of criteria, the organization should translate its strategic objectives into decision rules. Some decision screens will be financial and quantitative (e.g., "hurdle rates" of return on investment or the length of time until the break-even point). Other decision criteria will be subjective and value-driven (e.g., any new venture must be consistent with the mission statement of the organization).

Exhibit 17-1 Decision Matrix for Strategic Deal Making

Criteria	Strategic Factor Rating										Total
	1	2	3	4	5	6	7	8	9	10	
Financial performance											
Indirect financial benefit											
Marketing											
Demand and utilization											
Resources											
Product maturity											
Medical staff											
Strategic significance											
Ethics											

Financial Performance

Of all decision criteria for investment in new ventures, financial criteria are most widely used. Even so, many entrepreneurial initiatives have foundered as a result of ignoring financial danger signs evident before the project was launched. Here are five of the most common financial decision screens for new ventures.

Return on Investment (ROI)

A standard rule of thumb is that a rate of return on capital of 2–2.5 times the cost of capital (16–20 percent at current interest rates) should be achievable. Investment capital includes both startup (preoperation) and working capital. It is usually estimated at a level sufficient to cover operating costs for the first 6–12 months of operation. Capital needs should be projected over a three- to five-year period, including capital for startup, an operational subsidy (working capital), and expansion capital to fund the growth that the organization plans to achieve in the first two or three years of operation. Complex projects with a substantial market risk, such as urgent care centers, need careful capital analysis and planning, as the recent sale by Humana of its national network of ambulatory centers attests.

Net Revenues

Ideally, every venture produces a profit. The net contribution to the organization's bottom line is an important financial criterion. Some organizations use a threshold level of $50,000 to $100,000 annual net profit for any new enterprise. If a new activity is not going to generate what the organization deems a sizeable profit, then other investments will be preferred.

Growth

There are two kinds of growth that may function as decision screens for venturing: market growth (discussed below under "Marketing") and the growth of revenues and projected earnings. As in the case of ROI, many organizations set a rate of 2–2.5 times the prime interest rate as the level of annual growth that any new enterprise should achieve within two or three years of initiation. High-growth ventures are often higher risk! There is considerable entrepreneurial activity now in bundling behavioral medicine or occupational medicine packages and capitating these to major employers or insurance companies. The growth and profit potential is excellent, but this is a new and potentially dangerous business, since the provider is fully at risk.

Break-Even Point

A new health care venture should reach the break-even point within 18 to 24 months if it has low to midrange capital requirements ($25,000 to $250,000) and within 36 months if it has high capital requirements ($250,000 to $500,000 and over). Some high-capital projects may take longer to break even (e.g., the acquisition of a lithotripter) but be considered worthwhile for other strategic reasons (e.g., to preempt a competitor's move).

Cash Flow

Cash flow is a significant decision factor in strategic deal making. High cash needs may discourage an organization from a new venture like home care, where days in receivables can be a significant factor. An enterprise like a PPO may be a better investment, because it will be a major source of new revenues, even if profitability is low. The demands on the organization for working capital or periodic cash infusions must compete with other needs for capital. Projects are often rated high simply because they require little or no cash to initiate, another consideration which may offset low profitability.

Indirect Financial Benefits

There are other financial aspects to consider in the evaluation process. These are usually less obvious, but from a strategic deal-making perspective they may rank as high as some direct financial aspects.

Contribution to Overhead

New enterprises may be highly ranked if they help subsidize the overhead of another program or business. For example, a durable medical equipment business might complement an existing home care service.

Synergy

An important but hard-to-define objective of venturing is synergy. If two or more businesses are complementary and strengthen each other's market appeal or consolidate costs of operations, the synergy to be gained increases the ranking of these investments. For example, a mail order prescription service would probably complement and subsidize the overhead of a hospital or free-standing pharmacy.

Impact on Payer Mix

One of the most important strategic factors for health care organizations is payer mix. As discounting becomes widespread and government programs limit reimbursement, good payer mix will be an important key to limiting days in receivables, reducing cash flow demands, and achieving profit goals. New programs such as respite care, plastic surgery, and elder day care may be highly ranked because they are all-cash businesses with minimal delays in reimbursement. Occupational medicine may be considered a strategic investment because it is related to workers' compensation, a significant source of inpatient referrals.

Marketing

Market considerations are central in strategic deal making. Quantifying marketing criteria relies on a high level of marketing intelligence, a level that many medical practices, hospitals, and health care companies have indeed achieved. Product reputation, market image, and customer needs or wants can be rated with modern market research techniques.

Market Share

Market share is one of the strategic keys to success. In applying this criterion, the stage of the product in the product life cycle is critical. For a new product, early market entry can create a market leader. In a mature market, acquisition may provide an affordable market entry or a way to expand market share. Where only a few competitors exist, a 25–35 percent market share is desirable. In a competitive market with many producers, a 10 percent market share is the minimum.

Customer Value

The image of the product and the firm are often tied up with consumer perceptions of "value." Consumer perceptions must usually be tested using focus groups, telephone surveys, exit questionnaires, or other standard research methods. The organization may set a quantitative consumer rating (e.g., eight or above on a scale of ten).

Pricing

For established products, pricing tiers are well accepted and readily assessed. For new products or services, consumer ratings established by market research define whether the products or services to be ventured will garner a "premium" reputation and may be priced and positioned accordingly. Low consumer value, reflected in consumer ratings, implies a product will be a "commodity" (in market terminology) and will not command high prices or profits.

Impact on Competitors

This criterion is of great strategic consequence. The impact may be defined and measured in terms of market share or consumer ratings (e.g., reduce the competitor's market share by 10 percent or cut the competitor's consumer ratings by 5 percent).

Impact on Image

Any new venture will have an impact on the image of the firm. Again, the criterion may be set against a base-line rating established by market research. A minimum criterion would be to maintain the existing community perception and rating. As the new product or service gains wider market recognition, the impact on the firm's image will increase. More than one hospital has received very negative community publicity for demolishing housing to make way for a new facility. Such new ventures, regardless of profitability, may have a negative impact on other products and programs of the firm.

Utilization

Utilization and growth are important indicators of product vitality and have high symbolic value in defining "success."

Volume

This criterion is usually defined in terms of levels of volume to be achieved according to a preestablished timetable. Establishing volume criteria for a newly ventured product can be done by considering the existing volume levels of competitors. Alternatively, the volume criteria may be driven by other strategic considerations (e.g., the break-even point, profitability, and market share).

Growth

Venture capitalists prefer backing new products that will enter a market whose annual growth rate is expected to be 20–25 percent or more. As a general criterion, the market growth rate should be at least 10–15 percent per year, with the specific venturing criterion that the new product should at least match or exceed the market's growth rate.

Resource Investment

Resource criteria are an extension of the decisions the organization has made about financial performance. Following are the most significant of these criteria.

Investment Capital

Capital is always a top strategic priority. One important issue is whether the new project can be financed from existing resources (that is, out of operational revenues). If not, then additional criteria will be needed regarding the level of capital investment, interest rate, capital formation strategy, venture partners, and type of equity ownership.

Operational Capital

In addition to capitalizing the facilities of production in any new venture, capital will be needed to subsidize the working operations until the break-even point is reached. Criteria should be developed relating to sources and uses of working capital, especially as the capital demands of the new venture may lower the capital reserves of the organization.

Human Resources

Of utmost importance in new product or service development are the human resources. As always, strategic considerations are paramount. The selection of the project management team may be *the* most important task for the long-range success of the new venture. Human resource criteria may guide project selection with respect to use of existing staff resources, recruitment, need for retraining, and incentives and compensation. Since new ventures are often innovations, they may need new personnel policies. The impact of select policies on existing staff in areas such as incentive compensation should be part of the decision framework for any new venture.

Product Maturity

Applying biology to business has given us the concept of product life cycles. Every product or service can be located on a product life cycle curve. Product maturity should be an important strategic factor in the consideration of any venture. The underlying causes of product maturity are technological obsolescence and market saturation. Classic symptoms of product maturity include

- flattening of the growth curve
- saturation of the market (the majority of potential customers have already bought the product)
- increasing levels of competition
- arrival of new competitors

- price competition and discounting
- decline in customer loyalty
- vulnerability of sales to rumors of next-generation products
- decrease in new distribution outlets
- emergence of product substitutes
- exodus of top talent to new products

Product maturity is not the "Bermuda triangle" of market initiatives. It may provide special opportunities for venturing but can be risky. For example, any hospital considering the establishment of a cardiac bypass surgery program must recognize that this is a mature product with widespread market competition and whose price is already being substantially discounted. By 1995 Medicare may be purchasing bypass surgery in volume from selected providers, using a process of competitive bidding.

Medical Staff

Every marketplace has unique factors. In health care, the medical staff are a factor almost without parallel in any other industry. Their influence on every health care product is substantial, even if ownership is not involved. In many cases, physician support can make or break the product. Correctly anticipating the impact of medical staff participation is critical for success in any health care venture. Key criteria relating to the medical staff should include the following.

Medical Staff Benefits

For any new venture, it should be determined whether the venture will benefit the medical staff in terms of revenues, practice base and location, referrals, status, teaching, and research.

Medical Staff Reaction

Virtually every new venture must be acceptable to the medical staff. No health care executive should underestimate their ability to mobilize resistance. Physicians are influenced by a complex array of economic, professional, and personal factors. Medical staff acceptance will depend on such things as the manner in which the venture is presented, the terms of participation, validation and support by the physician leadership, and potential competition with existing staff practices. Often the location of the new venture is a key factor in medical staff support. The timing of physician involvement is also a strategic consideration.

Early involvement may increase acceptance but could telegraph strategic information to competitors.

Referrals

Any assessment of the feasibility of venturing a new program or service must include a review of the impact on referrals to and from key members of the medical staff. Most importantly, this review should determine the impact on the 20 percent of the medical staff who are responsible for 80 percent of the inpatient referrals in the average hospital. For any nonhospital project, the impact of the new service on physician ordering and utilization patterns is likewise of strategic importance.

Strategic Significance

The strategic implications of venturing are often hard to quantify, but often these are the overriding factors in the final "go or no-go" decision. Health care venturers should craft criteria for the following four related strategic variables.

Mission and Traditions

First and foremost is the organization's mission and traditions. A hospital's mission is the bundle of values and traditions that have made it a success. It is the essence of the organization. New ventures must be consistent with organizational values or they may not be accepted by key stakeholders—the board, the employees, the medical staff, and the community.

Development Opportunities

The second strategic significance criterion focuses on development opportunities. Engaging in new ventures opens some doors but closes others. It selectively draws on development capital and thus can impact other projects that are competing for that capital. The selection of venture partners will strengthen relationships with some stakeholders, but may distance others. The choice of development opportunities also sets priorities for the assignment of staff resources. Where staff with product development or marketing experience are in short supply, the decision to pursue one venture may preclude others being done concurrently.

Strategic Market Position

Beyond the issue of market share, venturing can sharpen or shift the hospital's market position. Acquisition of an MRI scanner may signal a hospital's expansion into specialized clinical high-technology markets. Development of an IPA signals the hospital's acceptance of a role in managed care. Selective provider contracting establishes a market price and a position for a hospital or medical group. All these ventures have strategic market significance.

Related Products

The strategic significance of related products should not be underestimated. Entry into new markets or development of new product lines often have substantial consequences for other programs and services. A new ambulatory surgery facility may reduce the surgical caseload (and revenues) in the hospital's inpatient operating suites. Other hospitals have found a synergistic effect can result from adding a free-standing surgery facility. Both inpatient and outpatient surgery thrive when physician convenience is improved. Acquiring all three laser modalities may attract new physician specialists and encourage existing surgeons to engage in new procedures.

Ethics and Values

Beyond the internal values and mission of the organization, there is a wider set of criteria relating to health care as a social institution. Few services are more basic to human survival than health care. Many people are convinced that health care is a right, not a market commodity. Health care venturing has a broader context and requires review of factors such as these.

Societal Expectations

This criterion goes back to the basics—the physician as healer and the hospital as a social institution to care for the sick and injured. This societal expectation is several thousand years old. The hospital's ownership or the tax status of the new venture make relatively little difference to the public. The state of Nevada just passed legislation rolling back profits at several of its largest investor-owned facilities. The state also enacted a requirement that nonprofit hospitals must demonstrate they have provided community service in reasonable balance with their tax forgiveness. Each new venture must be assessed against societal expectations regarding health care services.

Legal Requirements

Every venture must be consistent with legal requirements. Currently, one of the most difficult legal issues is the inurement of physicians involved in ventures with their hospital. Other aspects of ownership, capitalization, incentives, and financial participation will also need serious review. This is a difficult area abounding with "deal killers"—legal problems that could make or break new ventures.

THE DEAL MAKERS: THE NEW WAVE OF HOSPITAL ENTREPRENEURS

A new generation of health care entrepreneurs is reshaping the industry. These deal makers blend business expertise with tough negotiating skills. They don't rely on the old-boy network. Some of these "new wave" entrepreneurs have Ph.D.s or M.D.s. A growing number are women. Although many are based in hospitals or multihospital systems, an emerging group of elite deal makers operate as independents or consultants throughout the health care industry. What they share are an enthusiasm for venturing and a lack of regard for traditional rules.

• *Larry D. Shoemaker, M.D., M.B.A.*, typifies the new breed of physician entrepreneur. At the start of the 1980s, he saw that medicine would take an increasingly entrepreneurial direction. Selling his thriving medical practice, he went back to school for an M.B.A., then joined the Penrose Health System in Colorado Springs, Colorado, now part of the Sisters of Mercy of Cincinnati health system. His first ventures in chemical dependency were highly successful. He created new programs for adults, women, and adolescents that were eventually restructured into Interstate Health Services. One of Dr. Shoemaker's latest ventures is a temporary personnel agency. He converted Penrose hospital's nursing float pool into a nursing service agency. The new venture began to make money six weeks into operations.

• *Dennis W. Strum, Ph.D.*, although still in his thirties, is senior vice-president for the newly created UniHealth America, the result of the merger of the Lutheran Hospital Society of Southern California and HealthWest, both based in the Los Angeles area. His responsibilities cover the broad range of business development activities for this multihospital system, which takes in $600 million in annual revenues. While still in graduate school, Dennis became the founding director of the Center for Health Management Research for the Lutheran Hospital Society, raising more than $2 million in R & D grants in two years from the Kellogg Foundation, the ARCO Foundation, and the federal government. He provided strategic planning direction for the multistate expansion and for-profit conversion of Lutheran's HMO, Pacificare. The HMO's initial $18 million public offering sold out on the first day. Finally, he was one of the three senior executives who managed the merger negotiations between Lutheran and HealthWest, which created one of the largest nonprofit multihospital systems in southern California.

• *Katherine E. Johnson* is one of the most innovative and enterprising trade association executives in America. More than ten years ago she took over management of the Association of Western Hospitals in San Francisco. She quickly realized what this regional hospital organization needed if it was to survive in competition with national and state associations: (1) management (to strengthen internal operations), (2) diversification (to expand revenues beyond its limited membership base), and (3) an expanded niche (to avoid the erosion that was killing other regional hospital associations). Taking on the titles of president and chief executive officer, she restructured the organization, launched a number of diversification projects, created a series of corporate partnerships with Fortune 500 companies like 3M and Baxter, and took the association national, changing its name to the Healthcare Forum. Her organization has become a model for corporate renewal among industry associations, and her 1985 study "The Entrepreneurial Spirit," is widely read by association executives.

• *Ronn R. Kelsey* is vice-president of corporate marketing for Palomar Pomerado Hospital District of Escondido, California. Prior to moving to the San Diego area, Ronn headed corporate marketing for the Saint Agnes Medical Center of Fresno, and while there he infused this Catholic medical center with private sector marketing. It's working: Saint Agnes is the leader in virtually every category in the Fresno market. In conjunction with Baxter's Travenol Management Systems, Ronn established a computerized marketing data base that is now being sold to hospitals nationally by Baxter. The data base provided the springboard for a series of management agreements and affiliations between Saint Agnes and half a dozen rural hospitals in the outlying areas of the central California valley. Analysts from corporate marketing pinpointed market weaknesses and identified promising new programs to strengthen the local hospitals. The results are improved referrals to Saint Agnes and the creation of a strategic market network that counters multihospital system development by its competitors. Ronn's hot air balloon, "Tranquility", is in vivid contrast to his high-energy style.

• *Wayman Spence, M.D.*, inventor and innovator, is the paradigmatic entrepreneurial physician. He developed his first product, a clinical water bed, before completing his medical residency. His experiments with silicone gel as a hospital bed pad led to silicone insoles for arthritic and diabetic patients. Spence signed a royalty agreement with athletic footwear manufacturer Nike for the insoles in 1971. He sold his own company, Spenco, to the Kimberly Clark corporation in 1984 for $27 million. Today Dr. Spence is joint venturing Health Fair stores, retail mall shops carrying health-related products, with hospitals across the country. Baylor Medical Center built the first two pilot stores. Already the stores are paying for themselves through referrals to a number of Baylor medical programs. A mini-mall shop and Health Fair kiosk are being pilot-tested. As a spinoff, Spence is developing a franchised hospital gift shop with an upscale line of health-related products and a bedside consumer catalog.

• *Wanda Jones* is the founder and principal of her own consulting firm, H.O.M. She is one of the new generation of deal makers who facilitate venturing. Her clients are uniformly urged to operate outside of established boundaries and clear new ground. She is the architect of several hospital mergers and multi-hospital systems in California and the Northwest. Her clients, who have built off-campus ambulatory health centers and developed physician service bureaus, tend to share her philosophical commitment to health promotion and wellness. She is assisting the Planetree Foundation in San Francisco to develop their customer-centered Model Hospital Project into a marketable form. A major Catholic hospital client of H.O.M. has launched a biotechnology institute, the Advanced Biotechnology Treatment Center, which is the first such hospital-sponsored program in the nation. Under the leadership of Sister Gladys Marie of the Sisters of the Holy Cross, Mount Carmel Health in Columbus, Ohio, the new center has started 20 projects beta testing various genetically engineered products. Wanda is working to "clone" the biotech treatment institute in five other hospitals.

• *Ed Lagasse*, as a former marketing vice-president for Baxter Travenol, brought a solid private sector base of experience to the California Medical Center in Los Angeles. He conducted the hospital's first market image audit and established a marketing department and long-range plan. Within two years, the hospital had revamped its market image—it is now considered *the* hospital for downtown Los Angeles—and established strong links with the center city business community. These links were critical in positioning the hospital's PPO initiatives. Want to see successful marketing? The hospital signed over one hundred contracts with insurers, employers, and managed care organizations. Lagasse was a change agent. Nursing embraced marketing and launched its own customer service program. Several of the hospital's new product line managers and marketing representatives are nurses. Lagasse left the medical center to found the Diabetes Institute, a franchised program based in Glendale, California, which is targeting the diabetes market niche. Its pilot program at Downey Community Hospital in Downey, California, has been highly successful. Now Lagasse has returned to hospital marketing at MedAmerica Health Systems in Dayton, Ohio, where he is developing innovative strategies to increase the market dominance of this regional medical system.

• *John J. Buckley, Jr.*, is an executive who likes big challenges—tertiary care medical centers. Jack recently moved to the Midwest from his position as CEO of the second-largest medical center in Arizona. St. Joseph's Hospital and Medical Center in Phoenix is an inspiration for venture-minded executives of large urban hospitals who are "trying to teach the elephant to dance." Always looking for new ideas, Jack has taken the hollow corporation concept from private industry and applied it to the health industry. In the hollow hospital concept, small hospitals contract out for administrative and clinical services. The concept provides a new strategy for multihospital affiliation, and St. Joseph's has been pursuing it aggressively. The result is a network of affiliations, management agreements, and new business relationships that developed St. Joseph's into a heavyweight competitor that can challenge Arizona's largest health system, Samaritan Health Services.

● *Fred L. Brown and Jack Buckley*, besides sharing an alma mater (George Washington University's Graduate Program in Health Administration), share something else. Both operate hospital-based McDonald's franchises. In his first year at Christian Hospitals Northeast/Northwest, in St. Louis, Missouri, Fred launched a swarm of entrepreneurial ventures. After renovating the northwest hospital, he installed a new drug and alcohol abuse program, a new inpatient and outpatient psychiatric care program, and a new ambulatory surgery center. A new imaging pavilion houses state-of-the-art imaging technology, including MRI. There is also a comprehensive sleeping disorders center and the first "labor spa" facility in the Midwest. CH Video Theater is the first full-service hospital movie channel in the United States. A new media campaign pulled community awareness ratings up ten points. Now this two-hospital system is extending its domain by leasing a satellite hospital in rural Missouri and managing another County hospital, which brings the number of managed facilities up to six.

CASE STUDIES IN MEDICAL ENTERPRISE

Examples of innovation and enterprise abound. Enterprising physicians and hospitals are reshaping the delivery of medicine with new ventures in many sectors of health care.

● *Health Stop* of Boston, Massachusetts, purchased 34 Chicago-area MedFirst urgent care centers from Humana, making it one of the largest convenience care chains in the country. Health Stop already operates 33 centers in the Boston area. The new owners of the MedFirst centers plan to joint venture or affiliate them with local hospitals and physicians, hoping to achieve the success that eluded Humana. The sale ends a six-year experiment by Humana in ambulatory care. Humana once planned to create a national network of convenience care centers that would serve as a referral network for its hospitals. Humana's HMO was to provide a wrap-around financing package for hospital and ambulatory services. Health Stop is planning a managed care market initiative and hopes to link the MedFirst centers to HMOs and PPOs. It plans to cut overhead costs and thereby reduce the break-even point from 45 visits per clinic per day to 30. Allowing physician investment may offset the physician loyalty factor. Humana's MedFirst physicians were hourly employees, not stakeholders. The hospital affiliations will bring credibility and local reputation. The convenience care market has been tough on entrepreneurs. Perhaps Health Stop has hit on a winning formula.

• *The Mayo Clinic* of Rochester, Minnesota, continues to cut a wide swath across markets in Florida and Arizona. This is the first rollout of a national brand name by a major medical center. Accelerating its national expansion program, the clinic has taken over the St. Luke's Health System in Jacksonville, Florida. St. Luke's operates a 289-bed hospital, several nonprofit corporations, and three for-profit enterprises, with total assets of $105 million. This was a friendly acquisition. No cash changed hands, but Mayo agreed to assume $61.4 million of St. Luke's long-term debt. The new ownership should reverse the hospital's flagging fortunes. St. Luke's lost nearly $1 million in 1986. Although Mayo had announced it would not build or buy a hospital for its Jacksonville clinic, the demand has exceeded Mayo's projections. Mayo physicians already account for 25–30 percent of St. Luke's occupied beds. There is speculation that Mayo may next acquire one or more hospitals in Scottsdale, where its second expansion clinic is located. Mayo has developed a close relationship with Scottsdale Memorial. With its Mayo affiliation, Scottsdale Memorial has high levels of occupancy, and it is already building a satellite facility for expansion.

• *Aging Resource Centers* are being marketed by Age Wave of Emeryville, California. The resource centers are franchises intended to give hospitals a competitive advantage in the eldercare market. The heart of each resource center is a comprehensive library of health education materials oriented to older consumers. Information and referral, which are part of the resource center concept, are intended to link together a constellation of hospital-sponsored programs targeted at the senior market. Full-time staff in the centers are supplemented by volunteers. Most hospitals have funded their resource center out of foundation or development funds. More than 50 of the franchises have been sold. Most centers are located outside the hospital in storefronts or shopping malls. One hospital's Aging Resource Center is developing, in a joint venture with a local bank, a medical credit card for its senior consumers. The resource center franchise guarantees market exclusivity to the sponsoring hospital. Age Wave supports a "users' alliance" of clients by sponsoring a newsletter and tuition-free users' conferences held biannually. Aging Resource Centers are helpful in creating consumer loyalty among the elderly clientele of hospitals. No hospital can ignore the elder market. Age Wave estimates that a third of all health expenditures today are on behalf of the elderly, and it predicts that half of all health care will be consumed by the senior population by the year 2000.

MARKETING NEW VENTURES

Marketing will infuse the most successful new programs and entrepreneurial ventures. Here are examples of innovative marketing strategies brought to bear in health care enterprise.

Bricks-and-mortar marketing uses facilities as a central focus of marketing new health care ventures. In Cottonwood Hospital, Utah, the new Center for Women's Health is a villagelike complex in brick. The $2.5 million center was designed by Kaplan McLoughlin Diaz of San Francisco. The dedication to the woman customer is evident in the homey surroundings and thoughtful details. Seven birthing suites are at the heart of a complex of related treatment programs oriented to the women's market. In each birthing suite, a modern Victorian bed doubles as a birthing table. Women are responding: The hospital's occupancy has soared 30 percent in two years.

The spirit of the Old West flavors a successful series of TV and print ads for convenience care centers operated by the Penrose Health System in Colorado Springs, Colorado, a two-hospital multi owned by the Sisters of Charity Health Care Systems. The marketing campaign features a country doctor making house calls in a horse and buggy at the turn of the century. The general mood, engendered by images showing the country doctor's personal touch, is one of nostalgia. The marketing campaign was created by Dan Hudson of the Healthcare Marketing Group of Denver, with design and production by the Shubin Design Group of San Francisco.

Medical videos may be a trendy way to promote new health care programs and products. With VCRs in more than half of America's households, video "informercials" are a new way of reaching consumers. David Watts, M.D., is the producer of award-winning videos such as "Pregnancy: A Time for Change" and "The Hospitalized Adolescent." His San Francisco-based communications firm, David Watts Productions, works with the Hospital Satellite Network and a variety of health care organizations. Since consumers view video programs on their own televisions, the programs communicate information and a subtle marketing message in a personal setting. Videos may provide a way for health care marketers to cut through the morass of 2,500 ad images every American is exposed to daily.

LOOKING FORWARD: EVERY DEAL MUST BE STRATEGIC

Welcome to the future of health care enterprise. These are changing times for doctors and hospitals across America. Rule number one in this new era: Be strategic. Physicians and hospitals will make deals across a wide array of new and innovative ventures. All parties need to analyze which investments make the best strategic sense and which maximize their individual objectives. Only win-win deals should be pursued. There will be more opportunities than time. Pick strategically.

Health care is being radically reshaped today by enterprise. In today's intensely competitive marketplace, new ventures are driving the shift from inpatient to ambulatory care. The home care industry is highly competitive and alive with entrepreneurism. Few corners of the health industry are untouched by the spirit of enterprise. In venturing, the perspective must always be strategic: Will this initiative or investment benefit the organization over the long term? If there is a lesson from strategic deal making, it is to anticipate the future and manage the opportunities tomorrow's health care market will bring.

STRATEGIC IMPLICATIONS FOR PHYSICIANS

1. *As medicine becomes increasingly regulated and prices for medical services fail to keep pace with inflation, physicians must diversify their practices.* This means new patients, new services, and new ways of satisfying existing patients. It will be difficult for solo practitioners to diversify their practices on their own. These doctors may use physician extenders (e.g., nurse practitioners) in order to see more patients or they may develop a specialized service that is in high demand. For a number of doctors, the best strategy may be to join group practices or physician networks in order to develop an adequate organizational base for growth and diversification.

2. *Physicians should learn from the mistakes hospitals have made.* In their rush to diversify in the mid-1980s, hospitals made all the classic blunders: They had inadequate knowledge of the market, they were undercapitalized, and they relied on inexperienced management. Physicians should be mindful to avoid these common pitfalls as they start new ventures. Having a business plan, an experienced management team, double the amount of capital estimated, and market research data can greatly improve the chances of success.

3. *The most successful physicians of tomorrow will be those who have found a clinical niche with high patient demand.* The focus may be on a particular class of patients, (e.g., diabetics, arthritics) or on a type of procedure (e.g., lithotripsy). Although the Harvard RVS study will reduce fees for medical procedures, the growing number of elderly and chronically ill patients will drive demand for many procedures up in the next five to ten years. Doctors will provide two or more services other than average patient visits of the 1990s, including professional consultations, diagnostic tests, prescriptions, or therapeutic procedures. Doctors may even sell books, video tapes, and health education materials to their patients.

STRATEGIC IMPLICATIONS FOR HOSPITALS

1. *Hospitals should seek fewer but better deals.* Hospitals have slowed their heady rush into diversification. Today's ventures are better targeted and

capitalized. Market research, well-developed business plans, and tough-minded managers who know the territory will improve a hospital's ratio of successful to unsuccessful new programs and services.

2. *Deal making should strengthen the medical staff.* Hospital enterprise should have the twin goals of broadening the hospital's product portfolio with new revenues and enhancing the economic well-being of its medical staff. Of the two, strengthening medical staff loyalty may be the more important for the hospital's long-range future.

3. *Each hospital needs to identify and bond those key members of the medical staff who are essential to its strategic future.* It should use diversification and new ventures to enhance the clinical practices of these members and also build new programs and services around physician strengths.

BIBLIOGRAPHY

Coile, Russell C. Jr. 1987. "Second Wave of Entrepreneurship." *Hospital Entrepreneurs' Newsletter* (October): 1–8.

Foster, Richard. 1986. *Innovation: The Attacker's Advantage*. New York: Doubleday.

Johnson, Kathryn E., and Judith D. Berger, "The Entrepreneurial Spirit." *Future Perspectives*. Washington, D.C.: Foundation of the American Society of Association Executives, 133–147.

Ohmae, Kenichi. 1982. *The Mind of the Strategist*. New York: McGraw-Hill.

Porter, Michael. 1980. *Competitive Strategy*, New York: The Free Press.

———. 1985. *Competitive Advantage*. New York: The Free Press.

Chapter 18

Marketing Innovations

Innovation is the specific tool of entrepreneurs, the means by which they exploit change as an opportunity for a different business or a different service.
—Peter Drucker, *Innovation and Entrepreneurship*

In every industry, the market leaders are those who gain and hold the innovation advantage. Peter Drucker's *Innovation and Entrepreneurship* clearly establishes the *innovation imperative* as one of the driving forces in American enterprise. Innovation affects every product and service. In the product-life cycle, there are three types of innovation:

1. product innovation (creating the "better mousetrap")
2. service innovation (providing new ways of satisfying customer expectations)
3. marketing innovation (persuading potential customers of the value and benefits of the product)

Of these, successful marketing innovation may be the most difficult. Marketing is the vital link between product and consumer. In the health industry, marketing is the last major management technique to be applied from the private sector. Marketing's arrival in the medical offices of America and the executive suites of U.S. hospitals has not been without controversy. Health care marketing is encountering considerable skepticism—and just when the health industry is entering the most competitive era in its history.

DOES "MARKETING" FIT HEALTH CARE?

Marketing has drawn considerable heat in recent years from the health industry press and among health care administrators. Is the marketing concept appropriate to health care? (Super 1987). When a midwestern hospital closed its marketing department (saving $1.6 million), it sent a shockwave through the industry. Yet is marketing just another management hula hoop? In a recent poll for the *Healthcare Forum* (Coile and Grossman 1988), a national panel split (46.0 percent yes, 46.7 percent no) on the question, Is health care marketing a fad? The survival of health care marketing may rest more on marketing effectiveness than appropriateness. In many ways, the health industry and its marketing and advertising firms are just moving up the learning curve. Health care marketing is still in its infancy.

Among health care organizations, product and service innovation is very common. *Marketing* is the black box of health care competition. In the past five years, health care has discovered the world of marketing and invested heavily. Consumers are exposed to 2,500 commercials and advertisements each day. Health care joined the marketing fray. Virtually every familiar marketing strategy was applied—coupons, testimonials, image management, even celebrity endorsements. All media were utilized. Health care marketing and advertising doubled in 1986, and *Healthcare Forum's* expert panel predicted in late 1987 that the spending trend would continue to surge until 1990. Health care has become a major user of advertising media since the mid 1980s, despite qualms about advertising's appropriateness and cost (Droste 1988).

Not all health care executives share the panel's enthusiasm for marketing. Their concern became front-page news. *Hospitals* ran a cover story called "Time Out for Marketing"; *Modern Healthcare*'s cover read "Marketing, Take 2" (Super 1987). Too many hospitals invested heavily in marketing and advertising with too little research. Advertising agencies had to learn the health care business, usually from their clients. It was the classic story of the consultant's "borrowing the client's watch to tell the time."

MARKETING AN INTANGIBLE PRODUCT: HEALTH

In one of the *Harvard Business Review*'s best-read articles of all times, marketing guru Theodore Levitt tackled the real issue head on. The article, "Marketing Intangible Products and Products Intangible," posed the question health care marketers wrestle with daily: Is the marketing of "services" different from the marketing of "goods"? Levitt's answer was equivocal: The principles are the same but the outcomes differ profoundly.

Tangible products like automobiles, liquor, or clothing can be seen, touched, smelled, tasted, and tested. Intangible services like health care must be sold on promises of satisfaction. As an intangible product, health must be marketed symbolically, using analogies, metaphors, and surrogates to help customers anticipate before actual treatment how their needs would be satisfied.

Impressions are important in marketing intangible products, since customers can only imagine the ultimate outcome—return to health and positive well-being. Health care is not the only intangible product. Think of investment banking, auto repair, or travel. The less tangible the generic product, the more powerfully and persistently the judgment about it is shaped by packaging, and by metaphors, similes, symbols, and other surrogates for reality. How the promise is packaged becomes, in the mind of the customer, the essence of the intangible product or service.

Health care marketing, then, is not inappropriate, just very difficult! It requires intelligence and innovation and presents a challenge to every health care organization. At this early point, there are few successful marketing models for hospitals and health systems. One of the important goals of the fledgling field of health care marketing is to share the lessons of the innovators who are adapting marketing to the health industry.

HEALTH CARE MARKETING INNOVATIONS: THE NATION'S BEST

To inspire health care organizations, the Chicago-based Academy of Health Services Marketing conducts an annual competition for marketing innovations. The academy is a component organization of the American Marketing Association, which has 3,300 members representing thousands of hospitals and health-related organizations.

The 1988 competition was the academy's third annual search for the best and brightest in healthcare marketing. This year 13 health organizations competed for the national awards. Applicants were judged on the following:

1. *Overview.* The opportunity is well defined, the objectives are clearly stated, and the statement of results (benefits) is consistent with the entire outline.
2. *Situation Audit.* The planning and implementation of the program is shaped by the available research, audience attitudes and patterns, competitive forces, and financial issues.
3. *Objectives.* The program objectives are measurable, timely, and matched to the expected results.
4. *Execution.* The methods and processes for producing the marketing vehicle and conducting the program are appropriate, creative skills and ideas are reflected in the marketing vehicle, and the execution of the program is economical and effective.
5. *Results.* The evaluation of results focuses on whether the stated objectives have been met, and mechanisms for evaluation are built into the program.

6. *Excellence Factor*. The overall achievements or contribution to the practice of marketing in the field of health care are of a high level.

Gold Prize Winner: The Baptist Brigade

The Oklahoma Healthcare Corporation, whose flagship Baptist Medical Center is a 577-bed acute care hospital in Oklahoma City, was the gold prize winner for its Brigade program (Coile 1988). The concept of an employee "brigade" was inspired by Dupont's "Antron Army" campaign. Dupont recruited hundreds of employee volunteers to promote the company's special consumer credit program that was designed to increase sales of Dupont's new Antron nylon carpeting. Using the same idea, the Oklahoma Healthcare Corporation created an opportunity for all employees to volunteer as "marketers" of its "commitment to care" philosophy. The Brigade's first task was door-to-door promotion of the system's new Baptist Care Center, a primary care center in northwest Oklahoma City.

The organization hoped for 300 employee volunteers; more than 400 staffers came forward. The Brigade kicked off the campaign with a complimentary breakfast. There was plenty of hoopla at the rally held prior to the canvassing. Teams competed for a traveling trophy by performing an array of spirit cheers. A high school band played as 350 helium balloons filled the sky. Four teams canvassed a total of 3,325 households in neighborhoods surrounding the care center. Team spirit was boosted by a competition involving coupons that could be surrendered at the care center for free first-aid kits. The team with the highest percentage of redeemed coupons was eligible for a Hawaiian vacation.

Did it work? Yes! And it's still working. For openers, the system attained high-level visibility in local newspapers and TV. In the first week, more than 50 coupons were redeemed at the neighborhood care center, and visits jumped 5 percent. A second Brigade campaign knocked on 3,008 doors in neighborhoods surrounding the second care center in nearby Yukon, Oklahoma. This time 100 coupons were brought in for first-aid kits, and visits soared 72 percent over the next two weeks. Today, the Brigade has become a fixture at the Oklahoma Healthcare Corporation, and it staffs hospital exhibits, fun runs, and community services and publicizes new hospital programs.

Silver Prize Winner: Market Share Modeling

Rex Weston of Market Share Modeling, in Madison, Wisconsin, took the silver award in the academy's competition. His market share–modeling software package is a classic "better mousetrap" in a field dominated by national firms.

Weston's innovation was to create a microcomputer-based software package for market share analysis priced well below $5,000—and an astonishing 300 percent below the price of the nearest competitor.

The software runs off data from the 1986 National Hospital Discharge Study, which is based on a national sample of 418 hospitals and 193,000 discharges. The model yields a regional estimate of hospital market share by DRG. Several dozen packages have been sold to hospitals and marketing consultants.

Is it "user friendly?" Of course, since it was designed by a user dissatisfied with existing market alternatives. Market Share Modeling is just bringing to market a new ambulatory care module to complement the inpatient market analyzer. The ambulatory care package uses data from the 1986 National Health Interview Study and is universally applicable in estimating demand for ambulatory services.

Market Share Modeling follows in a rich tradition of marketing innovation. Look at the success of "better idea" companies that vaulted into the Fortune 500 and the INC 100 based on marketing innovation, companies like Compaq, Federal Express, and Chemlawn. All created niches, often in the face of sizeable competitors. Compaq outthought IBM in developing the first portable microcomputer. Federal Express outhustled UPS in introducing guaranteed overnight delivery. Chemlawn beat Scotts and Ortho to American lawns with home delivery. In every case, the initial competitive advantage came from marketing innovation.

Bronze Prize Winner: Endresen Research

The academy's bronze award went to a state-of-the-art contribution to health care marketing: a psychodemographic segmentation system, designed by Endresen Research of Seattle, Washington. This was not Karen Endresen's first time in the academy's winner's circle: Her technique for analyzing patient satisfaction won top prize in 1987 from the academy.

Endresen Research developed a typology of generic health styles as a way of translating broadbased demographic data into target segments for health care marketing. (The typology is called *HealthStyles*). Other consumer market research typologies exist, but none are specially oriented to health care. Using the HealthStyles matrix, the system assesses the potential utilization of proposed health services and products. The goal is to efficiently guide advertising and marketing to be most effective in reaching each target segment.

The benefits of the psychodemographic segmentation system are (1) that it identifies the segments by health style within the hospital's market area, (2) that it reduces product development expenses by more accurately predicting potential product use, and (3) that it maximizes the effectiveness of marketing and advertising investments by allowing marketing efforts to be tailored specifically to each market segment.

To date, three distinct systems have been created by Endresen Research using the HealthStyles methodology. The original system was based on a random sample of community residents over age 18. SeniorStyles and MaternityStyles were developed to meet the needs of specific demographic markets. HealthStyles segments are named "Avid Partners," "Fix-Me's," "Loyal Patients," and "No Timers." SeniorStyles segments are named "Healthy Traditionalists," "Active Independents," "Major Health Care Users," and "Uninvolved Nonconsumers." MaternityStyles segments are named "Young Starting Families," "Older Established Professionals," "Working Mothers," and "Passive Housewives."

The HealthStyles system is based on a factor analysis that revealed six primary factors which differentiated the four segments. The six factors are these:

1. *Quality*. High scores in this area indicate a strong desire to seek out high quality health care, even if it is more expensive and time consuming.
2. *Fitness*. This factor is linked to a strong personal concern for exercise, nutrition, and health maintenance.
3. *Loyalty*. Consumers with high loyalty scores have a strong inclination to trust physicians and stay with the same doctor.
4. *Involvement*. Some consumers express a strong desire to be personally involved in making their own health care decisions, including choice of specialists.
5. *Stress*. High scores here demonstrate consumers perceive themselves as living stressful lives.
6. *Self-Diagnosis*. Consumers with high scores have a strong tendency to diagnose their own illness before (or instead of) seeing a physician.

The HealthStyles system was pioneered at the Virginia Mason Medical Center in Seattle and has been applied in hospitals in Ohio and Texas and on the West Coast. The system brings modern market research from Madison Avenue and translates it into health care–specific segmented marketing applications.

MARKETING AN INTANGIBLE PRODUCT: QUALITY HEALTH CARE

"The purpose of a business is to get and keep customers," a piece of advice from Peter Drucker (1985), to which Ted Levitt (1983) adds, "Customers don't buy things, they buy *solutions to problems*" (emphasis added).

Of course, there is more to it than that. Which is exactly the lesson of Levitt's *The Marketing Imagination*, widely recognized as a classic management work on the essence of this black box called marketing. The business that intuits what customers need to solve their problems will have a competitive advantage. Levitt believes that the ''imagination that figures out what that is, imaginatively figures out what should be done and does it with imagination,'' will thrive (Levitt 1983).

The seven essays in Levitt's short book may be the most stimulating ever written about the mercurial concept of marketing. Below is a synopsis of his principles of innovative marketing.

1. *The CEO's Role.* A prime tenet of Levitt's marketing philosophy is that the CEO is the chief marketer of the organization and that every aspect of the business must contribute to the marketing effort.

2. *Global Markets.* Levitt asserts that the national corporation is obsolete. The future will belong to the corporations that can shift to a *global* perspective, recognizing that regional and national markets are just niches for the global enterprise. Certainly no ''local'' enterprise is safe anymore.

3. *Industrialization of Service.* This principle has special meaning for health care executives. The large, rationally managed service corporation is the new colossus that will affect the entire marketplace. No service sector— law, repair, brokerage, maintenance, or banking—will be safe from the market power of service companies organized on the industrial model.

4. *Differentiation.* In a competitive marketplace, differentiation is everything. Levitt believes that differentiation is the essence of competition. No matter what is to be marketed, from cement to cereal, the secret to gaining market share is differentiation from competing products. And it is relatively easy, Levitt suggests. In health care, the factors that consumers use to discriminate among providers include reputation, medical staff, high-tech equipment, nursing staff attitude, parking, and signage.

5. *Intangible Products and Product Intangibles.* Levitt's concept of ''intangibles,'' goes to the heart of the mystery about how to market health care. The fact is that ''service'' is a central part of even the most durable of tangible products (e.g., Caterpillar earthmovers). All products have tangible and intangible aspects whose images can be manipulated for marketing success.

6. *Relationship Management.* Don't call it sales but ''relationship management.'' This suggestion is based on Levitt's belief that each customer should be reconceptualized as a business asset. ''The customer asset has to be managed lest the equity you have in that account be dissipated,'' Levitt warns. Otherwise, the customer will ask, ''What have you done for me lately?'' This is particularly true as more of the world's work is done through long-term contracts or via supplier-customer links that stretch over years. Does this sound like ''managed care'' to the health executive?

7. *Marketing Imagination*. Dealing with so many illusions and intangibles is a creative task. That is the essence of marketing, illustrated by the private sector experiences of companies like American Express, Dupont, Apple, and the Dreyfus Fund. Each firm became a leader in its market niche by feats of marketing imagination. Take Apple, now a $400 million company but still described by its CEO as "the longest running venture company in the Fortune 500." Apple's success in invading the business market was due to its desktop publishing product, the most imaginative in the field. Apple's intangibles appeal to creative types and also bring out the creativity of average computer users with devices such as the hand-held "mouse" control device.

MEDICAL MERCHANDISING

Advertising is still considered unprofessional by many physicians, but 25 percent of medical groups reported they were advertising professional services. Medicine and health care are overcoming barriers to effective marketing and advertising. Health care is still moving up the learning curve when it comes to effective marketing.

Another euphemism for medical merchandising is "practice enhancement." Wayman Spence is launching *Practice Builders for Physicians' Offices*, a newsletter for doctors that is distributed by hospitals to their medical staff. Spence is the archetypal innovative marketer. A specialist in physical medicine, he sold his company Spenco Medical Products to Kimberly-Clark in 1984 for $27 million. In 1987 he launched a national chain of HealthFair stores retailing health care products. The stores are sold as franchises to hospitals, which cross-market hospital services through the stores' shopping mall locations.

Here are some successful examples of medical merchandising that suggest directions innovative medical marketing will take tomorrow.

- *Physician Office Concierge*. Why not? Just as a first class hotel always has a concierge who serves as a focal point for consumers, every busy doctor's office or group practice waiting room should have a patient relations person. A group of three family practitioners hired and trained a customer specialist. Her $18,000 annual salary was more than offset by the additional $36,000 in business attracted in the first six months of her employment.

- *Consumer Advertising*. America's consumers think doctors should advertise, even if doctors disagree. In a survey reported in *American Medical News* (Voelker 1988), a survey of doctors found that 86 percent do not have marketing plans to attract new patients or improve relations with existing patients. From the same news study a related survey of 100 consumers reported that 62 percent of younger consumers (under age 40) approved of physician advertising, as did 47 percent of all consumers regardless of age. Practice management consultant Keith Borglum of Professional Marketing and Management in Santa Rosa, California, recommends spending 3–5 percent of the medical practice budget for marketing just to maintain a stable base of patients; to expand the practice, 5–7 percent of the budget should be spent. To enter new markets, physicians will need to invest 7–10 percent of the budget in marketing (e.g., newspaper advertisements, radio spots, and publicity for special programs) (Borgland 1988).

- *"Let Your Fingers Do the Walking."* To see the rising level of physician advertising, look in the local Yellow Pages. Physicians are using the telephone book to publicize their services in ways many doctors consider appropriate. A growing number of physician practices are using "red ink" ads for extra visibility.
- *Medical Boutiques.* Physicians are focusing on medical niches to market their services, advertising state-of-the-art care for patients with bulimia, back problems, sleeping disorders, and stress. Some doctors are doing business as a "center" or "institute," that is, specializing in the care of particular diseases or types of patients, such as women, adolescents, or those with chronic pain.

CONTROVERSY SWIRLS OVER HEALTH CARE ADVERTISING

The battle for patients in the 1990s may be fought in the living rooms and on the television sets of America's consumers. In a 1988 article in the *Wall Street Journal*, "Drug and Alcohol Clinics Vie for Patients," there were numerous descriptions of expensive TV ad campaigns designed to fill beds in hospitals specializing in treating alcohol and drug abuse. The trend was begun by for-profit hospital chains but has spread to nonprofit hospitals and private clinics.

The number of alcohol and drug abuse programs has increased from 5,700 to 6,500 in the past six years. Critics complain that the growth is advertising induced. Some facilities, like the Betty Ford Center in Rancho Mirage, California, don't have to advertise, but most programs do, and the commercials are becoming more sensationalistic. A TV commercial for Beth Israel's Stuyvesant Square program in New York showed a young woman digging through a trash can to find a pill bottle. Comprehensive Care, one of the first companies to advertise, has run a commercial that opens with a shot of blue sky, followed by clumps of dirt falling on the camera lens. The perspective was that of an alcoholic lying at the bottom of a grave. Such scare tactics may be offensive but they are also effective.

This is a competitive marketplace. As many as 250 alcohol and drug abuse programs are competing for patients in southern California. Comprehensive Care, the largest advertiser in the field, spent $5.8 million on TV ads in the first half of 1988, 65 percent above the same period a year before. Celebrities like Patty Duke are making commercials for Psychiatric Institutes of America, a subsidiary of NME. Olympic gymnast Kathy Rigby has made commercials for an eating disorders program; olympic skater Elizabeth Manley has been filmed endorsing adolescent mental health programs. Celebrity endorsements are commonplace for most products. Medical care is not soap, but health services are clearly joining the shelf of consumer products that use widespread commercial marketing.

MANY INDUSTRIES ARE UNCOMFORTABLE WITH MARKETING

Health care is not the only industry to be discomfited by marketing. Everywhere, Levitt finds marketing under fire for its pushy, intrusive, and manipulative intrusions: "Nothing characterizes the successful conversion in the past two decades of so many companies to the practice of marketing concept than the rising criticism that they practice a baleful opposite." Is marketing a victim of its own success? Or is this the natural result of competing producers responding to the wants and wishes of the many segments of the consuming public? As Levitt observes, the fact is that "few of us actually need all of what we have." Or want all we might need (Levitt 1983, p. 145).

Levitt responds with the marketing counterpart of Adam Smith's "invisible hand" economic theory:

> When the marketing concept operates at full throttle, it generates products, services and communications that target the specifically discovered needs and wants of specific narrow best-fit customer segments. Each segment therefore has a better chance of getting what it really wants or needs, than in the bad old days when Henry Ford told people they could have any color model T they wanted so long as it was black (Levitt 1983, p. 142).

Health care marketing will get no better defense.

LOOKING FORWARD: FOSTERING INNOVATION

Who is an innovator? Are innovators born or trained? Can a hospital that seeks to raise its "IQ" (innovation quotient) identify these gifted individuals and provide the supporting environments in which new ideas flourish? What works—and what doesn't—in fostering innovation?

These are universal questions, and there is good news and bad news. First, the downside. There are not many "models" and the process of innovation seems highly person-dependent. When John Ketteringham and Ranganath Nayak of Arthur D. Little, Inc. began work on their book *Breakthroughs*, they searched for model innovative organizations and individuals. Sifting through hundreds of commercial breakthroughs of all types, the analysts were hard pressed to define *the* characteristics of innovative companies or those responsible for the breakthroughs.

Here is the brighter side. Innovation does not have to wait for the happy coincidence of genius and opportunity. Ketteringham and Nayak found that innovation in practice was more often a *team* process involving three types of people: innovators, inventors, and facilitators. Successful breakthroughs required input from all three types and often involved dozens or even hundreds of people to successfully transform a new idea into market reality.

The message for managers, marketers, and health care executives is that innovation can happen anywhere it is supported (and if necessary, even where it is opposed). Innovation is a cascading process that begins with an idea. The idea which is then nudged and prodded forward through the levels of organization, a process that may involve many "champions" of the idea at all levels. Most of all, innovation is driven by people. As Ketteringham and Nayak state, "Invariably, in a breakthrough, long before management has any idea of what's happening 'down there,' people start changing the system. They do it by themselves and they do it according to their own very specific vision" (1986, Introduction).

Good ideas are where innovations start, but they only become reality if there are people who are driven to see the ideas bear fruit. Marketing in health care has arrived; it will have an increasingly powerful influence on the future of medicine and health services in the 1990s. The appropriate employment of marketing and advertising in health care will be a challenge. But marketing is where forward-thinking physicians and health care executives will change the future of health care—one marketing innovation at a time.

STRATEGIC IMPLICATIONS FOR PHYSICIANS

1. *Every physician and medical group should have a practice marketing plan.*
   The plan should identify target markets of new and existing patients and specify strategies for communicating with them. Marketing goals should be clear and specific and progress should be tracked quarterly or annually. If the survey findings that only 14 percent of U.S. doctors have a marketing

plan are true, the other 86 percent need to get started before their patient base and market share erode.

2. *Physicians must select appropriate marketing tactics.* Tomorrow's question for medical marketing is not whether, but how. Marketing physician services is inevitable. The range of marketing approaches is very broad, from Christmas cards to direct mail and TV. Physicians should selectively utilize the techniques of marketing that are appropriate to their specialty, patients, and marketplace.

3. *Physicians need to understand the difference between marketing and advertising.* Physicians should avoid the mistake hospitals made when they embraced marketing. Don't confuse advertising with marketing. Advertising is just one of dozens of ways to effectively reach out to patients and potential customers. Marketing is a mindset as well as a portfolio of methods.

STRATEGIC IMPLICATIONS FOR HOSPITALS

1. *Hospitals are learning that the most effective way to bond physicians is to help enhance their practices.* This can be done through patient channeling programs (e.g., physician referral services), shared advertising that mentions the doctor's practice location, and physician directories mailed to local consumers.

2. *A growing number of hospitals are "detailing" their medical staff with a professional sales force.* The medical staff salespeople inform physicians of current hospital programs and new equipment and facilities. They also help solve any problems the physicians are experiencing with the hospital. Hospital sales people can also recruit new medical staff members from outlying areas and other hospitals in order to build up staff in needed specialties.

3. *Medical marketing committees can be useful in facilitating marketing efforts.* The appropriateness of hospital marketing and advertising can be a volatile issue. Some hospitals have formed a joint committee with the medical staff to review marketing and advertising. This anticipatory approach can do much to mitigate medical staff concerns about hospital advertising and marketing campaigns.

BIBLIOGRAPHY

Borgland, Keith. 1988. "How Much Should You Budget For Marketing Your Practice." *Practice Marketing and Management*, 6:5–6.

Coile, Russell C., Jr. 1988. "Marketing Innovations." *Hospital Entrepreneurs' Newsletter* (April).

Coile, Russell C., Jr., and Randolph M. Grossman. 1988. "Consumers Choice." *Healthcare Forum Journal* (March–April): 52–54.

Droste, Therese. 1988. "Ad Budgets Slow in the New Age of Accountability." *Hospitals*, 20 December, 32.

Drucker, Peter. 1985. *Innovation and Entrepreneurship*. New York: Harper and Row.

Jenks, Lyn. 1989. "Physician Bonding: A Key Marketing Component." *Health Care Marketing Report* (December): 20.

Jenson, Joyce. 1988. "Physician Liaison Programs—What's Working." *Healthcare Executive* (September–October): 39.

Ketteringham, John, and Ranganath Nayak. 1986. *Breakthroughs*. New York: Rawson Associates.

Levitt, Theodore. 1983. *The Marketing Imagination*. New York: The Free Press.

Perry, Linda. 1988. "Lack of Follow-Up Can Cost Hospitals Billions." *Modern Healthcare*, 14 November, 38.

Robertson, Marie. 1989. "Back to Basics Marks Competitive Approach in 1989." *Health Care Competition Week*, 2 January, 3–4.

Super, Kari, and Robert Muzzon. 1987. "Marketing: Take Two." *Modern Healthcare*, 10 April, 46–55.

———. 1987. "Services Should Be Linked to Practices' Life-Cycles." *Modern Healthcare*, 10 April, 57–58.

Voelker, Rebecca. 1988. "MDs Need More Marketing. MD-Consumer Survey." American Medical News 31 (21 October 1988): 13, 16.

Chapter 19

Outcomes Management

In medicine, we already have a consensus that our unifying goal is the good of the patient. To support this philosophy, I propose that we adopt a technology for collaborative action. Since one of my proclivities is giving old ideas new labels, let's label this technology "outcomes management."
                    —Paul M. Ellwood, *"Outcomes Management"*

Health care's next hot button is outcomes management. Physicians are relieved to learn that the pendulum is swinging back to quality. All of health care's major players are placing quality at the top of their priorities, each for different reasons:

- For hospitals, quality is the goal of patient care and a competitive advantage that will differentiate them in a high-competition market.
- For physicians, quality is the goal of medical practice and the standard by which they will be measured by peers, patients, regulators, and malpractice attorneys.
- For major employers and insurance companies, quality is the primary criterion for selecting doctors and hospitals when price is not a factor.
- For government regulators, quality is the means of protecting the public welfare and responding to voter blocks.

OUTCOMES MANAGEMENT: THE ELLWOOD CONCEPT

Paul Ellwood's Shattuck Lecture to the Massachusetts Medical Society in May 1988 presented the idea of managing quality with a new technology Ellwood called "outcomes management" (Ellwood 1988). If Ellwood's concept catches on, it could change the way health care is provided and purchased. The goal of outcomes management is to help patients, payers, and providers make rational choices regarding medical care based on information about the effect of these choices on patients' health problems. The concept is simple but making it operational is not.

For outcomes management to work, Ellwood recommends the establishment of a national data base that contains information about and analysis of clinical, financial, and health outcomes for specific diseases and diagnoses. Two other components must be put in place: (1) standards that accurately reflect the relationship between medical interventions and desired outcomes and (2) widespread access to the data base for decision makers.

Operationalizing outcomes management is possible. It would draw on four technologies already well developed: (1) standards and guidelines that physicians can use in selecting appropriate medical interventions; (2) systematic measurement of the functioning and well-being of patients in order to track their clinical outcomes on a disease-specific basis; (3) a data base, ideally a national one, containing clinical and outcome information; and (4) analysis and dissemination of findings to decision makers.

QUALITY—THE ELUSIVE INTANGIBLE

Quality is a slippery concept. In *Zen and the Art of Motorcycle Maintenance*, the author muses, "Quality . . . you know what it is, yet you don't know what it is. But that's self-contradictory. But some things *are* better than others, that is, they have more quality. But when you try to say what quality is, apart from the things that have it, it all goes *poof*! There's nothing to talk about. But if you can't say what quality is, how do you know what is or how do you know it even exists?" (Pirsig 1974, p.342).

Dr. Philip Caper (1988), former staffer on the Senate Labor and Public Welfare Subcommittee on Health, suggests that quality has three components. *Efficacy* is the measure of the diagnostic or therapeutic procedure's ability to accomplish its purpose. *Appropriateness* is the degree of utility in the particular circumstances—the state of the patient, the disease, and the costs and benefits of alternatives. *Caring*, the third component, encompasses the interpersonal, supportive, and psychological aspects of the physician-patient relationship.

Quality is a word that implies preference. Dr. Grant Steffen (1988), writing in *JAMA*, suggests that quality be defined as the capacity of an object to achieve a goal. Dr. William Anderson, trustee of the American Osteopathic Association, observes that while professionals continue to argue about it, everyone else has their own definition of quality: "Employers define quality in terms of value obtained for their health care dollars. For the patients, quality means feeling better. To hospitals, quality is achieved when the patient goes home before he exceeds the DRG limit " (Caper 1988).

Credit goes to Avis Donabedian, M.D., author of two books on quality care, for defining quality in the context of medical care. Donabedian (1982) analyzed the literature on quality in terms of structure (organization), process (procedures), and outcomes (benefits and harms). Advocates of outcome measurement believe that if the goal is to assess medical care, nothing could matter more than the ultimate net benefit. Most of the history of quality assurance in America has focused on aspects of structure and process. The pendulum is now swinging toward outcomes.

BUYERS WILL CHOOSE ON QUALITY, NOT PRICE

Many health care providers and insurance companies say the current focus on quality is just rhetoric. Price is the key factor behind health care purchase decisions and will be for years to come. Not so, says Don Arnwine (1987), until recently the chairman of VHA, in a "viewpoint" article for *Modern Healthcare*. To understand the role of quality in the future of health care, VHA interviewed more than 50 experts and surveyed consumers, employers, and physicians through its Market Monitor project. The VHA research highlighted these factors as converging to push quality to the top of all priorities:

- reduced demand for inpatient care, which causes financial strain for hospitals and restricts the resources available to delivery quality
- a shift to outpatient settings, where care is not monitored as closely
- growth in alternative delivery systems, with financial incentives for participation in those systems
- employer and government initiatives to hold down health care costs

Consumers Are Willing To Pay More for Quality

Buyers accept having to pay more for health services from providers they believe are of the highest quality. The VHA research shows that 40 percent of consumers are willing to pay extra for quality. A similiar 42.1 percent of health executives surveyed for *Healthcare Forum* predicted that business and insurance would be willing to pay more for higher quality.

The public has a keen interest in quality rankings. Quality surfaced as a major consumer issue in 1981, when a group affiliated with Ralph Nader published a hospital-specific study of mortality rates in Maryland for the ten most common surgical procedures. Lawsuits by consumer organizations brought under the Freedom of Information Act forced HCFA to release similiar data from Medicare cost reports. Journalists tended to sensationalize data from the first HFCA mortality rankings in 1986, as they had when the Maryland Cost Review Commission released quality data. Confronted regularly with such information, news coverage is becoming less extensive and more straightforward as journalists become more sophisticated in their understanding of how to interpret the crude HCFA data.

Major Employers and Insurers Screen for Quality

Major employers are working with their insurance carriers and third party administrators to develop "quality specifications" for purchasing health care. These criteria include patient satisfaction, health outcomes, hospital and physician credentials, and state-of-the-art facilities.

Expert consultants are devising review criteria to identify patterns of substandard quality in physician or hospital outcomes. Employers and insurers will periodically screen their data looking for quality problems and poor provider performance. Becoming a preferred provider in tomorrow's health care marketplace will depend on a combination of factors: cost, consumer satisfaction, and quality outcomes.

Suzanne Mercure of Honeywell Bull, in an interview in the January 6, 1989, issue of *Managed Care Outlook*, stated, "The coming year will see an increased emphasis on managed care programs overall, with a specific movement towards more active selection on the part of employers. They'll be looking more carefully at their options for developing their own plans or choosing one in the market. And they'll have tougher criteria for selection." Josephine Kaple of Corporate Cost Management in Gaithersburg, Maryland, added, "While efficiency measurement tools have been refined, quality assessment tools are now desired by purchasers and payers, as well as by hospitals. 1989 will see the development of provider assessment tools with a 'value' orientation—including efficiency and quality—and more aggressive use of those tools in implementing managed care strategies."

Government Targets Provider Quality

Media attention is a high-visibility weapon in government efforts to advance quality of care. HCFA has twice released rankings of hospitals based on institutional mortality rates. The 1988 release included separate mortality rate rankings for heart disease, stroke, lung disease, and orthopedic problems, which account for about 35 percent of all deaths nationwide. Hospitals roundly criticized HCFA in 1986 for releasing the mortality data without allowing a prior opportunity to review the findings.

As part of its drive toward quality assurance, the Department of Health and Human Services will establish a national "incompetents" data bank containing information on physicians and dentists who are sued for malpractice or disciplined by state licensure boards. A five-year, $15.9 million contract has been let to Unisys Corporation to establish the data bank. The data bank, which will not be accessible to the public, will be open by 1990. The program was authorized by Congress in 1986 to catch health professionals who try to hide their problems by moving from hospital to hospital or state to state. The system will be used as a screening tool by state licensing officials, hospitals, and others who hire health professionals. Federal officials plan to expand the data bank in the future to include disciplinary actions against nurses.

States Take Lead in Regulating Quality

The Maryland Cost Review Commission has been releasing quality data to the public since 1984. In response, the Maryland Hospital Association established a special Council for Quality Healthcare. The council has been sending diagnosis-specific and institution-specific mortality rate data to hospital executives and trustees. With the data, the council supplied a list of questions to ask the medical staff in order to strengthen quality assurance programs. The council has been developing a set of quality indicators, including

- hospital-acquired infection rates
- surgical wound rates
- autopsy rates
- newborn infant mortality
- Cesarean section rates
- unscheduled returns to intensive care
- unscheduled returns to the operating room

OUTCOMES MANAGEMENT: THE NEW HEALTH CARE TECHNOLOGY

No one in government or corporate America really knows what will be the result of the dramatic changes sweeping the U.S. health industry today and whether these changes will make Americans healthier or sicker. Nor do physicians really know. In spite of their education, state-of-the-art technology, access to miracle drugs, and the highest incomes in society, doctors often do not know for certain which treatment works best for a particular illness.

THREE QUESTIONS BUT ONE ANSWER: OUTCOMES MANAGEMENT

Three questions neatly frame the challenge before us. First, how do we improve our ability to make better and more cost-effective choices about health care options? Second, how do we collect and analyze the data necessary for validating our choices? And finally, how do we consolidate and share this information so that everyone in the health care system can benefit?

Dr. Paul Ellwood (1988) has advanced a system called "outcomes management," which would be based on a permanent and constantly updated computerized data base. This national data base would contain detailed information on the medical experiences of patients and the clinical and quality of life "outcomes" of the treatments they received. It would also contain and correlate information on provider practice patterns and treatment costs. This data would be digested by high-speed computers to provide on-line feedback to a variety of users and give physicians the opportunity to take advantage of the experience of others and to enhance their own knowledge.

BETTER-INFORMED CHOICES

The outcomes management system would be buyer-driven. Providers, payers, and patients would contribute information to the data bank and share access. This would result in better-informed choices about the medical quality of life and the economic value of medical interventions.

Although there exists nothing on the scale of outcomes management now, many medical and governmental organizations are collecting some of the needed data. Data bases already exist for tracking results regarding cancer, head injuries, heart disease, arthritis, and other conditions. Local providers may become voluntary (or mandated) contributors to a national outcomes data base. Records located in hospitals, clinics, and medical offices could be collected, coded, and filed on a statewide, regional, or national basis. Universal record forms in hospital and ambulatory care are bringing the advent of such a national health care data base nearer.

Current computer technology could not handle the system's requirements, but a national outcomes data base will take five to ten years to develop, or more. Supercomputers using new architecture approaches may provide the data capacity and access capacity such a huge system would require. Local users would interface the system through networks of microcomputers. Intel is introducing new computer chips with a capacity of 150 MIPS (million instructions per second), a thirty-fold improvement over the 3086 chip that now powers the largest of today's microcomputers.

SMART MEDICINE VERSUS COOKBOOK MEDICINE

One major problem, according to Ellwood, is that outcomes management would rely on standards of assessment for medical interventions. Using such standards is controversial and may be labeled "cookbook medicine" by critics. Some physicians will argue that such standards will be impractical and restrictive. They believe standards would take away a doctor's initiative to creatively prescribe medicine.

The battle over standards is just beginning. Ellwood believes that outcome standards will be flexible and constantly changing: "They would not be rigid laws to be followed blindly forever. They would be used as a starting point—data elements and recommendations that respond continually to what is learned from application and subsequent research." This will not be a technology that thinks better than human beings but one that can keep track of more data and store them more efficiently than even the most highly trained medical mind.

JOINT COMMISSION AGENDA

Clinical and organizational performance measurement will be the focus of a new evaluation methodology now under development at the Joint Commission (Jacobs, Christoffel, and Dixon 1987). The innovative concept of performance evaluation is centered on measures of health care quality as derived from clinical and organizational standards. Advancing its proposal to measure outcomes has thrust the Joint Commission into the high-visibility role of catalyst for industry change.

Developing patient-centered performance evaluation is a long-range project (Williamson et al. 1982). It will take five years or more to develop and test new criteria that will ultimately cover more than a dozen and a half clinical service categories. Johns Hopkins University Hospital is one of 17 hospitals pilot-testing the new standards. The initial testing focuses on three sets of clinical indicators: hospitalwide, anesthesia, and obstetric indicators. The clinical indicators and covariates will provide evidence of poor quality of care as well as patient risk, and poor ratings could be cause for losing Joint Commission accreditation. Because of the heavy weight given to Joint Commission accreditation by HCFA and state licensing agencies, losing it could mean losing Medicare certification and even the state license.

THE FIVE D'S

One classic list of outcome measures comprises the five Ds: death, disease, disability, discomfort, and dissatisfaction. This list captures as well as any the range of outcomes upon which hospital and physician performance will be judged in the future. Kathleen Lohr (1988), writing in *Inquiry*, suggests hopefully that payers and regulators will adopt a set of standards framed more positively: survival rates, states of physiologic, physical, and emotional health, and satisfaction.

FEDERAL GOVERNMENT REGULATION OF LONG-TERM OUTCOMES

The federal government is taking a new direction in regulating quality by focusing on "long-term outcomes." HCFA administrator William Roper, M.D., announced the new strategy. Inspired by the concept of outcomes management, Roper is launching a federal initiative to assess the long-term medical benefits of Medicare treatments. The assessment will investigate the results of treatment over an extended period of time (five to ten years) and will take into consideration other variables, such as quality of life.

The federal effort to monitor long-term results of Medicare payments will link together activities and the massive data bases of several Health and Human Services organizations, including the Public Health Service, HCFA, and the National Institutes of Health. According to Dr. Roper, "Federal health programs will no longer focus only on financing services, conducting biomedical research, implementing laws and administering bureaucratic rules. Federal agencies will also be involved in the collection of data and distribution of information about health care itself—information on health outcomes that will influence medical practices."

This is not the beginning of a new federal "rascal hunt" for low-quality Medicare providers. Julie Hopkins, editor of Aspen Publishers' *QRC Advisor*, believes the HCFA activities are designed to improve the quality of information that guides medical practice and thereby improve the general level of medical practice. Individual providers will not be singled out.

HCFA's outcomes initiative will include four types of activities: (1) use of data from Medicare claims processing and peer review systems to monitor trends and assess the effectiveness of specific interventions; (2) development of a data resource center that will provide access to Medicare files for research while ensuring patient confidentiality; (3) funding of research intended to evaluate the effectiveness and appropriateness of various medical procedures; and (4) improvement of data analysis methods used to monitor and measure health outcomes.

In addition to the HCFA program, the National Center for Health Services Research is designing a "national program for the assessment of patient outcomes." The purpose of this program is to evaluate patient outcomes and determine the appropriateness of treatments and surgical procedures. The program will assemble data bases and develop research methods to identify clinical areas in which costs, risks, and uncertainties are particularly high.

The goal of the HCFA intiative is to improve the effectiveness of medical care in the long term. Linking data bases will certainly be fraught with difficulties. The development of effective national standards can only result from research using national data bases. The development of a long-term outcomes program will easily require five to ten years of effort by HCFA.

Establishing a national outcomes system is a long-range project. Startup funding will require contributions from the federal government and from private foundations. Several prototype programs are already underway. HCFA could significantly advance the project by requiring standardized data from all federally paid health care providers. It is already moving in this direction, and it recently began collecting hospital death records to assess mortality. On HCFA's agenda is the evaluation of nursing home and other medical treatments. HCFA has funded the development of an outcomes management system in ten managed care organizations located in Missouri, Illinois, and Kansas.

WHAT IS OUTCOMES MANAGEMENT? AND HOW WILL IT WORK?

Outcomes management goes beyond quality assurance. Every hospital in America has a quality assurance program. Outcomes management would include quality assurance but also many other types of programs (Figure 19-1).

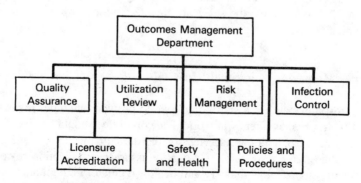

Figure 19-1 The Outcomes Management Department

Restructuring for Outcomes Management

By restructuring all hospital activities relating to quality and improved patient outcomes, management will gain a better focus on quality issues. There may be staff savings by co-locating and connecting efforts now spread across a number of different departments. More importantly, coaligning these activities may produce synergistic patient care improvements as outcome managers see opportunities for problem solving that were previously in other departments. Overcoming turf problems can make a substantial difference. Tom Peters (1988) states that 60 percent of the problems relating to quality and productivity lie at the boundaries of organizations whereas most quality control systems only function inside departments and work units.

Restructuring to establish an outcomes management department is more than a paper exercise. In most U.S. hospitals, there is a belief that "everyone is responsible for quality." The reality is that, although everyone is theoretically responsible, no one is actually in charge and accountable for ensuring that quality outcomes actually result from the patient care process. In the average hospital the most knowledgeable professionals whose work relates to quality of care seldom see each other or coordinate their efforts. The key to gaining improvements in outcomes is to bring together subunit managers and relevant medical staff across organizational boundaries, give them the information necessary to solve the problems identified, and assign them the responsibility of solving these problems.

Fitting Outcomes Management into the Hospital Organization

Think of outcomes management as a "superdepartment" reporting to the vice-president for patient care services (Figure 19-2). Does every hospital in America need an outcomes management department? Only midsize and larger hospitals, those over 200 beds, have the scale of related activities to provide the needed management focus.

Outcomes Management in Small Hospitals

Small hospitals can use a staff committee to provide outcomes management. This is "matrix management" at work. The committee should be chaired by the vice-president for patient care services or the director of nursing. Membership should include those responsible for quality assurance, utilization review, risk management, environmental safety and health, regulatory compliance and Joint Commission certification, and policies and procedures.

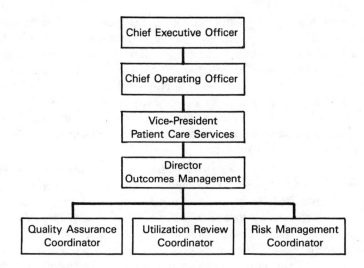

Figure 19-2 Outcomes Management Program Organization Chart

The development of hub-and-spoke referral networks may provide another mechanism for outcomes management. Multihospital systems and larger hospitals are developing networks to channel patients to tertiary care. Smaller hospitals are affiliating through management and clinical agreements. It may be desirable for a major medical center to develop a regional medical staff for monitoring quality, providing continuing education, and promoting better medical practices in the smaller and more rural facilities. A regional medical staff can aid in solving the problems of conducting peer reviews in small facilities with few physicians. There would also be economies of scale to be gained through monitoring quality and supporting a quality assurance process, conducting a regionalized risk management program, sharing biomedical engineering services, and obtaining consultations via telecommunications.

NEW OPPORTUNITIES IN OUTCOMES MANAGEMENT

Paul Ellwood may have created a new profession. New jobs, titles, job descriptions, and organizational charts will certainly come next as hospitals and health systems begin to operationalize the concept of outcomes management. And new programs and health professionals will be needed:

- *Vice-President for Outcomes Management.* This senior health care management position is most likely to be found in multihospital systems or major medical centers with teaching and research programs. At this level, the position is probably filled by a physician, nurse, or scientist with doctoral training. An outcomes management program in an academic medical center setting would involve active coordination with teaching and research programs for standard setting and data base development. In a multihospital system, the vice-president for outcomes management would oversee the monitoring of quality of care across the hospitals and other facilities in the system. Outcomes criteria would be among the primary criteria for monitoring care in system subunits.

- *Assistant Administrator or Assistant Vice-President for Outcomes Management*. Larger hospitals and small multihospital systems may create a position at the assistant administrator level to take charge of the various activities and positions relating to quality of care. These health care professionals should have a background of three to five years in quality assurance or risk management as well as management experience. They will be responsible for directing the activities of quality assurance, risk management, utilization review, and related efforts (e.g., certification, licensure, and accreditation). An assistant vice-president for outcomes management will most likely report to the vice-president for patient care services but in some cases may report directly to the CEO.

- *Director of Outcomes Management*. Creating a specific directorship for outcomes management will provide a management point of coordination for all quality assurance, utilization, and risk management efforts in the hospital. This is the likely strategy in smaller and midsize hospitals, where the function integrates existing activities and job responsibilities relating to the management of quality. In many hospitals this position may be located in the nursing department or affiliated with support offices of the medical staff.

COMPETITION, ENTREPRENEURS, AND VENTURE CAPITAL

The concept of outcomes management may engender a national competition among systems of patient care assessment. Payers and patients will increasingly demand more information about treatment alternatives and medical costs, especially when they realize that better-informed choices will save money and improve quality of care. New specialty companies may evolve to meet this demand. If existing organizations such as insurance companies do not respond, expect entrepreneurs and venture capitalists to fill the void.

LOOKING FORWARD: OUTCOMES MANAGEMENT IS A CONCEPT WHOSE TIME HAS ARRIVED

The American health care industry is changing. Rising costs, technological breakthroughs, government intervention, cost containment, managed care, and increased competition are all catalysts. The changing interplay between interdependent market segments is turning the health care industry upside down.

One thing seems certain today. Now that the box labeled "outcomes" has been opened, there will be no closing it. Hospitals and doctors will be graded and reimbursed based on their performance. Despite the difficulty of measuring health care outcomes equitably, the era of outcomes management is beginning. The health industry will not be the same.

What is clear is that outcomes management is a concept whose time has arrived. Hospitals can anticipate that all of their customers—patients, major employers, insurance companies, managed care plans, and government—will all be measuring and monitoring the outcomes of care.

STRATEGIC IMPLICATIONS FOR PHYSICIANS

1. *Quality is returning as a top priority.* Quality will be the primary criterion used by patients and major purchasers to choose physicians in the 1990s. Its importance will be especially evident once all payers adopt the Harvard RVS scale and the price for medical care becomes standardized.
2. *Preferred providers will be chosen based on outcomes.* Health care in the 1990s will be a managed care world. If a physician wishes to be a preferred provider in the future, that will mean demonstrating superior performance in terms of comparable outcomes. Doctors will be measured against their peers as well as national standards.
3. *The standards of practice (and payment) will be redefined.* The concept of outcomes management provides a way of bringing together all those interested in health and giving them a common basis for deciding which medical treatments, health care costs, and employee and insurance benefit investments are worthwhile.
4. *The art of medicine is becoming standardized.* Although many physicians lament this trend towards cookbook medicine, all doctors can anticipate that the standards of accepted practice will become much more precisely defined in the next five to ten years.

STRATEGIC IMPLICATIONS FOR HOSPITALS

1. *Competition among hospitals* will develop regarding the effective use of the information that outcomes management will produce. Health plans and hospitals will be rewarded for their ability to analyze the data contained in the national data base and to demonstrate their competitive advantage based on better medical outcomes and patient satisfaction.
2. *Preferred providers will have better outcomes.* Preferred providers in tomorrow's managed care marketplace will be judged on outcomes, not just costs. Hospitals and health plans will be rewarded for their ability to market products and services in response to the needs of their customers, including patients, physicians, government, employers, and a wide array of specialty companies.
3. *It is essential that hospitals begin to plan and organize their own outcomes management programs.* This may mean restructuring functions to coordinate all of the widespread hospital activities relating to quality. It is not too soon to begin thinking of the medical staff implications of outcomes management and of its marketing potential.
4. *Consider developing a regional medical staff to standardize a process for quality assurance and outcomes management across the hospital's hub-and-spoke network of smaller hospitals and outlying physicians.* If peer review and quality assurance are extended into physician offices in the 1990s, regionalizing the medical staff will be an important strategy for coping with this extension of regulation into ambulatory care by government, managed care organizations, or insurance carriers.

BIBLIOGRAPHY

Arnwine, Don. 1987. "Buyers Are Smarter, Looking for Quality." *Modern Healthcare*, 27 February, 32.

Berwick, Donald M. 1987. "Monitoring Quality in HMOs." *Business and Health* (November): 9–12.

Billings, John, and David Eddy. 1987. "Physician Decision Making Limited by Medical Evidence." *Business and Health* (November): 23–28.

Brook, Robert H., et al. 1977. "Assessing the Quality of Medical Care Using Outcome Measures: An Overview of the Method." *Medical Care* 15, supplement. (September).

Burda, David. 1988. "Providers Look to Industry for Quality Models." *Modern Healthcare*, 15 July, 24–32.

Caper, Philip. 1988. "Defining Quality in Medical Care." *Health Affairs* (Spring): 49–61.

Carter, Kim. 1987. "Severity Plays Crucial Role." *Modern Healthcare*, 27 February, 27.

Cassidy, Judy. 1987. "Assessing the Quality of Health Care Services." *Health Progress* (June) 28–31.

Coile, Russell C., Jr., and Randolph Grossman. 1987. "Quality: An Idea Whose Time Has Returned." *Healthcare Forum* (March-April): 21–27.

Davies, Allyson Ross, and John E. Ware, Jr. 1988. "Involving Consumers in Quality of Care Assessment." *Health Affairs* (Spring): 33–48.

Donabedian, Avedis. 1982. "The Quality of Medical Care." In *Quality Assurance in Hospitals*, edited by Nancy O. Graham. Rockville, Md.: Aspen Publishers.

Droste, Therese. 1988. "Quality Care: Elusive Concept Deserves Defining." *Hospitals*, 5 June, 58–59.

Ellwood, Paul M. 1988. "Outcomes Management." *New England Journal of Medicine* 318:1549–56.

Faurer, Susan. 1987. "A Quality Assurance Program." *AORN Journal*, 45:1384–89.

Fitch, Helen. 1986. "JCAH Standards for Quality Assurance: The Basics." *Nursing Management* 17 (October): 68–69.

Fletcher, Robert H., and Timothy S. Carey. 1987. "Seeking Good Care in an Outpatient Setting." *Business and Health* (November): 18–22.

Gonnella, Joseph S., Daniel Z. Louis, and John J. McCord. 1982. "The Staging Concept: An Approach to the Assessment of Outcome of Ambulatory Care." In *Quality Assurance in Hospitals*, edited by Nancy O. Graham. Rockville, Md.: Aspen Publishers.

Graham, Judith. 1987. "Quality Gets a Closer Look." *Modern Healthcare*, 27 February, 20–31.

———. 1987. "Hospitals Should Develop Plan for Presenting Mortality Data to the Public, Experts Warn." *Modern Healthcare*, 14 August 66–68.

Hays, Michael D. 1987. "Consumers Base Quality Perceptions on Patient Relations, Staff Qualifications." *Modern Healthcare*, 27 February, 33.

Henderson, Mary G., and Anne Collard. 1987. "Measuring Quality in Medical Case Management Programs." *Quality Review Bulletin* (February): 33–39.

Jacobs, Charles M., Tom H. Christoffel, and Nancy Dixon. 1987. *Measuring the Quality of Patient Care: The Rationale for Outcome Audit*. Cambridge, Mass.: Ballinger Publishing Company.

Jensen, Joyce. 1988. "Patient Surveys Help Measure Satisfaction." *Modern Healthcare*, 22 April: 40–41.

Kane, Rosalie A. 1988. "Case Management: Ethical Pitfalls on the Road to High-Quality Managed Care." *Quality Review Bulletin* (May): 161–66.

Lehmann, Ronald D. 1987. "Joint Commission Sets Agenda for Change." *Quality Review Bulletin* (April): 148–50.

Lohr, Kathleen N. 1988. "Outcome Measurement: Concepts and Questions." *Inquiry* 25 (Spring): 37–50.

Lohr, Kathleen N., Karl D. Yordy, and Samuel O. Thier. 1988. "Current Issues in Quality of Care." *Health Affairs* (Spring): 5–18.

Maxwell, Ian. 1986. "Quality Assurance: Simple, Rational and Desirable." *Dimensions* (October): 36–37.

Merry, Martin D. 1987. "What Is Quality Care? A Model for Measuring Health Care Excellence." *Quality Review Bulletin* (September): 298–301.

Micheletti, Julie, Thomas J. Shlala, and Ann T. Freedman. 1988. "Restructuring Quality Assurance Programs in HMOs and Other Competitive Medical Plans." *Quality Review Bulletin* (March): 80–85.

"Monitoring and Evaluation of the Quality and Appropriateness of Care." 1987. *Quality Review Bulletin* (January): 26–30.

Moore, Randy. 1988. *Outcomes Management: The Next Healthcare Technology?* San Diego, Calif.: Miller and Moore.

Osinski, Elsie. 1987. "Developing Patient Outcomes as a Quality Measure of Nursing Care." *Nursing Management* 18 (October): 28–29.

Payne, Susan. 1987. "How to Set Up a Focused Utilization Review Effort." *Business and Health* (November): 32–36.

Perry, Linda. 1988. "The Quality Process." *Modern Healthcare*, 1 April, 30–34.

Peters, Tom. 1988. *Thriving in Chaos*. New York: Harper and Row.

Pirsig, R. M. 1974. *Zen and the Art of Motorcycle Maintenance*. New York: Bantum Books.

Powills, Suzanne. 1987a. "Defining Quality: Jacobs Tackles It Head-on." *Hospitals*, 5 February, 56–57.

———. 1987b. "Quality, Not Ads, Increase Physician Loyalty." *Hospitals*, 20 June, 56.

Rhee, Kenneth J., Avedis Donabedian, and Richard E. Burney. 1987. "Assessing the Quality of Care in a Hospital Emergency Unit: A Framework and Its Application." *Quality Review Bulletin* (January): 4–16.

Roberts, James S., Jack G. Coale, and Robert R. Redman. 1987. "A History of the Joint Commission on Accreditation of Hospitals." *JAMA* 258:936–40.

Robinson, Michele L. 1988. "Sneak Preview: JCAHO's Quality Indicators." *Hospitals*, 5 July, 38–43.

Rosenberg, Stephen N. 1982. "Health Care Assessment: Choosing a Method." In *Quality Assurance in Hospitals*, edited by Nancy O. Graham. Rockville, Md.: Aspen Publishers.

Schroeder, Steven A. 1987. "Outcome Assessment 70 Years Later: Are We Ready?" *The New England Journal of Medicine*, Vol. 316, No. 13, 15 January 1987, 160–162.

Steffen, Grant E. 1988. "Quality Medical Care: A Definition." *JAMA* 260:56–61.

Steiber, Steven. 1988. "How Consumers Perceive Health Care Quality." *Hospitals*, 5 April, 84.

Sturm, Arthur C., Jr. 1988. "Healthcare Providers Would Be Wise Not to Promise More Than They Can Deliver." *Modern Healthcare*, 1 April, 36.

Summer, Steven J. 1987. "Maryland's Experiment with Quality Measures." *Business and Health* (November): 14–16.

Super, Kari E. 1987. "Providers Tout Quality to Get Edge in Marketing." *Modern Healthcare*, 27 February, 27.

Virapongse, Chat, Forrest Clore, and Richard Walker. 1987. "Setting Up a Quality-Assurance Program: Issues with Impact on Patient Care." *Applied Radiology* (February): 26–66.

Vuori, Hannu. 1987. "Patient Satisfaction: An Attribute or Indicator of the Quality of Care?" *Quality Review Bulletin* (March): 106–8.

Wan, Thomas T. H., and Ramesh K. Shukla. 1987. "Contextual and Organizational Correlates of the Quality of Hospital Nursing Care." *Quality Review Bulletin* (February): 61–64.

Williamson, John W., et al. 1982. "Health Accounting: An Outcome-based System of Quality Assurance: Illustrative Application to Hypertension." In *Quality Assurance in Hospitals*, edited by Nancy O. Graham. Rockville, Md.: Aspen Publishers.

Wyszewianski, Leon. 1988. "Quality of Care: Past Achievements and Future Challenges." *Inquiry* 25 (Spring): 13–22.

Chapter 20

Health Care as a Designed Experience

During the 1950s and the 1960s we mass-marketed the products of that industrial era—products whose regimented uniformities mirrored their industrial base. High tech was everywhere—in the factory, in our communication, transportation, and health care systems and, finally, even in our homes. But something else was growing alongside the technological invasion. Our response to the high tech all around us was the evolution of a highly personal value system to compensate for the impersonal nature of technology. . . . We must learn to balance the material wonders of technology with the spiritual demands of our human nature.

—John Naisbitt, *Megatrends*

DESIGNED EXPERIENCES

The "designed experience" is a phenomenon of the modern marketplace (Kotler 1984). Take a dream and give it to a marketeer. What results? Forty-year-olds play baseball with childhood heros from the diamond. The dream is real. The team could be the Chicago Cubs or Los Angeles Dodgers. The uniform is the real thing, too, and is included in the $3,000 price tag for the week-long fantasy come true.

Health care consumers have dreams too—quick and convenient appointments, accommodating attitudes, responsive service, a pleasant setting and a short wait, the best equipment, and someone to listen who cares. Better yet, the medical encounter results in therapy that works, or at least makes the patient feel better. Disney World is an environment that fulfills fantasies, but so is an ambulatory care center. Family Health Plan of Long Beach, California, is building senior health centers that look like private clubs, not clinics. They are competing hard for Medicare enrollees, and it is working. Family Health Plan has the largest

Medicare HMO market share in the hotly contested southern California HMO-PPO marketplace. (Richman and Baldwin 1986)

For physicians and hospitals, satisfying customers is the front line of market warfare in health care today. The battle for customer loyalty and retention will be fought here. If doctors and hospitals are to succeed over the long term, they must deliver not just on price but on customer service and satisfaction.

The Marketplace of Designed Experiences

There are many designed experiences available. Most cost a pretty penny. Price is not a problem. Today's upscale consumers have the disposable income. What they lack in our bureaucratic world is a sense of personal control. They seek mini-escapes from routine and are willing to pay for quality—and for getting "their burger made their way."

Choices abound. How about a champagne brunch as your balloon floats over vineyards? Feel like Marco Polo? Try a trek across Nepal. Want to play soldier? Bring your camouflage outfit—or rent one—and be a member of the Special Forces in the outlands of San Bernadino, California. Air guns shoot paint bullets: Bang, bang, you're dead! Except that you get to drive home at the end of the day. Like mysteries? Join other weekend sleuths as they play detective in "Hot Pursuit," a murder mystery pseudoadventure being staged around the country in hotels and aboard cruise ships. The cost is between $500 and $2,500 per couple depending on accommodations and is available from companies such as Murderous Mystery Tours in New York or The Plot Thickens in Los Angeles (Lippincott 1986).

And what about the fantasies of health care customers? Want to feel like Queen Victoria delivering a baby in the Royal Chambers? That fantasy is fulfilled daily at the Center for Women's Health at Cottonwood Hospital, near Salt Lake City, where a Victorian parlor becomes a labor-delivery-recovery room with all the high-tech equipment of modern delivery (Davis and Greenberg 1986).

What does this have to do with the future of medicine? Think of medical care as a designed experience from the customer's perspective, a total experience designed to satisfy the customer's every whim when he or she visits a doctor, a clinic, or a hospital emergency room. Who is better positioned to bring the designed experience concept into ambulatory care than doctors and hospitals—the most prominent providers in the health care industry.

Health Care Fantasy or Nightmare

The designed experience concept is badly needed to improve the deteriorating consumer image of medical care. For consumers, the reality is that a trip to the clinic, hospital, or health plan these days is a nightmare, not a fantasy. Too often, patients are depersonalized, made to wait, stripped of their clothing (and their dignity), manipulated by cold and strange hands, examined in haste, and finally sent home like errant schoolchildren with a note for their parents.

One consumer guide advises wary health care customers *How to Stay out of the Hospital* (Anastas 1986). For those patients who make the mistake of taking their "urgent care" problem to a hospital emergency room, the negative experience is probably multiplied. The wait is likely to be longer and the staff less tolerant of claimants for scarce (and pricey) emergency aid.

Today, most of these customers would have to pay in advance for the privilege of the indignity that doctors call the patient's "visit." They have hardly been treated like guests. It is high time that physicians and hospitals learned to be hospitable (Carey, Buckley, and Smith 1985). Something vital is missing from American medicine, and it is not research or technology. Customers want the "care" back in health care. (Switzer 1985).

RECONCEPTUALIZING HEALTH CARE AS A DESIGNED EXPERIENCE

Is this critique an exaggeration? Perhaps, but it is well intended. The point is that "health care" gets it backwards. It should be "care to restore health." Caring comes first. Now, what would medical care be like if it were a true "designed experience" provided through a customer-driven health care organization or physician office?

Constraint-Free Care

First, there is no "model" health care visit under the concept of the designed experience. Ideally, every patient would be treated uniquely. The doctor's office or hospital would sense and respond to the patient's wants and needs—and one patient at a time. There should be a seamless creation of service designed to please that single individual. This process would happen over and over.

Under the concept of the designed experience, there would be no rules that could not be broken, no policies that could not be waivered, and no stone that would remain unturned to satisfy a customer. In this market-driven environment, rule number one is, Please the customer. There is only one valid definition of business purpose: to create and satisfy a customer (Drucker 1954). The customer is king (or queen) for a day—every day. Health care providers live to serve customers. Consumer satisfaction is a health care provider's raison d'être. There are no constraints or boundaries when it comes to true customer service. With this attitude, there is hope for restoring customer trust in the patient-physician relationship.

Designed Experience Scenario

Janet Wilson was in heaven—or at least somewhere close to it. She could not believe this had really been a trip to the doctor. It had all started when she had switched health plans six weeks before. Her employer had recommended Preferred Providers, Inc., as one of a select group of hospitals and physicians in the area. Before Janet's visit, she received a letter of welcome from her new doctor, in his own handwriting, asking her how long it had been since she'd had a checkup. "How are you?" his note had asked. His letter was timely. How could he have known her back had been bothering her? "I should go see a doctor," she thought, but had done nothing about it. A day later the Preferred Providers office called to schedule an appointment. She would go to the doctor, Janet decided. Saturday was fine, and he was available evenings, too. On the telephone, the nurse ran through a short list of health questions. She seemed genuinely interested in Janet's health.

When Janet arrived at the physician's office a week later for her appointment, she was surprised by the ambiance. The office looked like a living room instead of a waiting room. The receptionist sitting at a small writing desk offered her coffee. The coffee was better than she expected, and in a china cup, too. She was soon summoned into the doctor's examination room. Janet settled into a comfortable wing chair, and the doctor began his examination—by asking her questions. They talked for 20 minutes about her job, any discomfort she might have experienced during routine activities, eating habits, and family matters (to see what stresses she had been under). Janet had been having headaches she attributed to stress. The doctor suggested the cause might be an allergy. They would do a few preliminary tests right in the office.

When it was finally time for the examination, the doctor slipped out and the nurse checked her vital signs and took blood and urine specimens. Janet dressed and returned to the doctor's study. He had the results of her tests already. Her back was fine. The headaches were probably the result of stress and a mild allergy. His advice surprised her: a 30-minute walk every day. Even more astonishing was his prescription. She was given a Walkman with a relaxation tape she could listen to as she did her "walk therapy."

As Janet was leaving the office, the receptionist told her that the visit would be billed automatically to Preferred Providers, Inc., her new health plan. She did not need to sign or pay anything. Janet walked out in a daze. Somehow the entire visit had taken only an hour. A few moments later Janet was back in her car and on her way to do some shopping—for a new pair of walking shoes.

DESIGNED EXPERIENCES BEGIN WITH THE ENVIRONMENT

Think of the health care setting—doctor's office, clinic, emergency room, hospital lobby—as a stage set for a drama. The "star" will soon arrive—the patient. The office environment is designed to make the patient feel important and the patient's needs seem significant. The impression to be created is that an entire organization has been poised at the ready to serve the patient.

Customer-centered design in health care has fought an uphill battle since being pioneered by Lindheim in her radical design of a Massachusetts children's hospital in the early 1970s (Lindheim 1972). Her concept was simple: Design the hospital around the children. This flew in the face of hospital architectural tradition. At that time hospital interiors had all the ambiance of a train station or college dormitory. Today's hospitals may have trendy pastel color schemes and carpeting to replace the miles of linoleum floors, but their design is still dictated by the mindset of the producer. It is time to reinvent the hospital and the medical office (Gaskie 1985).

Form Follows Function To Please Customers

Of course, the surroundings should fit the technical needs of health care. Not all waiting rooms need to look like the sitting room of an English country estate. Some patients like high-tech. The setting can emphasize the function of medical care in its highest form. Customers want to believe in the quality and worthiness of health care services. There are many ways to demonstrate that.

For a women's health center in New York, a San Francisco health care architectural firm engaged in extensive market research and design testing before developing the plan (J. Diaz, telephone interview, 1986). The results were surprising. The architects were told to design three spaces—each unique—for the three primary functional areas within the center. The reception area was for business, and the service there was intended to be efficient. The "waiting area" need not be sumptuous because the waits would be brief. In this ambulatory care center, design followed function as defined by the customers. The customers felt the examination and procedure rooms should be modern. The look the customers wanted was high-tech. However, in the postsurgery recovery and lounge area, customers wanted the feel to be warm and cozy—a caring environment.

The Comfort Zone

Forget coordinated carpeting and wallpaper. The goal of a health care setting from the designed experience perspective is for the setting to please the customer, not the designer. The customers want design concepts that most appropriately match their varying needs and expectations as they go through the process of ambulatory care. A southern California designer uses the concepts of "comfort zone" and "confidence zone." Design consistency is less important than functional fit (J. Thomas, telephone interview, 1986).

A new ambulatory care center designed for the Henry Mayo Newhall Memorial Hospital in Valencia, California, incorporates many aspects of the designed experience concept. Designed by a Los Angeles health care architectural firm, this 40,000-square-foot facility will house a number of ambulatory care "boutique centers." Each minicenter has its own customers, design, floor plan, and decor, even its own entrance (J. Thomas, telephone interview, 1986).

Just as every customer is different, so is every health care service. The surroundings of a diagnostic imaging center might be very different from those of an ambulatory surgery center. Pediatrics obviously serves a special population, just as a geriatrics program is focused on older patients. Segment the design and the facilities to match the customers. The surroundings must work to support the service process, but the point of departure is the perspective of the customer, not the producer.

In designing the setting, do not be swayed by the fashions of interior design. It is the customers who must be pleased. Ask customers what would most appeal. A sensitive designer can facilitate this process and translate customer desires into a stage set for preferred ambulatory care.

Location, Location, Location

The importance of location is equally characteristic of real estate and health care. The location of the service setting is no small matter. It could make or break utilization and profitability. Some health care organizations are testing the location-pull theory of retailing by creating "medical malls." Hospital diversification has been the driving force. HCA is building three medical malls to retail a cluster of ambulatory care services. Evanston Hospital in suburban Chicago has under construction an 80,000-square-foot medical building wrapped around a five-story atrium. The ground floor will have 10,000 square feet of retail space for pharmacies, maternity boutiques, and health-related products.

THINK LIKE RETAILERS

Medical offices and hospitals could benefit from the retail perspective and its focus on how to lure and hold customers. Especially important are entrances and exits. Entrances should be marked with a distinguishing canopy. First impressions are critical. Service begins at the initial contact a customer has with the provider. That first contact may determine whether the customer has a successful experience—or ever returns—regardless of the outcome of care.

The customers of each health care service should be asked their preferences, beginning with the front door—or even the parking lot. More impressions may be created in the parking lot than in the examining suite. If parking is a problem, provide valet service. Pioneered by Humana's Sunrise Hospital in Las Vegas, valet parking works well, at least in this town where no one walks. Again, there are no rules except rule number one: Please the customer.

50,000 Moments of Truth

The true character of service in any business is tested countless times each day. These are the 50,000 moments of truth when employees—often out of sight of supervision—are in contact with customers. These encounters determine the quality of service. They are the critical determiners in creating and maintaining customer satisfaction. From the successful experience of SAS airlines, health care organizations can learn the secret to successful customer relations: service management (Albrecht and Zemke 1985).

Good service is no accident. It occurs when all aspects of the customer environment are managed: setting, staff, and service (the "service triangle"). Think of ambulatory care as a designed experience from the customer's perspective. Ambulatory care has generally ignored the service dimension. Seeking care is an intensely personal experience. Customers want their needs and expectations taken seriously. Santa Monica Hospital Medical Center, a test site for a service management program, has rewritten its mission statement, incorporates customer ratings into employee incentive pay, and tracks customer satisfaction with a full-time manager (Albrecht and Zemke 1985).

REDEFINING THE PATIENT-PHYSICIAN RELATIONSHIP

In an idealized patient visit, customer needs would be anticipated fully in a way that would redefine the traditional patient-physician relationship—beginning with who is in charge. It is the customer. The physician should play the role of consultant, diagnostician, therapist, and advisor. The patient is a partner, client, and customer. Today's patients may or may not be patient or compliant. They know little about the aspects of quality that are central to a provider—the process of care and its outcome. But customers are excellent judges of *service*, and the success of an ambulatory care provider may rise or fall on the service dimension alone.

When customers describe their ideal health care visit, they use terms such as *courteous, prompt, direct, solicitous, sympathetic, responsive, and caring*. An attitude of caring and consideration should be demonstrated at the first contact—with the receptionist, clerk, or nurse—and extend through the physician visit and aftercare to the last polite goodbye. The "kid glove" treatment, unflagging courtesy, and attention to detail, must be repeated countless times each day. At Santa Monica Hospital, the ten principles of service management are prominently posted in every nursing unit and hang on the walls of all of the hospital's department managers (see Exhibit 20-1). The hospital's customer-first ethic is highly visible.

Since satisfying customers is the goal, each health care visit should be uniquely appropriate to each customer. Patients unsure of whether their condition is sufficiently acute to deserve professional attention must be taken seriously. Where cost is a customer's concern, the business arrangements should be completed quickly and unobtrusively. Busy customers are attended to promptly. Customers who are seeking a friendly face and sympathetic ear are listened to in an unhurried manner. Inarticulate or embarrassed customers are politely probed until their real concerns surface. Repeat customers are remembered. Adults are treated like adults, using surnames with respect. Privacy is honored and respected. Health information and aftercare instructions are clear and written out. Professional and support staff deal with customers in a friendly and forthright manner. Their attitude demonstrates the first principle of any business relationship: We are here to satisfy customers.

The Sheraton Grande Experience

Sound ideal? It could be even better. In 1983, the Sheraton Grande Hotel opened in Los Angeles. The hotel market was crowded and competitive, and

Exhibit 20-1 Code of Quality Service

1. Greet each person immediately.
2. Give each person my full attention.
3. Make the first 30 seconds count.
4. Be natural, show warmth and concern.
5. Be energetic and cordial.
6. Be each person's advocate.
7. Think for myself, use common sense.
8. Bend the rules sometimes.
9. Make a good last impression.
10. Stay "up," take care of myself.

Source: © 1986 Santa Monica Hospital Medical Center and Karl Albrecht.

most hotels operated at 70 percent occupancy. In its first year, the Sheraton Grande broke every record for year-one financial performance by a hotel in the Sheraton chain. One clue to its profitability can be gained from its customer satisfaction rating: 99 percent excellent. The hotel's general manager uses the "theater concept" to stimulate the highest levels of customer service. At the Sheraton Grande, employees are "members of the cast" and their locker rooms are "dressing rooms"—with a star on the door. When on duty, hotel employees are "on stage" every time they are in contact with a customer. Employee performance appraisals include a customer service rating, and bonuses are linked to customer satisfaction. This is a customer-driven organization, and its success is obvious.

Marriott has written the book on customer service, literally. Every job in this hotel chain is extensively defined in terms of customer service, right down to the number of seconds a waiter or waitress is given to make eye contact with a new customer. Managers get the same training and come back for frequent refreshers. Marriott has a passion for excellence in customer service (Peters and Austin 1985).

THE HOSPITAL OF THE FUTURE

The hospital of the future exists today, at least from a customer-service perspective (Jenner 1986). The San Francisco-based Planetree Foundation took its customer-centered concept of health care to Pacific Presbyterian Medical Center. The result is the Model Hospital Project, a 13-bed pilot program that combines environmental design with new rules for patient service (see Chapter 15). Information is at the core of the Planetree concept. All Planetree patients have complete and open access to their health records, and they are helped by staff to fully understand their condition and treatment. A mini-library and kitchen are at the physical center of the unit. Patients can enjoy their favorite foods and socialize fully with friends and family. There are no visiting hours. All staff are volunteers. Nurses are handpicked, and physicians have to apply for admitting privileges and to accept the Planetree principles of customer-centered care. This med-surg unit is consistently run at above 85 percent occupancy, and the model is being extended to the San Jose Hospital in San Jose, California.

Is health care a suitable candidate for such a complete focus on customer service? Without a doubt. The trend is starting already—with training programs to reorient employee attitudes and strengthen customer skills. In the health care field, guest relations consultants like Rita Fritz and Kristine Peterson are training hospital and HMO employees. The huge HMO, Kaiser Foundation Health Plan, and the Medical Center of University of California San Diego have guest relations programs. A few large private group practices are signing up, but the trend stops there. Smaller clinics, group practices, and solo practitioners are still not part of this trend. The opportunity just in group practices is enormous. Between 1980 and 1984, the number of group practices increased nearly 50 percent, and groups see more patients per doctor.

This is just the tip of the iceberg. Health care organizations will compete to capture and control ambulatory care. Ambulatory care is one of the high-growth markets in the health care industry, with 10–15 percent annual growth in ambulatory visits in the next three years (Coile 1988). The federal government is encouraging the shift. Since 1983, Medicare has identified more than 200 procedures it will pay for only if provided on an ambulatory basis. Ambulatory care will be a competitive battlezone in the 1990s with hospitals, physicians, and entrepreneurs competing intensely on price, service, and location.

REDESIGNING HEALTH CARE FOR A "31 FLAVORS" MARKETPLACE

Sears Roebuck used to offer its merchandise to its catalog shoppers in three price-quality levels: good, better and best. No longer. Today Sears is competing with discount chains like K Mart to offer 16 models of lawnmowers and 20 different televisions, including brand names and discount bargains, not all under the Sears brand name. America's customers want choices and are willing to pay for them.

Medical care has been a homogenous product. Professional norms have dictated standards of community practice from which few providers stray. Powerful mechanisms of government and major health care purchasers exist to ensure that the quality of care does not vary far from prevailing practice patterns. The only difference among health care providers in the past has been the size of the waiting room. In today's increasingly competitive market, the opportunity exists to differentiate ambulatory care based on the quality of the *service*.

The consuming American public is far from homogenized. America, the "melting pot," is still assimilating large numbers of new immigrants from around the world. The dominant white majority is losing ground to faster-growing ethnic groups. Major metropolitan areas such as Los Angeles and Oakland already have nonwhite majorities, and California will be the first state with an ethnic majority before the year 2000. In other bellwether states, Florida and Texas, the elderly and non-English-speaking populations are coming to dominate the political process (Naisbitt 1982).

As American as Apple Pie . . . or Salsa . . . or Sushi

Health care as a designed experience would respond to the unique cultural sensitivities of each customer segment in the market. Despite the leveling influence of television and the national marketing media, "born in America" still masks a high level of diversity. America, according to one view, consists of nine regional "nations" (Garreau 1983). From Ecotopia in the Northwest to the Heartland, every region has a distinctive local culture. Just as McDonald's has adopted its restaurant design and decor to reflect local traditions, so must aspiring ambulatory care chains and national health care organizations adapt to local patterns and preferences.

The ideal health care experience would be culturally apposite. Each customer would feel immediately at ease and be given subtle cues—decor, dress, cultural background of staff—to demonstrate cultural sensitivity. A fully developed staff training program would script the most culturally appropriate openings and responses for soliciting customer needs. In a multilingual marketplace, the medical care experience would be in the customer's language of choice.

THE CUSTOMER LIFE CYCLE

America in the 1990s is a complex marketplace. Age, gender, economics, and education are powerful differentiators in the marketplace. Ideally, the health care wants and service desires of each market segment would be planned and programmed for response.

Marketing and service management strategies in other industries have become increasingly sophisticated. Financial service companies like American Express and Security Pacific National Bank use the concept of "customer life events" to differentiate their products and services so they can be targeted at specific age-group markets.

SRI International's VALS (values, attitudes, life styles) market research has distinguished nine discrete American life styles, each with its own pattern of consumption preferences (Figure 20-1). The VALS data base has been used in developing marketing strategy for the California Lottery and hundreds of other products. It is now being used to shape new advertising and service strategies by Kaiser Foundation Health Plan, the nation's largest HMO.

THE DESIGNED EXPERIENCE CONCEPT AS A STRATEGIC ADVANTAGE

The strategic importance of the designed experience concept is clear. Customers may initially select health care providers on the basis of price but they will ultimately stay on the basis of service.

Satisfying customers is central to the long-range growth and development of every physician practice and hospital. Profitability depends in the long run on

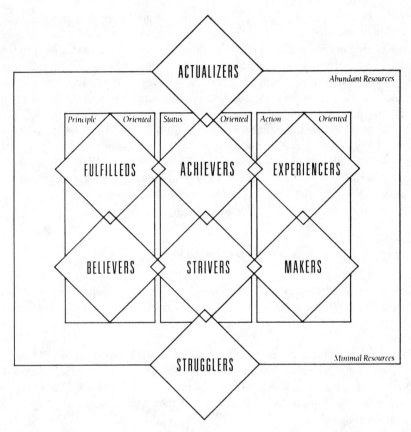

Figure 20-1 VALS®2 Typology. Reprinted with permission of VALS® Program, SRI International, Menlo Park, California.

capturing and holding consumer loyalty. As managed care becomes more prevalent, health plans must satisfy customers through the provision of ambulatory care services. That is where the war with health costs can be won. The designed experience concept can give consumer-oriented providers the competitive advantage over bureaucratic hospitals and clinics that treat patients as numbers instead of persons.

Putting "Preferred" Back into Preferred Provider Organizations

Today, PPOs are capturing a major market share and may cover a majority of Americans in the 1990s. By definition, PPO providers are "preferred," but that preference must be earned and maintained. Choice and convenience are factors in the selection of health plan and provider, but PPO customers have demonstrated their willingness to trade these amenities for more valued factors: quality and service. The designed experience concept is fundamentally an attitude about quality and service that is truly customer-driven.

The designed experience vision of quality in service and ambiance will not be easy to realize. It will drive the search by PPOs for the most service-oriented physicians. Both doctors and PPOs will need to make a significant investment in upgrading facilities and training staff. But a makeover of clinic waiting rooms or charm school for receptionists is not enough. The designed experience includes virtually everything that contributes to customer satisfaction. If successfully adopted and implemented, the designed experience could cause major changes in the process and outcome of ambulatory care. This commitment to service could provide a marketing boost for the PPO model that would allow it to eclipse its HMO and fee-for-service competition and become the dominant health care model.

COMPETING FUTURES FOR HEALTH CARE

There are many possible futures. Looking at health care from a customer service perspective, three scenarios can easily be visualized.

1. *A.M./P.M. Medical Care*. Picture health care as a mass-merchandised product available from convenience outlets like fast food. Price, quality, and service are predictable. The ambulatory care and minihospital operations fit the mobile life style of the many Americans who have no personal physician and who rely instead on a well-known brand name source for their health care.
2. *Boutique Medicine*. Imagine a specialized health care center for every customer segment, disease, and procedure. Every ambulatory care producer would find a niche. Every subgroup in the population would find a service catering to its needs and finances. Upscale customers might get limousine service or home visits or have their prescription drugs custom-compounded, paying the premium prices willingly. Other specialty health care centers would cater to women, the elderly, youths, or cultural population pockets. Diseases and procedures would be specialized. The Sloan-Kettering Institute could have a national chain of ambulatory cancer centers. Discount producers would provide care to those unwilling or unable to pay for frills.
3. *Contract Care Networks*. If health care conglomerates hold a dominant share of tomorrow's market, health care will be provided through a network of owned or contracted health care outlets. In this scenario, integrated health plans become the dominant health care organizations. The distinc-

tions between finance, payment, and health care delivery become blurred, since very large companies perform all three functions on a regional and national basis. Many companies have brand names that consumers recognize and identify with. In this "managed care" future, the formation of regional and national medical corporations is stimulated—big sellers to match big buyers. Franchises and subsidiaries proliferate. Most health care providers are multispecialty groups with excellent locations, professional management, and cost-efficient services. Top specialist groups are niche players, contracting with one or more integrated health plans for consulting services and specialized procedures.

LOOKING FORWARD

Which of these futures are possible? All are conceivable, and signs of each are evident in the marketplace today. Which will be dominant? Most probably the last if managed care health plans continue their high growth, but that is only one opinion. These scenarios can coexist, and other scenarios are possible, for example, "Fed-Care", in which Congress enacts national health insurance and unleashes a government takeover of the nation's health plans.

Where is the customer in these alternative futures? At the center, of course, because each scenario is market-driven. Whatever happens, pleasing customers will play a critical role in all health care futures. Look at the influence of the American Association of Retired Persons on health care policy making in Washington. In each alternative future, health care must be designed around the needs, expectations, and values of customers. Health care providers who fail to heed this advice will not meet the test of tomorrow's competitive market.

STRATEGIC IMPLICATIONS FOR PHYSICIANS

1. *Physicians should redesign the practice environment to make it more satisfying for consumers.* Rethink, redesign, and remodel physician offices and medical clinics from the consumer perspective. Market research can help, including surveys of current and former patients. Some market research firms even provide "test patients" who anonymously seek care, then critique it for the provider.
2. *Ultimately, consumers will stay on the basis of service.* Consumers may come to a physician for a variety of reasons, including word-of-mouth referrals, reputation, location, or the uniqueness of a treatment. Consumers, correctly or incorrectly, assume that providers will be competent, and they

expect technical quality from their doctors. Ultimately, consumers will be loyal when they are satisfied on the service as well as on the technical quality of the care.

3. *Physicians should collaborate in hospital guest relations programs.* Physicians are advocates for patients as well as their therapists. The quality of caring that a patient receives in a hospital is a direct reflection on the physician, since it was the physician who admitted the patient and selected the hospital. If the hospital's care is good—or bad—the patient will hold the doctor responsible.

STRATEGIC IMPLICATIONS FOR HOSPITALS

1. *In health care, a hospital's reputation among patients, physicians, payers, and the general public is everything.* Reputation depends on satisfying customers, one at a time, all year long.
2. *In a managed care environment, the designation "preferred provider" will mean the difference between success and failure.* Hospitals must win and hold that designation from a wide array of insurance companies, HMOs, PPOs, employers, and third party administrators. These can select virtually any hospital in the marketplace based on price. Since all hospitals will discount on price, quality and customer satisfaction are the criteria that will be used by major buyers.
3. *Hospitals must manage the 50,000 Moments of Truth.* Superior service is no accident. It needs service management (see Chapter 15). For health care to be a "designed experience," the coordinated effort and commitment of the hundreds of hospital employees is required. Service is a 24-hour-a-day responsibility and needs sustained attention from the hospital's top management. The loyalty of customers will be won with the little things, the details of patient care. And who says tomorrow's health care consumers will be patient?

BIBLIOGRAPHY

Albrecht, K., and R. Zemke, 1985. *Service America! Doing Business in the New Economy*. Homewood, Ill.: Dow Jones-Irwin.

American Hospital Association. 1985. *Hospital Statistics: 1985 Edition*. Chicago: American Hospital Publishing.

Anastas, L. 1986. *How To Stay Out of the Hospital*. Emmaus, Pa.: Rodale Press.

Anderson, H. J. 1986a. "Ambulatory Care Centers Offer Broader Range of Health Services." *Modern Healthcare*, 6 June, 142–52.

———. 1986b. "Outpatient Services Contributing to Total Hospital Revenues." *Modern Healthcare*, 18 July, 50–52.

Carey, J., J. Buckley, and J. Smith. 1985. "Hospital Hospitality: Health Workers Learn to Treat Patients with Kindness." *Newsweek*, 11 February, 78–79.

Coile, Russell C., Jr. 1986. *The New Hospital: Future Strategies for a Changing Industry*. Rockville, Md.: Aspen Publishers.

Coile, Russell C., Jr. 1988 "Health Care 1989: Top 10 Market and Management Trends." *Hospital Strategy Report* (December): 1–6.

Davis. D., and N. F. Greenberg. 1986. "The New High Style Hospital." *Newsweek*, 28 July, 62–63.

Drucker, P. F. 1954. *The Practice of Management*. New York: Harper Brothers.

Garreau, J. 1983. *The Nine Nations of North America*. New York: Harper and Row.

Gaskie, M. 1985. "Reinventing the Hospital." *Architectural Record* (October): 121–37.

Henderson, J. A. 1986. "Surgery Center Growth Slows: More Procedures Done." *Modern Healthcare*, 6 June, 132–37.

Jenner, J. K. 1986. "Towards the Patient-Driven Hospital." Parts 1, 2. *Healthcare Forum* 29 (May-June, July-August): 52–59.

Kotler, P. 1984. "Dream Vacations: The Booming Market for Designed Experiences." *The Futurist* 18:7–13.

Lindheim, R., et al. 1972. *Changing Hospital Environments for Children*. Cambridge, Mass.: Harvard University Press.

Lippincott, C. 1986. "Mystery Weekends Make Crime Pay." *Wall Street Journal*, 26 August, 24.

Naisbitt, J. 1982. *Megatrends: Ten New Directions Transforming Our Lives*. New York: Warner Books.

Peters, T., and N. Austin. 1985. *A Passion For Excellence: The Leadership Difference*. New York: Random House.

Richman, D. 1986. "Enrollment Soars 291% in HMOs Sponsored by Hospital Chains." *Modern Healthcare*, 6 June, 132–37.

Richman, D., and Mark F. Baldwin. 1986. "Government Spending Cuts Force HMOs to Walk Payment Tightrope." *Modern Healthcare*, 12 September, 64–68.

Switzer, E. 1985. "Whatever Happened to Caring? The Failure of America's Hospitals." *Ladies Home Journal* (June): 45–48.

Part IV

Epilogue

Chapter 21

Alternative Scenarios for the Future of Medicine in the Year 2000

The 21st century will be here in barely a decade, and there are many possible futures for medicine. Some are more likely than others. As old patterns break down, the trends are shifting to form new arrangements and relationships that will shape the future of medicine and health care's response in the 1990s.

Don't forget the "wild cards," those low-probability but high-impact occurrences that could change the course of events. In meteorology, these are unpredicted shifts of weather that can dump six inches of rain in an hour or restrict a region to six inches in a year. In politics, they are dark horse candidates like Harry Truman and Jimmy Carter. In sports, they are the pennant-winning teams that finished fifth in the division the year before. In science and medicine, breakthroughs can win Nobel prizes. In today's global economy, a natural disaster or political upheaval could trigger a chain of "falling dominoes" and worldwide recession. A depleted ozone layer or the third world debt crisis could be just such a catalyst for disaster. Remote but possible futures deserve assessment and some contingency planning.

When futurists and forecasters look to the future, they often use scenarios to explicate alternative possibilities. The term *scenario* comes from drama and means a synopsis of a play. For our purposes, think of scenarios as sketches of the future. Scenarios are most useful in illuminating the potential interaction of future events. One more thing about scenarios. As Herman Kahn (1980), the late futurist noted, "Remember, they're only scenarios, so don't take them too seriously."

There are at least four potential scenarios for medicine's future, as illustrated in Figure 21-1.

MEDICAL BREAKTHROUGHS SCENARIO

This is the high-tech scenario. Two driving forces contribute to the medical breakthroughs future: sustained economic prosperity, which allows a high level

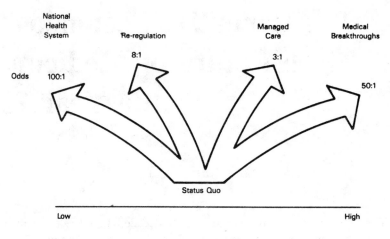

Figure 21-1 Alternative Scenarios for the Future of Medicine

of investment in biomedical research and health care services, and significant medical advances in cardiac, cancer, and AIDS care. In this scenario, health spending reaches 15 percent of the GNP by the year 2000. National health levels rise and the population gains an immediate one to two years of life extension through a combination of medical technology and improved life styles. With major advances against several of the leading causes of death, lifespans of between 100 and 120 years will be possible in the 21st century.

Physicians sort themselves into two groups: hospital-based specialists and community-based primary care practitioners. Most of medical specialists and subspecialists (75 percent) are located in a hospital or medical office building on a hospital campus. The concentration of specialists increases. By the year 2000, half of all specialists are affiliated with academic medical centers and teaching hospitals. Research activities enhance the specialist physician's practice and referrals. Primary care physicians are essential to the system of patient referrals. Few primary care doctors admit directly to hospitals; most refer patients who need hospitalization to specialists. Only small and rural hospitals still allow primary care physicians to admit directly and to keep responsibility for their patients. Protocols for care coordination by primary care doctors and specialists have been developed that protect the roles of all parties.

Science and technology flourish. R & D spending by government and the private sector rises 10–15 percent. Key medical breakthroughs occur in cardiac care with the arrival of artificial heart pumps that use an implantable space-age power source. The ventricular assist device (VAD) is now permanently installed; some patients with no prior heart attacks are given a VAD as precautionary therapy. Artificial lungs are being developed. Prototypes of artificial kidneys and livers are being tested. Artificial intelligence is widely used in medicine for diagnosis and therapy. Neurosurgery is now routinely computer guided using robot surgeons. Genetics is opening new doors in cancer therapy. Genetic probes can identify risks for a number of types of cancers, and new pharmaceuticals are proving successful in the treatment of liver, cervical, and colon cancer. An AIDS vaccine has been developed and is being administered worldwide by the turn of the century. AIDS treatments involving new drugs began to gain ground on the epidemic by the mid-1990s.

Reimbursement for physicians and hospitals is a mix of case-based and capitation, with some fee-for-service. Medicare blended hospital and physician payment in the mid-1990s, and hospitals have structured a variety of approaches to physician reimbursement. An innovative array of incentives reward doctors for efficiency and quality outcomes.

Health spending reaches 15 percent of the GNP by the year 2000. Physician incomes rise 5–8 percent as the aging of the population drives up the number of office visits and hospitalizations. Given the strong high-tech orientation of the health system, specialists outearn primary care physicians by 30–50 percent. Hospital stays are expensive. The cost of a hospital admission has doubled in the 1990s, reflecting the growing number of implants, bionics, and other high-tech treatments.

Hospitals are becoming sorted into two categories: low-tech community hospitals that provide routine medical treatment and high-tech specialized facilities. Access to capital is the critical factor. Smaller facilities that could not afford to keep pace with technology have drifted into a secondary status. A few have downlicensed to skilled nursing, psychiatric, or rehabilitation. Larger hospitals with strong operating margins and capital reserves are building specialized facilities for their centers of excellence. Projects costing more than $100 million are not unusual. In the medical breakthroughs scenario, academic medical centers are the most successful hospitals. They are magnets for patients, physician specialists, and research dollars.

MANAGED CARE SCENARIO

In the 1990s, managed care becomes the dominant form of health care financing and delivery. By the late 1990s, more than 90 percent of the population are enrolled to some form of managed care plan. Medicare shifts to a managed care strategy in the early 1990s, converting the last major segment of fee-for-service patients to Medicare HMOs and PPOs. As the economics of medicine are restructured by managed care, new patterns of physician and hospital service take hold. Health care inflation drops below 10 percent per year, satisfying government and major employers that more stringent regulatory controls were not needed to keep health care affordable. Managed care engenders a new pattern of compromises that alters medical utilization. Distinctions between HMOs and PPOs blur and disappear in the 1990s as each kind of plan adopts the other's most successful features. There is more control, but there is also more patient choice.

Physicians become reluctant supporters of the managed care movement. Managed care is the only alternative that still protects any vestige of fee-for-service medicine. Not without a price—physician autonomy in clinical decision making is now limited by the need for prior approval for many treatments by the managed care plan. Physician office visits increase, but fees for diagnostic and surgical procedures are cut. Discounting is so widespread that "usual and customary charges" is a meaningless phrase. Quality assurance invades the physician's private office. To monitor quality and use levels, managed care plans insist on utilization review and quality assurance for a sample of in-office care. In the managed care scenario, specialists work under more constraints, see fewer patients, and perform fewer procedures. Primary care physicians are "gatekeepers" who control physician referrals for one-half of all patients, a pattern established by 1995.

Science and technology achieve gains in the 1990s, but not as many as in the medical breakthroughs scenario. Managed care puts a premium on drugs and treatments that are efficient and effective. Experimental therapies and devices are slow to gain payment acceptance by managed care plans. R & D spending is moderate. Government continues to fund basic research but only at existing funding levels. The private sector shifts emphasis to applications of proven technologies. The price of new technologies is a major factor in market acceptance and marketing strategies. The market for "big ticket" diagnostic equipment and expensive drugs shrinks 10–15 percent. Foreign competition increases, and a growing number of Japanese and European companies gain major market shares in the pharmaceutical and medical devices industries.

Reimbursement shifts to capitation under managed care. All payment levels and prices are prospectively set. Hospitals and physicians sign two-year or three-year contracts with managed care plans. Preferred physicians and hospitals win volume guarantees. Many managed care plans require providers to share at least part of the financial risks for providing services within the prenegotiated ceilings.

Health spending slows to below 10 percent annual inflation by 1992 under the influence of managed care—just in time to forestall more regulation. Health care exceeds 12 percent of the GNP by 1993 but then levels off, with expenditure growth more closely tied to the rise of consumer spending (CPI).

Hospitals adjust to managed care. Some health care executives breathe a sigh of relief. At least patients and revenues are somewhat predictable! Hospital length of stay ratchets downwards again, and by 1995 it is another half day shorter for both those over and those under age 65. Hospital admission rates stabilize. The managed care plans use about 400–450 patient days per 1,000 enrollees under age 65 and 1000–1200 days per 1,000 enrollees over 65. The aging of the population drives up admissions throughout the nation. There is no widespread "shakeout." Contrary to many predictions, U.S. hospital closures continue at a rate of 75–100 per year through 1995, then to 50 per year—the same rate as in 1980. Managed care forces physicians to cut costs and become even more efficient. Some hospitals tighten up the number of beds in operation, but others experience bed shortages. Better hospitals experience rising occupancies. There is a small building boom in the 1990s, led by major medical centers and well-utilized suburban hospitals.

REREGULATION SCENARIO

Stung by rapidly rising health costs of 10–12 percent and more, a wave of reregulation sweeps the U.S. health industry. Hospital rate review programs are enacted in a dozen more states. Certificate-of-need review programs are revived by 15 states, including several that had eliminated them in the 1980s. States cannot keep pace with expanding budgets for Medicaid. Forced to choose between reducing services, restricting eligibility, or regulating providers, the states choose regulation. At the national level, Congressman Pete Stark convinces Congress to reenact "Section 1122" review of hospital capital expenditures under Medicare. A national price schedule for physician services (based on the Harvard RVS study) is approved in 1991, despite physician protests. Although reregulation is uncoordinated and patchwork, it makes enough of an impact to cut health inflation back under 10 percent by 1995.

Physicians are a major target of regulation. The imposition of the Harvard RVS on physician reimbursement creates a national price schedule for medical services. Medicare assignment is now mandatory (the relevant law was enacted by Congress in 1992 under pressures from AARP). Physicians may not charge their Medicare patients for more than the government payment. Insurance companies and managed care plans adopt similar price schedules, and physician incomes fall by 15–25 percent before leveling off. Cardiac surgeons, ophthalmologists, and neurosurgeons are particularly hard hit. Some doctors lose 40–50 percent of their revenues.

Science and technology are dampened by the tightening of the regulatory belt. Hospitals cannot add new technology or purchase capital equipment without an extended review and approval process. High-cost equipment acquisitions and major building projects are slowed or shelved. In crisis there is also opportunity. Small-scale technology designed for ambulatory care environments or physician offices flourishes. Pharmaceuticals are another beneficiary of reregulation. Payers prefer medical therapies such as tPA to high-cost surgical interventions such as cardiac bypass surgery.

Health spending comes back under control under reregulation, ending a five-year run of double-digit inflation. Health care may now only reach 12 percent of GNP by the year 2000. Reregulation is only partly successful. Despite the numerous state and federal regulatory programs, health spending continues to rise at 6–8 percent annually, at least 2–3 points above the CPI. Some blame the fragmented regulatory approach; others point to the built-in inefficiences of regulation itself. Both explanations are right in this scenario.

Hospitals must again cope with more regulation, turning the clock back 20 years to the 1970s. Certificate of need for new facilities is not a major deterrent to hospital decision making. Few new hospitals are needed in any state in the 1990s. The limitation on capital expenditures is more of a strategic handicap. Reimposition of capital expenditures review benefits those hospitals that rebuilt in the 1980s. Hospitals that waited for environmental stability missed their opportunity to build or buy. Now any major capital investment can take years to gain approval.

NATIONAL HEALTH SYSTEM SCENARIO

This is the scenario physicians have feared since the 1950s. Imposition of a Canadian-model national health system occurred in 1999, when it was becoming clear that neither managed care nor reregulation could effectively slow health spending. Inflation continued to run at 10–14 percent throughout the 1990s, triggering Congressional action. By the mid-1990s a coalition of major employers, labor unions, seniors, and reform-minded physicians was loudly calling for a national system. When another federal budget crisis loomed in 1998, Congress was finally forced to act. Despite a protracted and costly debate, the National Health System (NHS) was enacted, with implementation scheduled for the year 2000. A new era was about to begin.

Physicians would not become federal employees under the NHS, but the government would basically become the only payer. A single set of standard physician prices was established, extending the Harvard RVS system adopted by Medicare in the early 1990s. The AMA estimated that physicians would lose 10–15 percent of their incomes under the NHS. The coming of the system hastened the growth of group practices as physicians pooled their overhead and incomes out of self-defense. A national system of gatekeepers was to be established. Each participating internist, family practitioner, and pediatrician would be assigned a number of patients from the community and paid limited fees each month to provide and coordinate their routine medical care. Specialized services, consultation, and hospitalization would be channeled by the gatekeepers.

Science and technology could expect a gloomy future under the NHS. Private R & D spending fell by 50 percent when it became clear that the NHS act would pass. Government research could not fill the gap, putting a chill on medical and technological innovation. Europe and Japan were the beneficiaries of the U.S. cutbacks, because American pharmaceutical and biomedical firms shifted their focus to foreign markets.

Reimbursement would eventually be simplifed under the NHS, but the transition was expected to be difficult. As passage of the NHS act became more likely, there was a sudden surge of demand for surgery and diagnostic procedures in the late 1990s. Patients wanted to take advantage of their insurance policies and managed care plans, fearing they might be denied the services under the new system.

Health spending surged in the three years before enactment, jumping 18–25 percent annually. Hospitals and physician offices were glutted with patients, and private insurers experienced a 25–40 percent jump in health costs. Medicare costs rose 15–25 percent. Transition costs added $150–$250 billion to health spending in the final two years before implementation of the NHS. Authors of NHS legislation intended to reduce health inflation to 5 percent per year by draconian cutbacks on hospitals and severe restrictions on physician services.

Hospitals will be realigned under the NHS into a three-layer system of federally designated facilities. The intent is to create regional networks of hospitals and physicians controlled by appointed commissions. At the top of the regional pyramid are the regional care facilities. Only 15–20 percent of U.S. hospitals are expected to qualify as regional facilities. Another 50 percent of existing hospitals will be designated community care facilities, whose purpose is to provide routine medical and surgical services. The remaining hospitals, predominantly small and rural, will be designated medical assistance facilities. They are intended to provide emergency medical care and skilled nursing services. Conversion to the federal system is expected to take ten years. Regional health authorities will develop plans for allocation of specialized services and equipment and will control regional health budgets in a manner similar to their counterparts above the U.S.-Canadian border.

LOOKING FORWARD

Do any of these scenarios sound far-fetched? Perhaps they all do. Yet each scenario could occur. It is the power of scenarios to create images of what could be. However, the actual future is not likely to be as simple or "pure" as the scenarios outlined here.

Yet strains of each scenario are very much in evidence today. Aspects of the scenarios are quite plausible. The benefit of illuminating possible futures is to avoid the threats and benefit from the opportunities that tomorrow will bring.

Think of the future as a resource to be managed. Physicians, hospitals, and the health industry can shape their preferred future. They will need a shared vision and a commitment to collaboration in order to achieve it. Above all, they will need a sense of optimism about the future and the patience to work for their desired scenario over a long time. The 1990s will be a period of transition to yet another future for medicine. Remember that the future begins today.

BIBLIOGRAPHY

Kahn, Herman. 1980. "The Future Isn't What It Used to Be." Public Broadcasting System, 1 May, television program.

Kahn, Herman, William Brown, and Leon Martel. 1976. *The Next 200 Years: A Scenario for America and the World*. New York: William Morrow and Company.

Wilson, Ian H. 1978. "Scenarios." In *Handbook of Futures Research*, edited by Jib Fowles. Westport, Conn.: Greenwood Press.

Index

About the Author

Futurist Russell C. Coile, Jr., is president of the Health Forecasting Group, in Alameda, California, which provides advanced market research to the health industry. He is the author of *The New Hospital: Future Strategies for a Changing Industry* (Aspen Publishers, 1986).